Frontiers in Myocardia

(*Volume 3*)

(Compendium on Cardiomyopathies - Basics, Therapeutics, and Perspectives)

Edited by

Jinfu Yang & Iroegbu Chukwuemeka Daniel

Department of Cardiovascular Surgery,
The Second Xiangya Hospital, Central South University,
Middle Renmin Road 139, Changsha, China

Frontiers in Myocardia

Volume # 3

Compendium on Cardiomyopathies - Basics, Therapeutics, and Perspectives

Editor: Jinfu Yang & Iroegbu Chukwuemeka Daniel

ISSN (Online): 2451-8352

ISSN (Print): 2451-8344

ISBN (Online): 978-981-14-3234-7

ISBN (Print): 978-981-14-3233-0

Bentham Science Publishers Pte. Ltd.
80 Robinson Road #02-00
Singapore 068898
Singapore
Email: subscriptions@benthamscience.net

BENTHAM SCIENCE

CONTENTS

PREFACE

Cardiomyopathy is a complex and a multifactorial pathogenetic group of diseases affecting the heart muscle having a high morbidity and mortality rate. Over the past fifty years from 1956, several definitions, revisions, and classifications of cardiomyopathies have been postulated. With the rapid increase in literature and knowledge of cardiomyopathies both in clinical findings, basic research and clear evidence during clinical settings, the gap from the very onset of cardiomyopathies in the field to present and where we are heading to in the future is ever increasing. However, applying these new revisions during day to day clinical practice is complex such as the advances and contemporary upcoming medical information including genetic mutations and their specific organ involvements. The abundance of basic, clinically applied, and new insights in cardiomyopathy as a single entity has outsourced and further enhanced the diseases complexity. However, with the currently reviewed system encompassing all updates including new classifications and criteria's to be added and reviewed right from the morphological standpoint to its specific phenotypes only further creates overlaps, gaps and the laxity to memorize and employ from family practice to outpatient and inpatient visits and other emergency scenarios.

Rather than follow a classical interdisciplinary division, the entire cardiovascular system here in this book is presented as a functional unit, and the contributors explore pathophysiological mechanisms from different perspectives, including genetics, molecular biology, electrophysiology, invasive and non-invasive cardiology, imaging methods, and surgery to provide a balanced medical view. This book will keep clinicians and post-graduates updated about what to expect by taking a quick overview as a whole from the past to the present with the possible future directions of cardiomyopathies from bases to therapeutics, thereby, applying up to date treatments obtained from serial clinical investigations.

This book also covers important imaging methods, especially echocardiography; cardiac magnetic imaging is used in various types of cardiomyopathies and also provides a vivid presentation of the current state of cardiomyopathies from genetics to management to cardiologists, cardiovascular intensivists, and cardiac emergency specialists. As a compendium, it will encompass all the new terms describing the groups of cardiomyopathies, providing practicing physicians the advantage of applying modern clinical management in patients and their families. It will also give medical practitioners a complete image and understanding of the disease for each patient, making it possible to identify the familial pattern of inheritance. It will include history, genetics, etiology, varying time courses of the disease when diagnosed in the respective time frame of its natural history and the highly variable effects of the acquired conditions affecting the course of cardiomyopathies.

Finally, Vol. 3 of the book series "*Frontiers in Myocardia*" comprises eleven articles written by leading researchers in this field. We the editors would further like to express our gratitude to the entire team of the Bentham Science Publishers particularly, Mr. Mahmood Alam (Director Publications), Mr. Shehzad Naqvi (Editorial Manager Publications), and Ms. Fariya Zulfiqar (Manager Publications) for their professional and efficient handling of this book at all stages of its publication.

Jinfu Yang & Iroegbu Chukwuemeka Daniel
Department of Cardiovascular Surgery,
The Second Xiangya Hospital, Central South University,
Middle Renmin Road 139, Changsha,
China

FOREWORD

Cardiomyopathy refers to diseases of the heart muscle causing cardiac myocyte injury and myocardial dysfunction, which impair structural and functional ventricular filling or ejection of blood in the absence of other structural or vascular heart diseases. As a compendium on cardiomyopathies, it hence, provides a superb amalgamation between basic/translational science and clinical medicine on a wide variety of expertise in the field of both cardiology (therapeutics) and cardiovascular surgery by two renowned talented practicing surgeons and academicians alongside carefully selected contributors who are also recognized authorities in the field of medicine and surgery. Both Professor Jinfu Yang and Iroegbu C Daniel are distinguished scholars who have both made a significant impact in the field of cardiology and cardiac surgery (adult and pediatric) over the years. They both have special surgical interest in aortic surgery, coronary artery bypass grafting, valve repairs, and valve replacements, maze procedure for atrial fibrillation, lung and chest wall diseases, heart failure, heart transplantation, and basic/translational research (basic medicine, biomolecular science, cardiac biochemistry and physiology, experience pathology, molecular biology, molecular epidemiology and pathology). These two expert editors have both thoroughly revised and combined their expertise and unique perspectives with a group of highly experienced specialized contributors to present a comprehensive book on cardiomyopathies from basic to therapeutics, and the possible future developments/outlooks to reflect the current knowledge and practice in the field today. This book provides a comprehensive, state-of-the-art concise view of the current knowledge and understanding of cardiomyopathies. The essence of excellence in cardiology and cardiac surgery strongly relies on a massive collaborative effort from the family physician, epidemiologists, geneticist basic/clinical science researchers to therapeutic physicians and surgeons themselves which this book, "*Compendium On Cardiomyopathies - Basics, Therapeutics, and Perspectives*" extensively and thoroughly discusses. The editors and their selected authors have to be thanked for their combined effort to present practitioners, a concise, clear and detailed current knowledge of the discussed cardiomyopathies with respect to both basic/translational science and clinical science. This book significantly adds to in-depth knowledge of practitioners and medical students at large and will be a valuable bedside reference for us all.

Professor Liu Li Ming
Vice Chair/Director, Department of Cardiovascular Surgery
The Second Xiangya Hospital, Central South University,
Middle Renmin Road 139, 410011 Changsha, Hunan
China

DEDICATION

To my wife Hong Feng, for her "old fashioned" devotion, support, and sacrifice to myself and our family. To our daughter, Danni Yang for her understanding and tolerance.

Jinfu Yang

I want to acknowledge my loving parents Rev, Engr. Iroegbu Chidozie Joseph and Bishop Iroegbu Agnes Benedicta for their loving support, encouragement, and guidance throughout my medical school days and career till date. To my siblings, Dr. Engr. Iroegbu Udochukwu Frank, Dr. Engr. Iroegbu Paul Ikechukwu, and Miss Iroegbu Chioma Phoebe, they are the bright stars of my world and a source of constant encouragement to me.

To my mentors Professor Zhongming Zhang, Professor Guoxiang Wang, Professor Zhongxin Zhou, Professor Liu Jindong, Professor Yang Jinfu, and Li Ming Liu, I genuinely feel blessed and honored to have been one of their students. Special thanks to my assistants, and my warm gratitude to all of those who helped in one way or the other in the success of this book.

Iroegbu Chukwuemeka Daniel

List of Contributors

Chengming Fan	Department of Cardiovascular Surgery, The Second Xiangya Hospital, Central South University, Middle Renmin Road 139, 410011 Changsha, China
Iroegbu Chukwuemeka Daniel	Department of Cardiovascular Surgery, The Second Xiangya Hospital, Central South University, Middle Renmin Road 139, 410011 Changsha, China
Jiarong Li	Department of Cardiovascular Surgery, The Second Xiangya Hospital, Central South University, Middle Renmin Road 139, 410011 Changsha, China
Jinfu Yang	Department of Cardiovascular Surgery, The Second Xiangya Hospital, Central South University, Middle Renmin Road 139, 410011 Changsha, China
Jiang Bo	Department of Thoracic and Cardiovascular Surgery, Affiliated Hospital of Xuzhou Medical University, Xuzhou, 99 Huaihai Road West Xuzhou, Jiangsu Province 221000, China
Jindong Liu	Department of Anesthesiology, Affiliated Hospital of Xuzhou Medical University, Xuzhou, 99 Huaihai Road West Xuzhou, Jiangsu Province 221000, China
Jeremiah Ong'achwa Machuki	Department of Biochemistry, University of Nairobi, P.O. Box 30197-001000, Nairobi, Kenya
Liu Jingsong	Department of Thoracic and Cardiovascular Surgery, Affiliated Hospital of Xuzhou Medical University, Xuzhou, 99 Huaihai Road West Xuzhou, Jiangsu Province 221000, China
Luo Cheng	Department of Cardiovascular Surgery, The Second Xiangya Hospital, Central South University, Middle Renmin Road 139, 410011 Changsha, China
Ming Wu	Department of Cardiovascular Surgery, The Second Xiangya Hospital, Central South University, Middle Renmin Road 139, 410011 Changsha, China
Qing Guan	Department of Cardiovascular Surgery, The Second Xiangya Hospital, Central South University, Middle Renmin Road 139, 410011 Changsha, China
Song Long	Department of Cardiovascular Surgery, The Second Xiangya Hospital, Central South University, Middle Renmin Road 139, 410011 Changsha, China
Sheng Tang	Department of Thoracic and Cardiovascular Surgery, Affiliated Hospital of Xuzhou Medical University, Xuzhou, 99 Huaihai Road West Xuzhou, Jiangsu Province 221000, China
Shiyuan Tang	Department of Cardiovascular Surgery, The Second Xiangya Hospital, Central South University, Middle Renmin Road 139, 410011 Changsha, China
Xiaoming Wu	Department of Cardiovascular Surgery, The Second Xiangya Hospital, Central South University, Middle Renmin Road 139, 410011 Changsha, China
Xin Chen	Department of Cardiovascular Surgery, The First Affiliated Hospital of Nanjing Medical University, Jiangsu, PR, China
Xun Wu	Department of Cardiovascular Surgery, The Second Xiangya Hospital, Central South University, Middle Renmin Road 139, 410011 Changsha, China

Wangping Chen Department of Cardiovascular Surgery, The Second Xiangya Hospital, Central South University, Middle Renmin Road 139, 410011 Changsha, China

Wasti Binaya Department of Respiratory Internal Medicine, The Second Xiangya Hospital, Central South University, Middle Renmin Road 139, 410011 Changsha, China

Zhang Hao Department of Thoracic and Cardiovascular Surgery, Affiliated Hospital of Xuzhou Medical University, Xuzhou, 99 Huaihai Road West Xuzhou, Jiangsu Province 221000, China

Zhou Zhongxin Department of Thoracic and Cardiovascular Surgery, Affiliated Hospital of Xuzhou Medical University, Xuzhou, 99 Huaihai Road West Xuzhou, Jiangsu Province 221000, China

CHAPTER 1

The Dynamics and the Continual Pursuit for an In-Depth Understanding of the Genetics of Cardiomyopathies

Iroegbu Chukwuemeka Daniel*

Department of Cardiovascular Surgery, The Second Xiangya Hospital, Central South University, Middle Renmin Road 139, 410011 Changsha, China

Abstract: Cardiomyopathies are a complex and essential group of heart muscle diseases with diverse etiologies and heterogenous phenotypic expressions, often leading to progressive heart failure (muscular or electrical dysfunction) of the heart with significant morbidity and mortality. In some cases, cardiomyopathies can be asymptomatic in the early stages of the disease with symptoms (fatigue, shortness of breath, paroxysmal nocturnal dyspnea, orthopnea, edema, and cough) characteristically similar to any heart failure. Estimated to occur in 3% of the general population worldwide, knowledge and the understanding of these diseases in both the general public and the medical communities have historically been impaired by periodic confusion surrounding definitions and terminologies. Cardiomyopathies may be primary (*i.e.*, genetic, acquired, or mixed) or secondary (*e.g.*, toxic inflammatory, and infiltrative). Major types include hypertrophic cardiomyopathy, restrictive cardiomyopathy, dilated cardiomyopathy, and arrhythmogenic right ventricular cardiomyopathy. Relieving symptoms of heart failure and decreasing hospitalization rates of cardiac failure are therapeutic aims of cardiomyopathy.

Keywords: Arrhythmia, Arrhythmogenic cardiomyopathy, Cardiomyopathy, Classification, Dilated cardiomyopathy, Heart failure, Heart transplantation, Hypertrophic cardiomyopathy, Implantable cardioverter defibrillator, Myocardial diseases, Restrictive cardiomyopathy, Sudden death.

INTRODUCTION

Cardiomyopathy is a complex and a multifactorial pathogenetic group of disease which affects function, structure, ventricular filling and the ejection of blood as they are either circumscribed to the heart or being part of a generalized systemic disorder affecting the heart muscles. Cardiomyopathies have a high morbidity and

* **Corresponding author Iroegbu Chukwuemeka Daniel:** Department of Cardiovascular Surgery, The Second Xiangya Hospital, Central South University, Middle Renmin Road 139, 410011 Changsha, China; E-mails: dr.iroegbu_daniel@yahoo.com and dr.iroegbu_daniel@csu.edu.cn

Jinfu Yang & Iroegbu Chukwuemeka Daniel (Eds.)

mortality rate, frequently leading to progressive heart failure-related disability in the absence of coronary artery disease, hypertension, valvular disease, or congenital heart diseases [1]. As the condition worsens, it damages muscle tone of the heart and reduces its ability to pump blood to the rest of the body and maintain a normal electrical rhythm as a result can either be heart failure or irregular heartbeats. Compared to other cardiac-related issues, it is remarkably seen in young individuals as a weakened heart and may also cause other complications, such as heart valve problems. For the heart to properly function, it requires the synchronous electrical and mechanical activity of each cardiomyocyte to ensure the coordinated excitation and contractile performance of the heart, like an organ. The heart's proper function is supported by a unique membrane structure (intercalated disk) forming at the edges of mammalian cardiomyocytes [2] which allows the secure transmission of both electrical and mechanical activities between neighboring cells [3, 4].

Being one of the essential heterogeneous group of diseases, its all-around insight which also includes its knowledge, awareness, and its related pathologies to the public and as well the medical community is impaired by the persistent confusion surrounding its nomenclature, definition(s), therapeutics and diagnosis. This heart muscle disease is so dangerous, and most often goes untreated as many adults are affected and may not even know they have the condition as it is a well-known cause of heart failure and also the most common reason for the need of a heart transplant. Over the years, significant progress has been achieved in getting explicit knowledge about the physiological, molecular, and genetic aspect of cardiomyopathies with novel discoveries being made. The tremendous achievements made in molecular genetics of inherited cardiomyopathies allowed the establishment of hypertrophic-restrictive cardiomyopathies (as sarcomeric, force generation disease) dilated cardiomyopathies (as the cytoskeleton, force transmission disease), and arrhythmogenic cardiomyopathy (as desmosome, cell junction disease). Channelopathies (Brugada, short and long QT,) are also additions considered cardiomyopathies because of electric myocyte dysfunction.

Palliative pharmacological and invasive therapies have been the gold standard for treatments of cardiomyopathies. However, curative treatment made it possible to target critical mechanisms responsible for the onset and progression of cardiomyopathies with a clinical understanding of the involved molecular pathogenesis. The advances made by researchers and clinicians to interpret this disease only goes to show how vital and intricate cardiomyopathy as a complex entity is. Knowledge of the genotype, etiology, pathophysiology and the clinical course is pivotal to diagnosis and prevention of cardiomyopathies as new approaches for its clinical and prognostic assessment are based on contemporary knowledge of its mechanism and the gene-phenotypic complex clinical evaluation and management strategies which invariably improves its clinical evaluation.

The translations and interpretations of cardiomyopathies discussed here are in line with the current concept of cardiomyopathies and have direct clinical applications and implications for cardiac diagnosis. Furthermore, presented classifications of cardiomyopathies herein are not intended to provide precise methodologies or strategies for clinical diagnosis. Instead, its classification rather serves as a scientific and an objective demonstration that offers new insights, aiding in the understanding of this complex and heterogeneous group of diseases, and the underlying disease mechanisms.

DEFINITIONS

The term cardiomyopathy was used in 1957 for the first time. In the original World Health Organization (WHO) 1980 classification, cardiomyopathies were defined only as "heart muscle diseases of unknown cause," reflecting a general lack of available information about underlying disease mechanisms [5]. WHO in 1968, defined cardiomyopathies as "diseases of different and often unknown etiology in which the dominant feature is cardiomegaly and heart failure" [5]. The final WHO classification published in 1995 proposed "diseases of the myocardium associated with cardiac dysfunction" and included for the first time arrhythmogenic right ventricular cardiomyopathy (ARVC), as well as primary restrictive cardiomyopathy (RCM) [5].

However, the American Heart Association (AHA) expert consensus panel proposed definition of cardiomyopathies is as follows: "Cardiomyopathies are a heterogeneous group of diseases of the myocardium associated with mechanical and/or electrical dysfunction, which usually (but not invariably) exhibit inappropriate ventricular hypertrophy or dilatation, due to a variety of etiologies that frequently are genetic. Cardiomyopathies are either confined to the heart or are part of generalized systemic disorders, and often lead to cardiovascular death or progressive heart failure-related disability" [6]. This definition of cardiomyopathies, similar to that reported by the European Society of Cardiology (ESC), under the auspices of the Working Group on Myocardial and Pericardial Diseases, excludes myocardial involvement secondary to coronary artery disease, systemic hypertension, and valvular and congenital heart disease [1].

CLASSIFICATION OF CARDIOMYOPATHIES

In general, the proper distinction of cardiac diseases is an important and essential one to make, as cardiac diseases with similar phenotypes can have a diverse origin and may need different types of management. However, as for cardiomyopathies, its classification is difficult, as the background or its pathophysiology is not always understood. The classification of these cardiac diseases has been based on morphofunctional phenotypes, but it has been changed according to molecular genetics in recent years. As we know, the traditional classification proposed by the WHO (Table **1**) is easy to differentiate between various cardiomyopathies in a couple of functional and structural phenotypes, which help us to define common treatment strategies [5]. New classification-orientated genomic and molecular science also help us understand the heterogeneity and complexity of these diseases [6]. To promote a consistent terminology and well-defined clinical patient groups, new knowledge on underlying causes and pathophysiology of cardiomyopathies has been implemented in a cardiomyopathy classification system both on behalf of the AHA and of the ESC (Table **2**). The AHA divided cardiomyopathies into two major groups based on predominant organ involvement. Primary cardiomyopathies (genetic, nongenetic, acquired) are those solely or predominantly confined to the heart muscle and are relatively few [6].

Table 1. Classification of cardiomyopathies by World Health Organization (WHO).

Restrictive
Dilated
Hypertrophic
Arrhythmogenic
Unclassified (mitochondrial diseases, fibroelastosis)
Specific
Valvular Ischemic Metabolic Peripartum Hypertensive Inflammatory Muscular dystrophies General systemic disease Neuromuscular disorders Sensitivity and toxic reactions

Secondary cardiomyopathies show pathological myocardial involvement as part of a large number and variety of generalized systemic (multiorgan) disorders [6]. According to the ESC guidelines, cardiomyopathies are grouped into specific morphological and functional phenotypes; each phenotype is then sub-classified into familial and non-familial forms [6]. The last classification system (MOGES) proposed by the World Heart Federation (WHF) (Table **3**) includes all characteristics: morphofunctional phenotype (M), organ(s) involvement (O), genetic inheritance (G), etiology (E), and functional status (S) [7]. From the clinical perspective, the essential objective is the diagnosis of the mechanism of heart failure and delivery of the appropriate, effective treatment.

Table 2. American Heart Association (AHA) Classification for Cardiomyopathies.

1. Primary (Predominantly Involving the Heart)
a. Genetic
Conduction defects Hypertrophic cardiomyopathy Mitochondrial myopathies Glycogen storage (PRKAG2, Danon) Arrhythmogenic right ventricular dysplasia Ion channel disorders (Brugada, SQTS, LQTS, CVPT, Asian SUNDS)
b. Acquired
Peri- or postpartum Tachycardia-induced Inflammatory (myocarditis) Stress-provoked (Takotsubo) Infants of insulin-dependent diabetic mothers
c. Mixed
Dilated cardiomyopathy Restrictive (non-hypertrophied and non-dilated)
2. Secondary Electrolyte imbalance Inflammatory = granulomatous (Sarcoidosis) Cardio-facial (Noonan syndrome; Lentiginosis) Toxicity (drugs, heavy metals, chemical agents) Infiltrative (Hurler's disease; Gaucher disease; amyloidosis; Hunter's disease) Storage (Fabry's disease; Hemochromatosis; Glycogen storage disease = type II Pompe; Niemann-Pick disease) Nutritional deficiencies (Beriberi, pellagra, scurvy, selenium, carnitine, kwashiorkor) Endomyocardial (endomyocardial fibrosis; hyper eosinophilic syndrome = Loeffler's endocarditis) Endocrine (Acromegaly; hyperthyroidism; pheochromocytoma; diabetes mellitus; hypothyroidism; hyperparathyroidism) Neuromuscular/neurological (Myotonic dystrophy; Emery-Dreifuss muscular dystrophy; Friedreich's ataxia; Tuberous sclerosis; Duchenne-Becker muscular dystrophy; neurofibromatosis) Autoimmune/collagen (systemic lupus erythematosus; dermatomyositis; Rheumatoid arthritis; scleroderma; polyarteritis nodosa) A consequence of cancer therapy (Radiation, doxorubicin, Adriamycin, anthracyclines, daunorubicin, cyclophosphamide)

SPATIOTEMPORAL DISTRIBUTION OF INTERCALATED DISK COMPONENTS

During maturation and the developmental stages of cardiomyocytes, significant changes occur in the structures associated with the intercalated disk. During the early developmental periods in human myocardium, adherens junction, and desmosomal organization follow that of gap junctions [8]. However, at the postnatal developmental phase, proteins of the adherens and gap junctions appear to orient themselves at the intercalated disk simultaneously [9].

Table 3. World Heart Federation (WHF) MOGE(S) classification for cardiomyopathies.

Notation	**M** **Morpho-functional Phenotype**	**O** **Organ/system Involvement**	**G** **Genetic Inheritance**	**E** **Etiology**	**S** **Stage**
Characteristics	**Cardiomyopathy diagnosis** (DCM, HCM, RCM, ARVC)	**Clinical history and evaluation** -organ involvement -multi-disciplinary involvement evaluation	**Genetic counseling with pedigree** *-Familial inheritance* *-Non-familial sporadic* **Clinical family screening** *-affected and asymptomatic* *-with ECG and ECHO abnormalities* *-healthy family members*	**Genetic testing in the proband** -Positive -Negative	**Functional Status (ACA/AHA; NYHA)**
Subscript	**D.** Dilated **H.** Hypertrophic **R.** Restrictive **EMF.** Endomyocardial fibrosis *LV-left ventricle,* *RV-right ventricle,* *BV-biventricular* **A.** Arrhythmogenic right ventricular cardiomyopathy *M-major,* *m-minor,* *c-category,* *LV-left ventricle,* *RV-right ventricle,* *BV-biventricular* **NC** Left ventricular non-compaction **E** Early **NS** Nonspecific phenotype **NA** Information non- available **O** unaffected	**H** Heart *LV-left ventricle,* *RV-right ventricle* *BV-biventricular* **M** Muscle **N** Nervous **C** Cutaneous **E** Eye, ocular **A.** Auditory **K** Kidney **G** Gastrointestinal **L** Liver **Lu** Lung **S** Skeletal **O** Absence of organ involvement	**N** Family history negative **U** Family history unknown **AU** Autosomal Dominant **AR** Autosomal Recessive **XLD** X-linked Dominant XLR X-linked Recessive **XL** X-linked **M** Matrilineal **O** Family history not investigated **S** Phenotypically sporadic	**G** Genetic cause **OC** Obligate carrier **ONC** Obligate carrier **DN** De novo **Neg.** Negative genetic familiar mutations **N** no identified gene defect O no genetic test no reason **G-A-TTR** Genetic amyloidosis **G-HFE** Hemochromatosis Non-genetic etiologies: **M** Myocarditis **V** Viral infection **AI** Autoimmune/immune-mediated **A.** Amyloidosis (add type) **I** Infectious, non-viral **T** Toxicity (add cause/drug) **EO** Hyper-eosinophilic heart disease **O** Other	**A-D** [ACC /AHA stages] **NA** Not applicable **NU** Not used **1-IV** NYHA classes

ORGANIZATION OF THE INTERCALATED DISK

The direct communication between neighboring cardiomyocytic cells for the transmission of signals and an electrical current is mediated by *Gap junctions* ("hexagonal arrays") (Fig. **1**) due to the low resistance pathways formed [10]. A *gap junction* is composed of twelve connexin proteins, with connexin-43 being the most prominent, along with lesser amounts of connexin-45 and 40 [11, 12] (Figs. **2 A, B, C & D**). Each cardiomyocyte contributes six connexin molecules to form a hemichannel or a connexion; two connexons join to form a pore or gap junction channel, which is isolated from the extracellular space and connects the cytosol of two neighboring cells [13].

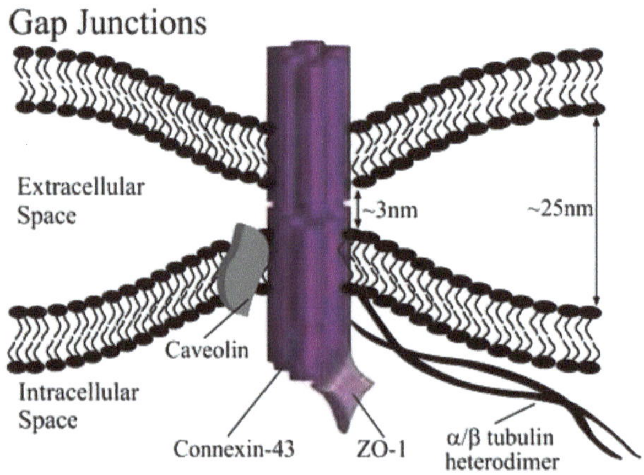

Fig. (1). Gap junctions in ventricular cardiomyocytes are composed of two homo-hexameric hemichannels.

Consequently, in the absence of connexin-43 channels, normal propagation of contraction is disrupted, and lethal arrhythmias develop [14, 15].

On the other hand, *Adherens junctions* composed of mainly transmembrane cadherins and cytosolic catenin's [16], helps in facilitating the transmission of contractile forces between cardiac cells and is also crucial in maintaining a uniform mechanical strength across the heart [17]. Adherens junctions serve as anchors between the extracellular space and the actin cytoskeleton [18] (Figs. **3 A & B**).

Desmosomes provide structural support to cardiomyocytes [19]. They are similar to adherens junctions and are composed of intercellular (desmosomal cadherins, desmocollin, and desmoglein) [20], and intracellular components (proteins of the armadillo/catenin- plakoglobin and plakophilin), and plakin (desmoplakin) families [21] (Fig. **4**).

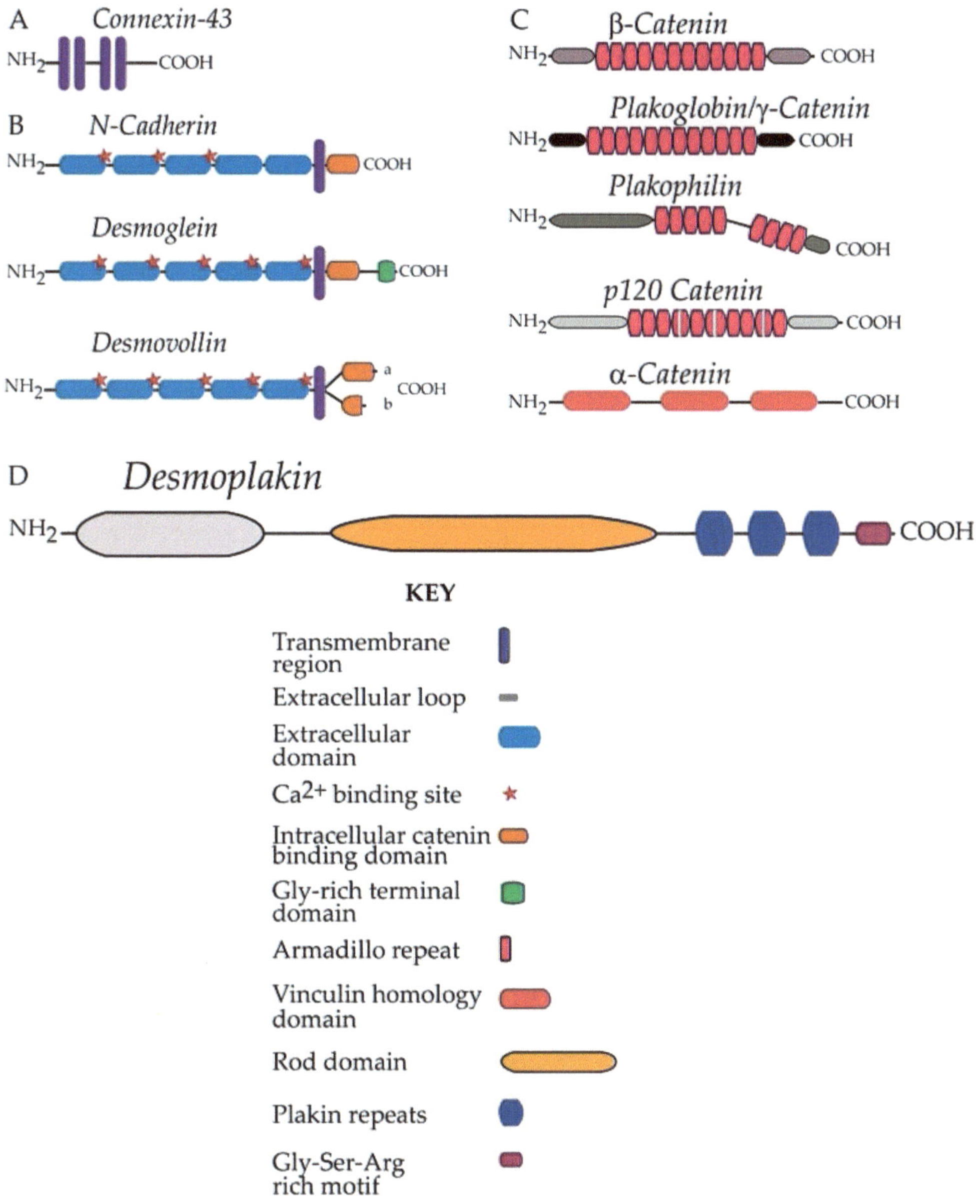

Fig. (2A, B, C & D). Schematic representation of the domain structure of major intercalated disk proteins. Grey ovals denote protein specific domains.

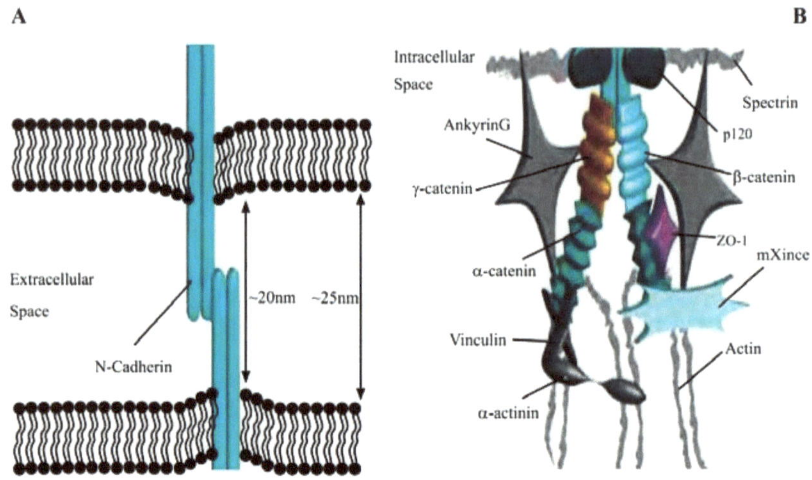

Fig. (3 A & B). Adherens Junctions connect neighboring cardiomyocytes through homophilic dimers of N-cadherin. Connections within the intracellular space link N-cadherin to the actin cytoskeleton (depicted in grey), via additional adherens junction proteins (shown in hues of teal). Adherens junctions did not consider proteins components traditionally but localizing to the intercalated disk are shown in grey. Proteins of other intercalated disk structures, ZO-1 (gap junctions) and.-catenin (desmosomes), are depicted in light purple and gold, respectively.

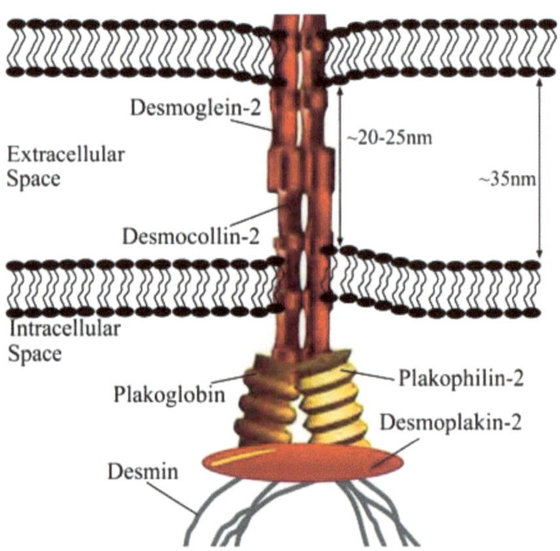

Fig. (4). Desmosomes connect neighboring cardiomyocytes through heterophilic dimers of desmocollin-2 and desmoglein-2 (shown in hues of orange) forming within the extracellular space. Interactions with plakophilin-2, plakoglobin, and desmoplakin-1 (depicted in shades of gold and orange) link the desmosomal complex to the intermediate filament protein desmin (shown in gray) in cardiomyocytes.

Both echocardiography and cardiovascular magnetic resonance imaging are complementary imaging modalities and powerful tools used in the diagnosis of cardiomyopathies. However, echocardiography is superior in the assessment of diastolic function and dynamic outflow tract obstruction while cardiovascular magnetic resonance imaging has several advantages over the former such as excellent resolution, demonstration of relationships between the heart and thoracic structures, three-dimensional visualization, can be repeated safely, tissue characterization (scar or infiltration), and the quantification of cardiac volumes and function [22]. Therapeutic options include pharmacotherapy, implantable cardioverter-defibrillators, cardiac resynchronization therapy, and heart transplantation alongside lifestyle changes.

CONCLUDING REMARKS

Cardiomyopathies represent an ideal translational model of integration between basic and clinical sciences. A multidisciplinary approach is, therefore, essential to ensure their correct diagnosis and management. Rather than affecting mostly the elderly like other heart diseases, it is now commonly found among young adults, directly damaging cardiac muscles, and hence impairing the heart's ability to pump blood to other parts of the body. However, the exact frequency of cardiomyopathy is still currently challenging to ascertain. Although, about five thousand new cases develop each year in the States with an estimated 3% in the general population worldwide. At present, and in the foreseeable future, clinical classifications of cardiomyopathies based on clinical presentation and morphological criteria would prove vital and serve as an essential tool for clinicians involved with these complex disease(s) while calling for a constant improvement and update in the light of the advances provided by imaging genetics and basic sciences.

CONSENT FOR PUBLICATION

Not applicable.

CONFLICT OF INTEREST

The author confirms that this chapter contents have no conflict of interest.

ACKNOWLEDGEMENTS

Declared none.

REFERENCES

[1] Elliott P, Andersson B, Arbustini E, *et al.* Classification of the cardiomyopathies: A position statement from the European Society of Cardiology Working Group on Myocardial and Pericardial Diseases. European Heart Journal 2008; 29(2): 270-6.

[2] Li J, Radice GL. A New Perspective on Intercalated Disc Organization: Implications for Heart Disease Dermatol. Res Pract 2010; pp. 1-5.

[3] Noorman M, van der Heyden MAG, van Veen TAB, *et al.* Cardiac cell-cell junctions in health and disease: Electrical versus mechanical coupling. J Mol Cell Cardiol 2009; 47(1): 23-31. [http://dx.doi.org/10.1016/j.yjmcc.2009.03.016] [PMID: 19344726]

[4] Delmar M, McKenna WJ. The cardiac desmosome and arrhythmogenic cardiomyopathies: from gene to disease. Circ Res 2010; 107(6): 700-14. [http://dx.doi.org/10.1161/CIRCRESAHA.110.223412] [PMID: 20847325]

[5] Richardson P, McKenna W, Bristow M, *et al.* Report of the 1995 World Health Organization/International Society and Federation of Cardiology Task Force on the Definition and Classification of cardiomyopathies. Circulation 1996; 93(5): 841-2. [http://dx.doi.org/10.1161/01.CIR.93.5.841] [PMID: 8598070]

[6] Maron BJ, Towbin JA, Thiene G, *et al.* Contemporary definitions and classification of the cardiomyopathies: an American Heart Association Scientific Statement from the Council on Clinical Cardiology, Heart Failure and Transplantation Committee; Quality of Care and Outcomes Research and Functional Genomics and Translational Biology Interdisciplinary Working Groups; and Council on Epidemiology and Prevention. Circulation 2006; 113(14): 1807-16. [http://dx.doi.org/10.1161/CIRCULATIONAHA.106.174287] [PMID: 16567565]

[7] Arbustini E, Narula N, Tavazzi L, *et al.* The MOGE(S) classification of cardiomyopathy for clinicians. J Am Coll Cardiol 2014; 64(3): 304-18. [http://dx.doi.org/10.1016/j.jacc.2014.05.027] [PMID: 25034069]

[8] Pieperhoff S, Franke WW. The area composita of adhering junctions connecting heart muscle cells of vertebrates - IV: coalescence and amalgamation of desmosomal and adhaerens junction components - late processes in mammalian heart development. Eur J Cell Biol 2007; 86(7): 377-91. [http://dx.doi.org/10.1016/j.ejcb.2007.04.001] [PMID: 17532539]

[9] Peters NS, Severs NJ, Rothery SM, Lincoln C, Yacoub MH, Green CR. Spatiotemporal relation between gap junctions and fascia adherens junctions during postnatal development of human ventricular myocardium. Circulation 1994; 90(2): 713-25. [http://dx.doi.org/10.1161/01.CIR.90.2.713] [PMID: 8044940]

[10] Rohr S. Role of gap junctions in the propagation of the cardiac action potential. Cardiovasc Res 2004; 62(2): 309-22. [http://dx.doi.org/10.1016/j.cardiores.2003.11.035] [PMID: 15094351]

[11] Beyer EC, Paul DL, Goodenough DA. Connexin43: a protein from rat heart homologous to a gap junction protein from liver. J Cell Biol 1987; 105(6 Pt 1): 2621-9. [http://dx.doi.org/10.1083/jcb.105.6.2621] [PMID: 2826492]

[12] Vozzi C, Dupont E, Coppen SR, Yeh HI, Severs NJ. Chamber-related differences in connexin expression in the human heart. J Mol Cell Cardiol 1999; 31(5): 991-1003. [http://dx.doi.org/10.1006/jmcc.1999.0937] [PMID: 10336839]

[13] Söhl G, Willecke K. Gap junctions and the connexin protein family. Cardiovasc Res 2004; 62(2): 228-32. [http://dx.doi.org/10.1016/j.cardiores.2003.11.013] [PMID: 15094343]

[14] Gutstein DE, Morley GE, Vaidya D, *et al.* Heterogeneous expression of Gap junction channels in the heart leads to conduction defects and ventricular dysfunction. Circulation 2001; 104(10): 1194-1199(a).

[http://dx.doi.org/10.1161/hc3601.093990] [PMID: 11535579]

[15] Gutstein DE, Morley GE, Tamaddon H, *et al.* Conduction slowing and sudden arrhythmic death in mice with cardiac-restricted inactivation of connexin43. Circ Res 2001; 88(3): 333-339(b). [http://dx.doi.org/10.1161/01.RES.88.3.333] [PMID: 11179202]

[16] Niessen CM. Tight junctions/adherens junctions: basic structure and function. J Invest Dermatol 2007; 127(11): 2525-32. [http://dx.doi.org/10.1038/sj.jid.5700865] [PMID: 17934504]

[17] Tepass U, Truong K, Godt D, Ikura M, Peifer M. Cadherins in embryonic and neural morphogenesis. Nat Rev Mol Cell Biol 2000; 1(2): 91-100. [http://dx.doi.org/10.1038/35040042] [PMID: 11253370]

[18] Franke WW, Borrmann CM, Grund C, Pieperhoff S. The area composita of adhering junctions connecting heart muscle cells of vertebrates. I. Molecular definition in intercalated disks of cardiomyocytes by immunoelectron microscopy of desmosomal proteins. Eur J Cell Biol 2006; 85: 69-82.

[19] Delmar M. The intercalated disk as a single functional unit. HRTHM 2004; 1: 12-3.

[20] Green KJ, Simpson CL. Desmosomes: new perspectives on a classic. J Invest Dermatol 2007; 127(11): 2499-515. [http://dx.doi.org/10.1038/sj.jid.5701015] [PMID: 17934502]

[21] Bass-Zubek AE, Godsel LM, Delmar M, Green KJ. Plakophilins: multifunctional scaffolds for adhesion and signaling. Curr Opin Cell Biol 2009; 21(5): 708-16. [http://dx.doi.org/10.1016/j.ceb.2009.07.002] [PMID: 19674883]

[22] Quarta G, Sado DM, Moon JC. Cardiomyopathies: focus on cardiovascular magnetic resonance. Br J Radiol 2011; 84(Spec No 3): S296-305. [http://dx.doi.org/10.1259/bjr/67212179] [PMID: 22723536]

CHAPTER 2

The Relationship Between Myocarditis (Viral, Autoimmune) and Cardiomyopathy (Infective, Inflammatory)

Iroegbu Chukwuemeka Daniel[1], **Jiarong Li**[1], **Xiaoming Wu**[1], **Zhou Zhongxin**[2] and **Jinfu Yang**[1,*]

[1] *Department of Cardiovascular Surgery, The Second Xiangya Hospital, Central South University, Middle Renmin Road 139, 410011 Changsha, China*

[2] *Department of Thoracic and Cardiovascular Surgery, Affiliated Hospital of Xuzhou Medical University, Xuzhou, 99 Huaihai Road West Xuzhou, Jiangsu Province 221000, China*

Abstract: Myocarditis, an inflammatory disease of the heart muscle, most often caused by an autoimmune process or viral infection is an essential cause of dilated cardiomyopathy worldwide and also, one of the most challenging diagnosis in cardiology today. Myocarditis of either viral or an autoimmune cause can lead to fatal, life-threatening arrhythmias and/or cardiogenic shock which in some patients, may progress to chronic myocarditis and dilated cardiomyopathy affecting both short- and long-term prognostic outcomes where rapid elimination of the infectious agent and rapid withholding changes of the inflammatory process in the myocardium are too small. Conceptually, the pathogenesis of myocarditis can be sub-divided into three stages: an initial viral proliferation phase, immunologic response and inflammation phase, and finally, a myocardial remodeling and fibrotic phase. Due to the long-term consequences, and the broad spectrum of factors (infectious, immunologic, toxic, among others) causing/leading inflammatory heart muscle diseases, it is imperative that diagnosis and appropriate treatments are done early. At present, due to the insensitivity of traditional diagnostic tests, no diagnostic gold standard is generally accepted, leading to the search for new diagnostic approaches/methods, resulting in the emergence of new molecular diagnostic techniques, and a more detailed immunohistochemical analysis of endomyocardial biopsies. Be it as it may, this chapter aims to discuss the unresolved issues faced with myocarditis (viral and autoimmune) and cardiomyopathy (Infective inflammatory), their relationship as single entities, associated autoimmune processes, old and new treatment options available for patients, recently proposed new general diagnostic approaches, diagnostic gold standard, setbacks, and pitfalls.

[*] **Corresponding author Jinfu Yang:** Department of Cardiovascular Surgery, The Second Xiangya Hospital, Central South University, Middle Renmin Road 139, 410011 Changsha, China;
E-mails: yjf19682005@csu.edu.cn, Dr.iroegbu_daniel@yahoo.com, Dr.iroegbu_daniel@csu.edu.cn

Jinfu Yang & Iroegbu Chukwuemeka Daniel (Eds.)

Keywords: Autoimmune mechanism, Biopsy, Cytokine, Consensus, Cardiomyopathy, Contrast media, Cardiovascular magnetic resonance imaging, Diagnosis, Endomyocardial fibrosis, Heart failure, Inflammation, Infective heart disease, Immunosuppression, Immunomodulation, Immunoadsorption, Myocarditis, Management, Polymerase chain reaction, Pediatric Cardiology, Therapy, Virus.

INTRODUCTION

Myocarditis as a term was first coined and introduced by a German physician Joseph Friedrich Sobernheim in 1837 [1] although, individual cases of myocarditis were documented as early as the 1600s [2]. Pathologically and clinically defined clearly as "inflammation of the myocardium". the term has since been a center of controversy over the past decades as it has continuously been confused with other cardiovascular conditions such as ischemic heart diseases and hypertension [3]. Acute myocarditis is a potentially lethal disease and in most cases it leads to sudden death and usually progresses to dilated cardiomyopathy (DCM) in 10 to 15% of patients either by a progressive autoimmune myocardial injury or as a result of a persistent viral infection. Also, issues of sudden cardiac death prevalence in young people reported in some autopsy studies are highly variable, ranging from 2 to 40% [4].

Similarly, biopsy-proven myocarditis is reported in 10–18% of adult patients with unexplained non-ischemic DCM and in 48% of children with an identifiable cause [5]. However, in 20% of biopsy-proven cases, myocarditis can progress to DCM [6, 7]. Excess amount of cytokine-induced by inflammatory stimuli contributes to the progression of myocardial damage in myocarditis. However, various published studies have shown that cytokines generated by activated immune cells cause an increase in nitric oxide (NO) *via* induction of NO synthase, which eventually results in a direct negative inotropic effect and a modulation of inotropic responsiveness [8 - 10]. Myocarditis is a challenging heart disease to diagnosis due to its heterogenic clinical presentations. In the pursuit for a global standardized diagnostic criterion for myocarditis, the Dallas classification [11] was introduced in 1987 although, the designation had several pitfalls, being susceptible to variation in pathological interpretation, sampling errors, and not considering the exact cause of pathological findings.

The actual incidence of myocarditis is also challenging to determine due to the infrequent use of endomyocardial biopsy (EMB) as the gold standard for diagnosis [12, 13]. With this in mind, EMBs is, however, no longer recommended for the determination of autoimmune or viral myocarditis, mainly due to its lack of additional immunostaining for inflammation and polymerase chain reaction

(PCR) for viral diagnosis. Viral myocarditis presents with various symptoms, ranging from minimally symptomatic cases to fatal arrhythmia and cardiogenic shock, and may develop chronic myocarditis [14]. However, efforts made to redefine viral and autoimmune heart disease may eventually lead to the abolishment of the Dallas criteria as a diagnostic criterion for myocarditis [15]. Experimental Investigations in mouse models carried out described complicated relationship between myocarditis (viral) and cardiomyopathies (infective). The pathological cardiac changes that occurred as a result of the direct cell damage are caused by the virus which was evidently no longer detected (disappeared) in the myocardium as events other than direct myocardial cell damage and inflammatory processes. However, the concept supported by the ongoing damage occurs on an immunologic basis. Whereas in humans, the elevation of cardiotropic viral antibody titers in patients with cardiomyopathy provides evidence of the relationship between the two conditions since lymphocytic myocarditis, in most cases, are related to a preceding viral infection.

Furthermore, histological examination provides further links between myocarditis and cardiomyopathies, documenting definite acute inflammation in patients suffering from cardiomyopathies. Although, the exact prevalence of inflammatory changes in cardiomyopathy is still not apparent. Jean Nicolas Corvisart in 1806, further described a cardiac inflammatory disorder that could result in progressive abnormalities of cardiac function after all the evidence of the infective agent had disappeared [16]. These various infective agents cause functional and structural heart disorders with vast variety form of symptoms such as hypertrophy and dilatation of heart chambers, making a diagnosis of infective inflammatory cardiomyopathies (ICM) steep [17].

Myocarditis onset is often clinically challenging to recognize. Even when the diagnosis is made, the diagnostic procedures suffer from various limitations [18, 19], resulting in many cases diagnosed after congestive heart failure has occurred or only at autopsies [20]. Therefore, strategies to diagnose and depict small areas of myocardial damage in patients with suspected myocarditis is essential as postmortem studies show active myocarditis which causes small areas of myocardial necrosis [21]. Active myocarditis is characterized by inflammatory cellular infiltrate with evidence of myocyte necrosis. As a result of the various clinical features of the disease, Lieberman *et al.* [22] proposed a broader clinicopathological classification to incorporate these features. The classification divided myocarditis into fulminant, subacute, active chronic, and persistent subtypes. However, Borderline myocarditis demonstrates an inflammatory cellular infiltrate without any evidence of myocyte injury, unlike active myocarditis. The inflammation could be mild, moderate, or severe, and its distribution can also be focal, confluent, or diffuse, respectively. The extreme diversity of clinical manifestations has led to the development of molecular techniques to facilitate new insights into autoimmune inflammatory processes that affect the myocardium. Despite the well-established associated myocarditis morbidity and mortality rate, clinical practice guidelines about its evaluation and treatment are lacking caused as a result of the variety of etiologies and its various clinical presentations [23, 24].

Sampling error with EMB has remained a significant limitation to myocarditis diagnostic accuracy. Although three to six biopsy samples are performed routinely during diagnostic procedures, postmortem investigations proved that above ten samples were necessary to clinically and correctly give a definite diagnosis for myocarditis which is not feasible in clinical practice [25]. Intra-observer variability is also another significant limitation in the diagnosis of myocarditis. However, the treatment of many forms of myocarditis is symptomatic, but biological molecular analysis of EMB, autoantibody serum testing, and immunohistochemical analysis is essential in identifying patients for whom specific therapy is appropriate [18, 22, 26 - 28]. Myocarditis and cardiomyopathies are one of the most difficult and challenging diagnosis in cardiology as it is difficult to recognize, misdiagnosed, and its pathophysiology defectively understood.

Be it as it may, this scientific chapter aims to discuss the unresolved issues faced with myocarditis (viral and autoimmune) and cardiomyopathy (Infective inflammatory), their relationship as single entities, associated autoimmune processes, old and new treatment options available for patients, recently proposed new general diagnostic approaches, diagnostic gold standard (EMB's), setbacks and pitfalls.

NATURAL HISTORY

Myocarditis natural history is as varied (fulminant, acute, viral, bacterial, autoimmune, *etc.*) to its various clinical presentations (fever, fatigue, chest pain, clinical heart failure, dyspnea on exertion, palpitations, and subsequent viral prodromes), complete recovery, and long-term evolution to DCM [29]. Due to its asymptomatic course and its difficult diagnosis, D' Ambrosio *et al.* [29] reviewed the "history of histology-proven acute myocarditis." Once patients with acute fulminant myocarditis survive the severe illness, they tend to have a favorable long-term prognosis of 90-94% at an average of eight to eleven years with a one-year mortality rate of 20% [30] as compared to patients presenting with acute non-fulminant myocarditis [23]. Patients with a previous history of myocarditis, Kuhl *et al.* [31] showed that viral persistence in the myocardium leads to left ventricular deterioration (LV), whereas clearance of the viral genomes resulted in a significant improvement of LV function. Myocarditis masquerading as myocardial infarction usually results in a full recovery of cardiovascular function in previously healthy adults [32]. Patients with clinical features of heart failure may have a mildly compromised left ventricular ejection fraction [LVEF] of 42% to 50% which typically improves within weeks to months. Moderate to severe cases lead to a more advanced left ventricular dysfunction (LVEF 30-35%, left ventricular end-diastolic dimension 60 mm). Alternatively, patients with chronic ventricular dysfunction will need planned surgical heart transplantation, or will eventually lead to sudden death [33]. Patients follow-up of two to three years suffering from myocarditis is pivotal as reoccurrence even after years of its first episode is highly possible. However, the natural course of history in patients with newly diagnosed cardiomyopathy due to myocarditis remains unclear and problematic.

INCIDENCE AND ETIOLOGY

Myocarditis is reported to be one of the leading courses of the sudden death of young adults [34 - 37] and is also a primary underlying etiology of other myocardial diseases such as DCM and infective inflammatory cardiomyopathy [38, 39]. Infective ICM, however, may also be triggered by reversible and irreversible toxic, mechanical injury, ischemic or drug-related inflammation, transplant rejection or other immune reactions as the case of autoimmune myocarditis. The incidence of the infectious disease accounts for the majority of cases, in previously healthy patients typically due to either a direct viral infection or post-viral immune-mediated reaction. Viral myocarditis still remains the prototype for the disease study. Although, a broad array of etiologies is implicated as causes of myocarditis as a single disease entity and its evolution. The extensive testing of myocardial tissues for potential viral etiologies are facilitated by the use of polymerase chain reaction (PCR) [40]. The etiologies of myocarditis, infective inflammatory cardiomyopathies are manifold and include viral, bacterial, helminthic, fungal, rickettsial, and protozoal infections as well as other noninfectious causes (Table **1**). The histology of inflammation in the myocardium is nowadays characterized quantitatively by an infiltrate of $\geq$14 cells/mm^2. The respective subpopulations named as B- (CD 21-positive) and T-cells, whereby CD3 labels all, CD4 only helper, CD8 suppressor, CD45R0 activated T-cells and CD 68 macrophages and monocytes. The interplay between the myocardial injury by microbial agents and the different components of the patient's immune system determine the histological and clinical phenotype of the individual patient.

Table 1. Etiologies of Myocarditis, human infectious and non-infectious inflammatory cardiomyopathy.

Bacterial	Mycoplasma pneumoniae, Mycobacterial, Treponema pallidum, Streptococcal species
Viral	HCV, HIV, Adenovirus, Coxsackievirus
Toxins	Cocaine, Anthracyclines, Interleukin-2
Protozoal	Trypanosoma cruzi
Fungal	Candida, Aspergillus, Histoplasma, Cryptococcus, Coccidiodes
Parasitic	Larva migrans, Schistosomiasis
Immunologic syndromes	Systemic lupus erythematosus, Sarcoidosis, Churg-Strauss, Giant cell myocarditis, Takayasu's arteritis, Wegener's granulomatosis, Diabetes mellitus, Inflammatory bowel disease, Thyrotoxicosis
Hypersensitivity	Diuretics, Dobutamine, Tricyclic antidepressants, Cephalosporins Digoxin, Sulfonamides
(Auto-)Immune activation Giant cell myocarditis, Postinfectious, Sjögren's syndrome, Takayasu arteritis, Wegener's granulomatosis, Sarcoidosis, Churg- Strauss syndrome, Influenza vaccination, Inflammatory bowel disorders, Systemic Lupus Erythematosus	
Physical pathogens Irradiation, Heatstroke Arsenic, Lithium, Hypothermia	

MYOCARDITIS

The term myocarditis "inflammation of the myocardium" describes acute inflammatory disorders of the heart muscle of various infectious and non-infectious origin with subsequent disturbance of left or right ventricular function. This irresistible and non-infectious causes over a long period eventually lead to chronic inflammation of the myocardium. If, however, the immune system is overwhelmed and fails to eliminate the infectious pathogen, chronic infection develops, which in most cases, is accompanied by inflammation [41]. Lasting myocardial injury and persistent inflammatory process which does not spontaneously resolve even after elimination of the pathogen over time indicates chronic inflammatory cardiomyopathy is present [29].

INFLAMMATORY (INFECTIVE) CARDIOMYOPATHY

ICM is the inflammation of the heart muscle associated with impairment of myocardial function, which often takes the morphology of DCM. These inflammations of the myocardium may be as a result of infectious (bacterial, viral, and protozoal infections) or noninfectious (myocarditis accompanying autoimmune disease or hypersensitivity to certain harmful substances). It becomes evident due to LV dysfunction, which is also an integral part of the diagnosis of ICM. However, the contemporary view on its pathophysiology though based on animal models of an enterovirus which is believed to be in three-phase [42 - 45]. The first acute phase is associated with viral entry into myocytes over the virus-specific receptor [46]. The second phase usually starts two to four weeks after the onset of the disease and characterized by a specific immune reaction [47 - 50]. The third phase occurs several weeks to months as the inflammation might either subside with an improvement in LV function or a further persistence in LV dysfunction and DCM [29, 51]. Whether the described course takes place in all cases is still not entirely clear [52]. Chronic post-infectious or autoimmune inflammatory processes (chronic ICM's) with a duration of illness of more than six months do usually respond well to immunosuppression treatment with azathioprine or cortisone therapy by decreasing the pathogen persistence. Although, it uses remains controversial (reviewed in detail further in the chapter) [53 - 56].

EXISTING DEFINITIONS AND HISTORICAL CLASSIFICATIONS IN MYOCARDITIS AND INFLAMMATORY CARDIOMYOPATHY

Myocarditis: is an inflammation disease of the heart muscle (myocardium) (**Box 1**).

Box 1. World Health Organization and International Society and Cardiology definitions of myocarditis, and inflammatory cardiomyopathy

Inflammatory Cardiomyopathy: is both a functional and histological diagnosis characterized by myocarditis in association with systolic and diastolic cardiac dysfunction by quantitative immunohistological criteria for inflammation ($\geq$14 infiltrating cells/mm^2). The infiltrating cells could be T and B lymphocytes, their activated forms, and up to 4 monocytes or macrophages/mm^2 [42].

Viral Myocarditis: Myocardial histological evidence for myocarditis associated with positive viral PCR (Fig. **1**).

Auto Immune Myocarditis: Histological myocarditis with negative viral PCR, with or without serum cardiac autoantibodies (aabs).

Viral and Immune Myocarditis: Histological myocarditis with positive cardiac aabs and positive viral PCR. However, it is essential to note that follow-up EMB's may document persistent viral myocarditis, persistent virus-negative myocarditis, without serum cardiac aabs or histological and virological resolution, *e.g.*, a post-infectious autoimmune disease.

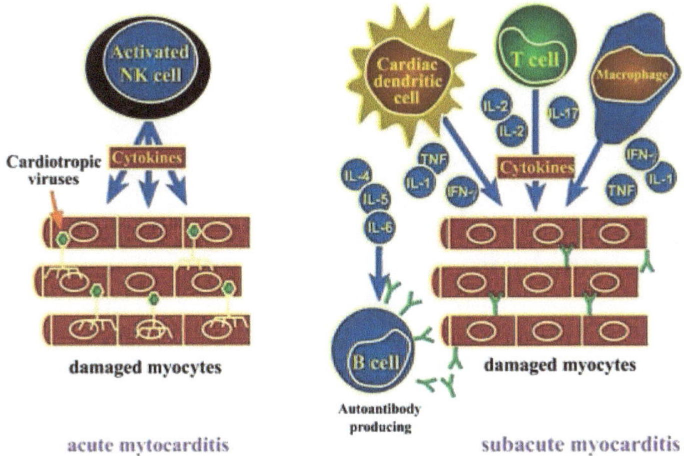

Fig. (1). Pathophysiology of Viral Myocarditis.

Hickie and Hall first used cardiomyopathies in the 1960s. The WHO/ISFC (World Health Organization/International Society and Federation of Cardiology) Task Force defined it as "heart muscle diseases of unknown cause." The WHO/ISCF classification of 1996 further expanded the term cardiomyopathies to all heart muscle diseases that lead to functional impairment of the heart which made DCM one of four main clinical phenotypes (dilated, restrictive, hypertrophic, and arrhythmogenic right ventricular cardiomyopathy). The 1996 task force also included inflammatory heart muscle diseases (peri-myocarditis, myocarditis), ischemic cardiomyopathy, hypertensive cardiomyopathy, and other forms of heart failure of known origin in the group of secondary cardiomyopathies.

PATHOGENESIS AND PATHOLOGY OF MYOCARDITIS

Myocarditis is a disease with both variable clinical progression and presentation [29]. To better understand its often unpredictable progress, addressing its underlying pathophysiological process is essential. In human myocarditis, there is evidence for autoimmune and viral mechanisms, acting in individuals with or without a genetic predisposition (sporadic or familial cases, respectively) [57, 58]. The destruction of the cardiomyocytes occurs by virus-mediated lysis during the first phase [59], degrading the structure of the cells, facilitating the entry of the virus into the cells with significant myocyte injury and cardiac dilatation [60]. This phase (initial phase) frequently goes unnoticed as the initial damage are often prevented by the innate immune response [23]. Two weeks later (post-infection), severe cytopathic effects can be noticed due to the enteroviruses which preferentially enter cardiomyocytes *via* specific receptors [61, 62].

CLINICAL PRESENTATIONS AND PATTERN OF MYOCARDITIS LESIONS

Clinical Pathognomic Signs and Associated Symptoms: Myocarditis presents in many different ways, often starting with flu-like symptoms, either of gastrointestinal or upper respiratory tracts. Cardiac symptoms appear ranging from mild chest pain, and associated palpitations with transient electrocardiography (ECG) which then progresses to life-threatening cardiogenic shock and ventricular arrhythmia, sinus tachycardia, gallops, murmurs of mitral or tricuspid insufficiency, a diminished first heart sound, and rarely but pathognomic, a pericardial friction rub. Typically, cardiac symptoms delay a few days to a few weeks after initial flu-like symptoms. Although, clinical cardiac signs and symptoms may be vague. It affects individuals of all ages and is most frequently seen in younger patients [63]. Myocarditis can also, produce variable effects on the cardiac conduction system. Ventricular tachycardia is a different initial manifestation of myocarditis but often develops during long-term follow-up. Cardiac involvement is often considered as the differential diagnosis only when cardiac symptoms, such as angina, palpitations, and exertional dyspnea, persist over a long period after the underlying infection has resolved. At this stage, the laboratory chemical findings and the ECG results that are characteristic of acute myocarditis such as raised cardiac enzymes and changes to the ST segment that are typical for severe myocardial involvement are no longer presents [33].

It's important to note that, diagnoses at this point can't pinpoint the cause of the existing disorder but can only collect data on the extent of myocardial injury. Even if imaging methods such as (ECG, angiography, and magnetic resonance imaging [MRI]) are used to exclude specific cardiac disorders such as (valve deficiencies, and ischemic cardiomyopathy); or provide clues for a suspected diagnosis of infectious myocarditis [29]. This only implies that clinical cases/scenarios for the determination of myocarditis require a high level of suspicion. In cases of suspected myocarditis, it is compulsory to exclude coronary artery disease and other cardiovascular diseases, *e.g.*, hypertension, or extra-cardiac non-inflammatory diseases. If the clinician strongly suspects this, the further specific investigation may be appropriate. In terms of therapeutic considerations, physicians should bear in mind that a positive treatment effect will only occur if treatable causes such as inflammatory processes, and viral infections, or cardio depressive autoantibodies are present and the myocardium still has the regenerative potential [64]. If, However, irreversible myocardial damage such as post inflammatory or post infectious DCM has occurred with no specific treatment available, the progression of heart failure or sudden death in the nearest future is inevitable.

The Pattern of Myocarditis Lesions: The tend to occur predominantly in the lateral free wall and originate from the epicardial quartile of the ventricular wall which is the preferred location of inflammatory lesions, clinically confirmed during postmortem studies [65]. Origins from the subendocardium are typical for myocardial infarction [20].

PROPOSED CRITERIA FOR CLINICALLY SUSPECTED MYOCARDITIS

The proposed criteria's bellow based on clinical presentations and patterns above, consistent with the diagnosis and the presence of one or more abnormalities on non-invasive testing (discussed in details further in the chapter).

Ancillary Features for Clinical Suspicion of Myocarditis

A. Family history of myocarditis (DCM)
B. Family and personal account of allergic asthma, other types of allergy, extra-cardiac autoimmune disease
C. Fever 38°C and above at presentation or within the previous 30 days with or without evidence of a gastrointestinal (nausea, vomiting, diarrhea, decreased appetite) and respiratory (general malaise, chills, muscle aches, headache) infection.
D. Previous clinically suspected or diagnosed myocarditis

Additional Investigational Clinics for Suspected Myocarditis

For patients fulfilling the above clinically suspected myocarditis criteria, selective coronary angiography alongside EMB is advisable. It also applies to patients with acute myocarditis masquerading as myocardial infarction (MI), increased cardiac troponins, and preserved ventricular systolic function with or without features suggestive of myocarditis on cardiac MRI [66].

DIAGNOSIS AND DIAGNOSTIC EVALUATION OF MYOCARDITIS

Diagnosis

Initial diagnosis of myocarditis involves a careful physical examination and a detailed history of the patient to help provide clues to its etiology. The inspections should include an ECG, chest X-ray, computed tomography (CT), blood studies, non-invasive imaging techniques, and EMB. The use of non-invasive imaging techniques such as CMR provides additional detailed clues to help support the diagnosis of myocarditis and also monitor the disease's progression. According to current guidelines, a determination made should be EMB's based although this remains controversial [44, 67], as the directions are also particularly helpful in only a limited number of clinical scenarios that do not include common myocarditis presentations, in particular, pseudo-infarction [68].

Diagnostic Evaluations

The diagnostic evaluations implored provides vital clinical clues on arrhythmias, systolic or diastolic heart failure, or injury to the heart valves which are quantitatively and qualitatively identified, easily differentiating the dominant clinical cardiomyopathic phenotypes (Dilated, hypertrophic, restrictive, and arrhythmogenic).

Electrocardiogram (ECG): It is usually abnormal in patients with myocarditis ranging from conduction delays to ECGs mimicking acute MI or acute pericarditis [32, 69]. Though ECG signs are neither non-sensitive nor non-specific [6, 70 - 72], some ECG readings could be more informative and suggestive of myocarditis, such as, ST-T segment elevation in myocarditis which is typically concave (rather than convex in myocardial ischemia) and diffuse without reciprocal changes.

Viral Serology: Peripheral viral cultures and traditional serological studies in the past have been used to identify the most frequent viral myocarditis. Although, these methods, unfortunately, lack sensitivity and specificity. However, at the presentation of cardiac symptoms, the presence of raised IgM, IgA, and low IgG suggest viral cardiac manifestation.

Biopsies

Generally reserved for patients with unexplained cardiomyopathy that is associated with progressive conduction system disease, progressive cardiomyopathy refractory to conventional therapeutic management or life-threatening ventricular arrhythmias. Biopsies should also be considered when cardiovascular signs or symptoms develop in a patient with a systemic disease known to cause LV dysfunction [73] (Table **2**).

Table 2. Indications for Endomyocardial Biopsy. DCM-Dilated cardiomyopathy, HF-heart failure, SLE-Systemic Lupus erythematosus.

Exclusion of potential common etiologies of DCM (familial; ischemic; alcohol; postpartum; cardiotoxic exposures) and the below:
Acute or subacute symptoms of HF refractory to standard management
Substantial worsening of EF despite optimized pharmacological therapy
Development of hemodynamically significant arrhythmias, particularly progressive heart block and VT

(Table 2) cont.....

Peripheral eosinophilia, fever, or concurrent rash
History of collagen vascular diseases such as scleroderma, SLE, or polyarteritis nodosum
New-onset Cardiomyopathy with known associated hemochromatosis, amyloidosis, or sarcoidosis.
IF "x_+3" "@008@012" "" @003@004@005
IF "x_-3" "@008@012" "" @003@005T

According to the American College of Cardiology (ACC) and American Heart Association guidelines (AHA) [68, 74], it supports the use of EMB for patients presenting with unexplained new-onset heart failure two to three weeks in duration associated with a normal-sized or dilated left ventricle in addition to hemodynamic compromise. Although, the standard timeframe for obtaining EMBs is still much debated. However, a maximum of two to three days has been made clinically justifiable and safe. It is of paramount importance that the EMB analysis should include immunohistological techniques for inflammation, routine light microscopy, and PCR for virus detection.

Biopsies (Viral Diagnosis): The current improvements with molecular techniques, such as in situ hybridization and PCR, new prevalent viruses (PVB19 and HHV6) have emerged recently [75 - 77]. The infections trigger pathognomic processes (long-term cardiac injury and dysfunction) similar in patients with acute myocarditis and DCM. Recent findings, however, indicate a shift of adenovirus and enterovirus to PVB19 and HHV6 as the most common viruses causing acute myocarditis.

Biopsies (Histological Evaluation): The presence of an inflammatory infiltrate with or without necrosis under light microscopy is necessary for myocarditis histological diagnosis. According to Dallas criteria [11], the absence of a sparser inflammatory infiltrate, and myocyte necrosis suggests borderline myocarditis. However, questions, whether the Dallas criteria are sensitive enough to identify viral cardiomyopathy, have been a concern among pathologist. Additional quantitative evaluation of the EMBs and immunohistological analysis is required to address the shortcomings. Immunohistochemical techniques allow identification, quantification, and differentiation of inflammatory cells, focusing on T-lymphocytes [78]. Also, criteria for immunohistological diagnosis in EMB of ICM is quantitatively specified as 14 infiltrating leukocytes/mm^2, preferably activated T-cells or T-lymphocytes. If foci of activated T-cells are present, active myocarditis can be diagnosed due to the nature of the infiltrate even if the critical number as quantitatively specified is not attained, as defined by World Heart Federation's Council on Cardiomyopathies [79].

Blood Studies

Cardiac Enzymes: Cardiac enzymes are elevated in patients with myocarditis, but lacking specific markers to detect acute myocarditis in routine blood studies are creating room for repeated questions about its reliability [80]. Apart from the conventional determination of creatine kinase levels, cardiac troponins serum levels are more sensitive in patients with clinically suspected myocarditis indicating myocyte injury [81]. Although cardiac troponin levels are also elevated in patients with familial and acute myocarditis, its prognostic values remain unclear.

Cardiac Auto-Antibodies: The pathophysiologic role of auto-antibodies in cardiac injury after a viral pathogen infection remains unclear. However, autoantibodies against contractile structures, ion channels transporters, proteins producing energy for metabolism and transfer, and sarcolemmal receptors have all been found to play significant roles in the pathophysiologic mechanism of myocarditis [82]. Below are indications for their role in the pathophysiology of myocarditis:

[I]. Auto-antibodies lead to the production of inflammation in the heart, which results in cardiomyocytes injury [83].

[II]. In a study by Schwimmbeck PL *et al.*, a human proven heart-reactive auto-antibodies lymphocyte transferred into a severely immunodeficient mouse caused myocardial inflammation, autoantibody production, and an impaired cardiac function [84].

[III]. Also, in another study by Okazaki T, *et al.*, the direct transfer of auto-antibodies against b-adrenoreceptors and cTnl in rodents resulted in cardiac dysfunction and dilatation [85].

[IV]. Active immunization with cardiac auto-antigens leads to auto-antibody production, cardiac dysfunction, and heart-specific inflammation [86].

These cardiac markers are present in about 55% of patients with active to borderline biopsy-proven myocarditis. Be it as it may, further studies on this is still much required [6].

Immunologic Approach

Characterization of infiltrating lymphocytes subtypes have been enabled with immunohistochemical staining allowing a more precise characterization of infiltrating lymphocytes subtypes which accurately help define and quantify significant histocompatibility myocyte-specific (MHC) antigens. Immunological advances have expanded the diagnostic capabilities of EMBs, using MHC antigen as an essential criterion in diagnosing ICM.

Imaging Tools

Echocardiography: Currently recommended in the initial diagnostic evaluation of all patients with suspected myocarditis. It helps rule out non-inflammatory cardiac disease such as valvular disease and also monitor changes in ventricular function, wall thickness, cardiac size, and pericardial effusions. It is also useful in distinguishing fulminant myocarditis from subacute myocarditis, as the former often presents with a non-dilated, thickened and hypercontractile left ventricle. Regional wall motion abnormalities, ventricular, and diastolic dysfunction with preserved ejection fraction (EF) occur in myocarditis [87, 88]. The use of ultrasonic tissue characterization is essential to as anatomic features on echocardiography (*i.e.*, wall motion abnormalities, chamber dimensions, and EF) are insufficient to differentiate myocarditis from other forms of cardiomyopathy. Transmission and reflection of ultrasound energy depend on tissue elasticity, density, and acoustical impedance. Changes in these factors (either one or more) lead to different ultrasonic backscatter and altered image texture.

Cardiovascular Magnetic Resonance Imaging: CMR supports the diagnosis of myocarditis by providing a non-invasive tissue characterization of the myocardium [89, 90]. Timing is crucial, but when remains debatable. Although, it's advisable to perform CMR in clinically stable patients, before EMB. It should, however, not be done on patients with life-threatening presentations where EMB is urgently indicated [68, 90]. Contrast-enhanced CMR imaging appears to be the most promising technique for diagnosing myocardial inflammation and myocyte injury based on clinical studies. Besides providing morphological and anatomic information, CMR imaging provides accurate tissue characterization by measuring spin densities and T1 and T2 relaxation times. As active myocarditis is associated with typical myocyte injury, including cellular swelling and edema, relaxation time assessment provides a sensitive measure for its detection [91] (Table **3**).

***Nuclear Imaging*:** Radionuclide evaluation, including anti-myosin antibody imaging, has been described as a screening method for myocarditis with high sensitivity (91–100%) and negative predictive value (93–100%) by detecting localized or diffuse myocardial necrosis [91]. Unfortunately, due to limited data on radionuclide evaluation, availability, the pronounced risk from radiation exposure, 48 h delay in obtaining images, and nuclear techniques, its use has been remained restricted and not routinely recommended, except sarcoidosis.

INDICATIONS FOR CARDIOVASCULAR MAGNETIC RESONANCE IMAGING, PROCEDURES, AND PROTOCOL

Indications for CMR: It is professionally advisable to perform CMR only in the following conditions:

[I]. Symptomatic (persistent, recurrent chest pain, increased troponin levels, *etc.*) including both current and persisting past symptoms.
[II]. Conclusive clinical evidence for myocarditis.
[III]. Results obtained would inevitably likely affect clinical judgment and management.
[IV]. Confirmation of suspected viral etiology (past and present).
[V]. Evidence of significant myocardial injury with the diagnostic help of ECG.

Table 3. Lake Louise Consensus Criteria.

Proposed Diagnostic CMR Criteria (LLCC) for Myocarditis
In the setting of clinically suspected myocarditis [a] CMR findings are consistent with myocardial inflammation if at least two of the following criteria are present: 1 Global or regional myocardial SI increase in T2-weighted images [b] 2 Increased global myocardial early gadolinium enhancement ratios between myocardium and skeletal muscle in gadolinium-enhanced T1-weighted images [c] 3 One focal lesion with non-ischemic regional distribution in IR-prepared gadolinium-enhanced T1-weighted images (" late gadolinium enhancement") [d].
A CMR study with myocyte injury and scar caused by myocardial inflammation is said to be consistent if: - criterion 3 is present.
A repeat CMR study between one and two weeks after the initial CMR study is recommended, if: - there is clinical evidence for myocardial inflammation, recent onset of symptoms, and none of the criteria are present. - one criterion is clinically present.
The presence of pericardial effusion or LV dysfunction provides additional, and supportive evidence for myocarditis.

An additional indication is also necessarily needed for a specific group of patients exposed to strenuous physical exercise. *e.g.*, for professional athletes or for a group of patients presenting with an unexplained new ECG finding which is consistent with myocarditis.

CMR Procedure: Patients are typically examined in a supine position. A cardiac surface phased-array coil is used to acquire functional images. For a qualitative and quantitative signal intensity analysis, a body coil or signal intensity correction algorithm should be used as an inhomogeneous sensitive field could give a false positive result (septum) and a false negative result (inferolateral wall). During the procedure, all LV segments of the heart should be covered to provide sufficient and adequate scan to support the diagnoses [92].

It is, however, essential to ensure all the below basic requirements are met before and during CMR procedures:

[I]. The process should only be carried out by a trained, certified physician in the field and should only be done in cardiac centers with vast knowledge and experience.
[II]. During the procedure, a physician trained in cardiac resuscitation should be available and on standby.
[III]. Drugs, equipment for immediate interventions, and other cardiac modalities should be within reach.
[IV]. Monitoring of patients throughout each session is mandatory, including breathing and oxygen saturation, blood pressure, and ECG's.

CARDIOVASCULAR MAGNETIC RESONANCE IMAGING DIAGNOSTIC TARGETS IN MYOCARDITIS AND CARDIOMYOPATHY

Apart from the morphological and functional targets of CMR for myocarditis and cardiomyopathies, it also includes tissue pathology as a diagnostic feature target of CMR for myocardial inflammation (discussed further in the chapter).

Morphological Abnormalities: It describes the transient increase of wall thickness and an increase in LV volume during myocarditis, providing additional and supportive findings in follow-up studies of the patient [93]. However, another significant morphological abnormality favorable finding provided by CMR in patients with suspected myocarditis and ICM is the decrease of LV mass as assesses by T2-weighted CMR imaging [94].

Functional Abnormalities: CMR asses both right and left ventricular dysfunction by quantifying and identifying functional abnormalities from mild to severe cases and any other underlying pathophysiology, both regional or global.

CARDIOVASCULAR MAGNETIC RESONANCE IMAGING DIAGNOSTIC ADVANTAGES FOR MYOCARDITIS

[I]. Visualizes the entire myocardium which is integral for a patchy process such as myocarditis.
[II]. Highly sensitive to changes in tissue composition in myocarditis and ICM, which is altered in inflammation.
[III]. The T2 relaxation time is an inherent indicator of tissue water content, and

possess a high sensitivity to cardiac inflammation, which is increased in inflammation or necrosis.

The mobilization of inflammatory cells, cytokine release, antibodies, and other foci activities enhances tissue remodeling, increases vascular permeability, tissue edema, and finally fibrosis. All these inherent tissue activities enable detection readily by CMR.

CONTRAST ENHANCEMENT AND MEDIA ACCUMULATION

Mechanism of contrast enhancement is facilitated as a result of myocyte rupture, which provides gaps for the contrast to diffuse into the cells resulting in an increased tissue level concentration of the contrast medium. Although, this mechanism is extremely slow as compared to infarcts, which usually have significantly larger extracellular space than usual, mostly due to its gaps been replaced by fibrous tissues [95, 96]. Contrast-enhanced associated myocarditis might not be as bright as infarcts, which are because inflammatory areas in infarcts usually still contain more living myocytes between necrotic islands. This method of detecting acute myocarditis and cardiac inflammatory processes with the use of noninvasive techniques that can be repeated several times without the application of radioactive materials or the use of radiation and other invasive methods is needed for follow-up and the better management of patients with acute myocarditis and ICM.

CARDIOVASCULAR MAGNETIC RESONANCE TISSUE CHARACTERIZATION

The use of CMR in diagnostic follow-up (Figs. **2** & **3**) of myocarditis and ICM is very much vital as it possesses excellent tissue changes in visualization qualities. These tissue pathologies include:

Intracellular and Interstitial Tissue Edema: Increased tissue permeability of the cellular membrane is an essential hallmark of inflammatory cell injury. The practical nature of membrane injuries is the influx of Na^+ which is followed by intracellular edema, whereas, a severe membrane injury such as myocarditis process initiates a more severe net flow of H_2O and other transmembrane leakages of larger molecules such as troponin which eventually lead to loss of cellular functions. Although Myocarditis progression is patchy like, the use of CMR T2-weighted imaging provides a distinct sensitivity separation between fat and the flowing blood for regional edema and the normal myocardium [97]. It is also however important to note that in some cases, some patients might present with global myocardial distribution, unlike its patchy nature. Hence, it is necessary to analyze the entire myocardium [98, 99].

Hyperemia and Capillary Leak (Early Gadolinium Enhancement): The increase of blood flow into the inflamed area leads to an increase re-uptake of gadolinium contrast in enhanced T1-weighted imaging to detect inflammatory processes and acute myocarditis especially in the early vascular phase as it disseminates faster into the interstitial space after its administration [99, 100].

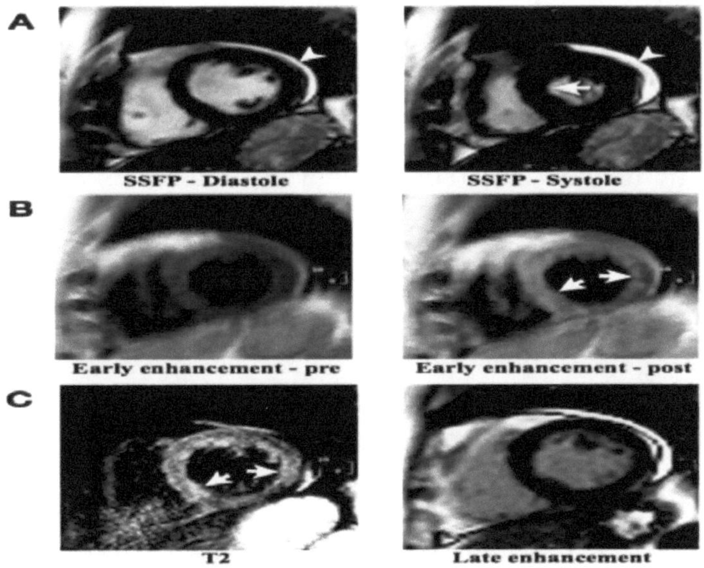

Fig. (2). Short axis CMR views in a patient with clinically acute myocarditis.
A: Still frames from a cine series at end-diastole (left) and end-systole (right), showing only very mild septal hypokinesis (arrow) with preserved EF. Small pericardial effusion is present along the lateral segments (arrowhead). These findings represent two supportive criteria for myocarditis.
B: T1-weighted spin echo images before (left) and shortly after (right) gadolinium administration with early gadolinium accumulation in the septum (arrows). Quantitative evaluation of the signal enhancement (skeletal-muscle normalized myocardial enhancement ratio of equal to or greater than 4.0 or an absolute enhancement of equal to or greater than 45%) is required to use information from this pulse sequence as a positive criterion.
C: Left: T2-weighted spin echo image with high signal intensity of the septum and lateral wall (arrows). Evidence for regional edema, or a signal intensity ratio of equal to or greater than 2.0 (signal intensity normalized to skeletal muscle in the same slice) renders T2 findings positive. Right: Late enhancement image without evidence for significant delay of gadolinium washout. The thin subepicardial layer of high signal intensity in the inferolateral region represents fat.

Necrosis and Fibrosis (Late Gadolinium Enhancement): Myocarditis-related necrosis is visualized as gadolinium enters the acutely injured cell membranes. Late gadolinium enhancement (LGE) imaging uses an inversion pulse to decrease the signal response from normal myocardium, thereby highlighting areas with increased accumulation of gadolinium as bright regions. However, LGE maybe insensitive in patients with symptomatic myocarditis with limited or non-focal irreversible injury as studies is needed to address the issue [65, 70].

EVALUATION OF CARDIOVASCULAR MAGNETIC RESONANCE IMAGING [FOLLOW-UP AND STANDARDIZED CONSENSUS REPORTING TERMS]

Reporting of CMR Results: It is essential to be aware that CMR results only depicts the status of the patient's at a given point in time and cannot, however, characterize acute, chronic and relapsing forms. These terms are somewhat based on the clinical course rather than imaging (or biopsy) findings. Based on the consensus group, its rather best to avoid the conditions acute, chronic, *etc.* concerning CMR findings, but rather comment on the presence or absence of "active" or "ongoing" inflammation. Bearing this in mind, the CMR imaging reports should therefore address the questions raised by the referring physician such as: LV function (size, weight, volume), inflammatory activity and other vital information, such as cardiac apex, pericardial effusion and the extent of scarring, if acquired should also be reported (Table **4**).

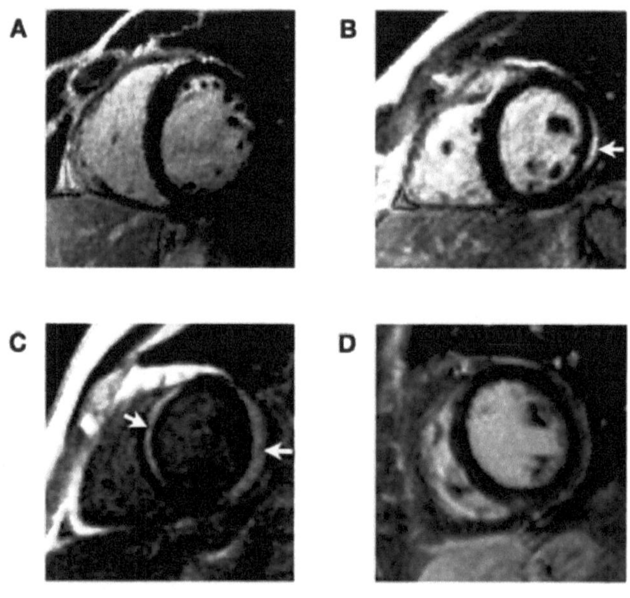

Fig. (3). Late enhancement patterns in myocarditis.
A: Normal myocardium with no evidence of irreversible myocyte injury.
B: Regional sub-epicardial enhancement of the lateral wall (arrow).
C: Subepicardial enhancement of lateral and mid-wall enhancement of the septal wall (arrows).
d: Subepicardial enhancement of lateral and mid-wall enhancement of the septal wall (arrows).

Follow-up by CMR: CMR studies and monitoring during the first day may be less sensitive when compared to those obtained 5 to 7 days after the initial clinical onset of the disease which could be as a result of the focal nature of the early stages of the disease. Although, the decision regarding when follow-up studies should be done is solely based on individual scenarios and the attending physician. Thus, in a patient with strong clinical evidence for myocarditis yet negative criteria in the initial CMR study, a repeat scan may be needed to establish the diagnosis. A follow-up study of at least 3 to 4 weeks after the initial onset of the disease is necessary as it would help differentiate uncomplicated systemic viral illness of the myocardium from a problematic course with autoimmune disease or viral persistence.

Table 4. *To avoid misinterpretation of artifacts; areas with abnormal SI should consist of at least ten adjacent pixels to be regarded as relevant. † Global high T2 signal is defined by an SI ratio between myocardium and skeletal muscle of ≥2.0.m‡. Increased myocardial early gadolinium enhancement ratio is determined by either ≥45% absolute myocardial enhancement or a 4.0 skeletal and myocardial SI muscle ratio enhancement.

Proposed Terminologies for Describing CMR Findings **Normal CMR findings consistent with myocardial inflammation**					
Capillary Hyperemia leak	Non-evident early myocardial gadolinium enhancement ratio		Increased myocardial early gadolinium enhancement ratio‡	Increased myocardial rapid gadolinium enhancement ratio‡	
Irremediable cell injury	Non-evident late myocardial gadolinium ratio enhancement	Patchy areas indicating focal injury	Septal layer or subepicardial of late gadolinium enhancement indicating regional injury	Transmural late gadolinium enhancement, consistent with but not specific for myocardial inflammation	
LV dysfunction	Normal LV function	Regional systolic dysfunction		Global systolic dysfunction	
Pericardial effusion	Lack of evidence for pericardial effusion	Small pericardial effusion	Moderately large pericardial effusion	Large pericardial effusion without hemodynamic relevance	Large pericardial effusion with hemodynamic relevance

LIMITATIONS OF ENDOMYOCARDIAL BIOPSY

[I]. Severe complications, such as tamponades and perforations, occur.
[II]. Reduced sensitivity due to sampling errors.
[III]. Poorly standardized markers and diagnostic criteria's for analyzing myocardial tissue specimens combined with inter-observer differences.

[IV]. Availability, cost, experts, centers and, standardized protocols have limited the widespread use of immunohistochemistry and viral genome analysis as it possesses a higher sensitivity than standard histopathology used in EMB's for the diagnosis of myocarditis.

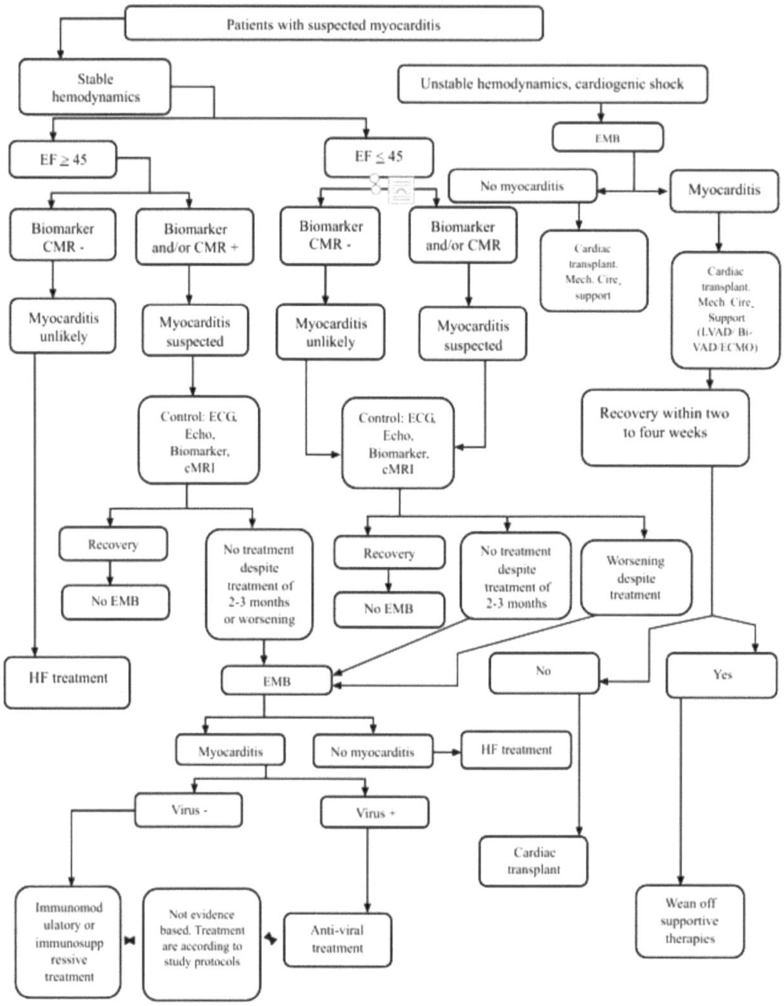

Fig. (4). Proposed Diagnostic and Therapeutic Algorithm for Suspected Myocarditis.
Bi-VAD- biventricular assist device; Circ- circulatory; ECMO- extracorporeal membrane oxygenation; LV- left ventricular; LVAD- left ventricular assist device.

CLINICAL MANAGEMENT

Outcomes and prognosis of myocarditis and cardiomyopathy largely depend on etiology, clinical presentation, and the stage of the disease. In about 50% of clinical cases, acute myocarditis resolves in the first 2-3 weeks of onset as 25-30% develop persistent cardiac dysfunction and 15-20% acutely deteriorate, die or progress to end-stage DCM with a need for heart transplantation (Fig. **4**).

Conventional Treatment

Hemodynamically unstable patients: Hemodynamically unstable patients presenting with heart failure should be managed immediately in specialized intensive care units equipped with respiratory and mechanical cardiopulmonary support facilities according to the current European Society of Cardiology (ESC) guidelines for heart failure [101]. Cases of cardiogenic shock and severe ventricular dysfunction, ventricular assist device or extracorporeal membrane oxygenation should be used to provide a bridge recovery or transplant.

***Hemodynamically Stable Patients*:** Asymptomatic or mildly symptomatic patients when myocarditis is suspected should be hospitalized and clinically monitored until a definite diagnosis is established since most cases evolve rapidly (life-threatening arrhythmia) and a cardiopulmonary emergency is possible and unpredictable, even if the systolic function is initially preserved. Exercise testing is contraindicated as it can precipitate arrhythmia. An angiotensin-converting enzyme inhibitor, diuretics, angiotensin receptor blockers, and beta-adrenergic blockers are recommended for patients with hemodynamically stable heart failure. However, in patients with persistent heart failure even after optimal treatment, additional treatment with aldosterone antagonist can be administered.

Arrhythmia: Its management should be based on the current ESC guidelines as there are no specific recommendations for its control [102 - 107]. Sinus bradycardia increased left ventricular hypokinesis on echocardiography, prolonged QRS duration, persistent or fluctuating cardiac troponin levels may precede a life-threatening arrhythmia. Temporary pacing may be needed for complete atrioventricular block. The use of cardioverter defibrillator is not recommended as myocarditis can heal completely.

Avoidance of Exercise: It recommended to restrict physical activities during the acute phase of myocarditis not until the disease has resolved entirely. However, differentiating strenuous activities from non-strenuous ones are based on therapist, physicians, and patient by patient case. Regardless of gender, age, treatment regimens or symptoms severity, Athletes should temporally be prevented from taking part in competitive or armature sporting activities. Clinical reassessment of the disease state, progression and general wellbeing of the patient after six months before sporting activities can be recommended though on a step by step level until the patient is back to full fitness [108, 109].

Immunomodulatory Therapy

Anti-Viral Therapies: In general, there is currently no approved antiviral therapy for the treatment of myocarditis and ICM. Although unproven myocarditis treatment; acyclovir, valacyclovir, and gancyclovir can be options for the treatment of patients with herpes virus infection [110]. However, it's advisable to manage and treat patients with an infectious disease specialist. Preliminary data on interferon beta treatment suggest that it eliminates adenoviral and enteroviral genomes in patients with LV dysfunction [111], and it is associated with an improvement in New York Heart Association (NYHA) functional class I and II [112] and, specifically in enteroviral infection, with a better ten-year prognosis.

High Dose Intravenous Immunoglobulin: High dose intravenous immunoglobulin (IVIG) is effective and have no significant side effects. Although IVIG modulates the inflammatory and immune response by a variety of mechanisms and is used in several systemic autoimmune diseases [113], it may be used in myocarditis refractory to conventional heart failure therapy, both viral and autoimmune forms, particularly if autoantibody-mediated [44].

Immunoadsorption: Although therapeutic strategies used in other auto-immune disorders [114], such as, neutralization or immunoadsorption of disease-causing aabs, might offer treatment options for autoimmune myocarditis and ICM, it's still not recommended as of yet not until proven clinical results are made available.

Immunosuppressive Therapy

Most data on the efficacy and safety of immunosuppression have been obtained from azathioprine and steroids alone. However, data from randomized clinical trials of immunosuppression in myocarditis has reported response to therapy mainly in chronic negative forms, and inactive myocarditis defined as autoimmune (*e.g.*, virus-negative and autoantibody-positive). Be it as it may, the use of immunosuppressive or antiviral treatment (corticosteroids, azathioprine, cyclosporine, an' interferon or immunoglobulins) remains controversial in the treatment of acute myocarditis.

Heart Failure Therapy

Basically, for now, treatment is solely symptomatic and based on clinical presentation as there is currently no pathogen-specific therapy for viral myocarditis to improve survival free of HF. HF pharmacological treatment should be initiated according to the current guidelines, NYHA, which includes beta-blockers, diuretics, angiotensin-converting enzyme (ACE) inhibitors or angiotensin-II receptor blockers (ARBS) [115].

Diuretics: Used to treat and prevent fluid overload.

Beta-blockers: Its use should be avoided in the acute phase of decompensated HF and early fulminant myocarditis treatment [53]. Its use, however, reduces hospital admission for worsening HF, improves ventricular function, and improves chances of survival.

ACE Inhibitors and ARBS: Early blockade of renin-angiotensin initiation, chronic attenuated maladaptive cardiac remodeling, and the progression to DCM can be reduced.

Aldosterone Antagonist: Administration of aldosterone antagonists is recommended for systolic HF patients with persistent NYHA functional class II to IV symptoms.

Calcium-Channel Blockers: They are not generally recommended in the management of acute HF [53].

Cardiac Glycoside: Digoxin may limit the maximally tolerated dose of beta blocker due to bradycardia or heart block. Therefore, cardiac glycosides should be avoided in patients suffering from acute HF induced by viral myocarditis.

CONTINUING CHALLENGES IN THE DIAGNOSIS OF MYOCARDITIS

The use of volunteers (healthy) as study controls have led to a spectrum bias and an unrealistic diagnostic performance of CMR (*i.e.*, the actual clinical utility of CMR) among patients with structural heart diseases that masquerade as myocarditis. Conversely, because these study cases were defined based on clinical criteria and other readily available biomarkers, its role in the routine clinical workup of suspected myocarditis, and the incremental diagnostic value of CMR requires further clarification. Because the distribution and extent of tissue changes detected by CMR evolve, whether the proposed diagnostic cutoffs and the optimal timing of this modality should be modified according to the time from symptom onset are among other practical issues. Finally, because myocarditis represents a heterogeneous disease, the most significant clinical utility of CMR lies in its ability to prognosticate patients. Those with good natural history are unlikely to benefit from aggressive treatments, whereas, those with less-favorable prognostic features duly need intense surveillance and may be enrolled in clinical trials evaluating novel therapies. We (the authors) are optimistic that, in concern with ongoing advances in genomic and proteomic technologies, future developments in molecular and cellular imaging using CMR will provide invaluable insights in the early diagnosis, pathophysiology, and the management of this intriguing disease.

CONCLUSION AND FUTURE DIRECTIONS

Myocarditis is an under-diagnosed cardiac disease with a variable natural history resulting from a broad range of infectious, toxic, and immune causes. Although it was first recognized a hundred years ago, myocarditis and cardiomyopathy still provide the medical community with significant conceptual difficulties. However, its diagnosis in the past was difficult due to the insensitivity of traditional diagnostic tests. It is the result of both myocardial infection and autoimmunity that results in progressive inflammatory destruction of myocytes. Its natural history and precise characterization have been limited by the extraordinary variability of its clinical presentations, diverse etiologies and, laboratory findings. Acute myocarditis suspected patients should undergo a complete cardiological workup and detailed history. The workup and the history should include ECG's, blood analyses, and serum tests for anti-heart aabs, EMBs for both PCR and immunohistochemical analysis, and imaging techniques (echocardiogram and especially CMR). Although, detailed history, clinical examinations, and serological test in some cases have been unsatisfactory in the diagnostic accuracy of myocarditis. However, biopsies, including immunohistochemistry, have played vital roles in the disease diagnostic accuracy but may, however, not be appropriate for many patients, especially those with less severe disease. Also, consideration should be given to patients who lack evidence of pathophysiological etiologies such as takotsubo syndrome or coronary atherosclerosis.

Remarkable advances and progress over the years in understanding the pathophysiological mechanisms, diagnosis, and the treatment of myocarditis and cardiomyopathy have been achieved. Although, standard treatment strategies remain limited to evidence-based HF therapy in most cases. Currently, the standard of care for acute myocarditis (viral, autoimmune) and severe cardiomyopathy (infective, inflammatory) remains cardiovascular and hemodynamic support, including the use of ventricular assist devices and transplantation when necessary. Apart from antiarrhythmic and heart failure therapies, there are no other alternatives to an etiologically driven specific treatment. Their prerequisites are invasive and noninvasive biomarkers, including PCR for cardiotropic agents on EMB, immunohistochemistry and, immune serology. Immunosuppressive therapy has proven beneficial for fulminant, acute, and chronic autoreactive myocarditis (acute myocarditis associated with autoimmune diseases, for example, lupus myocarditis). However, the use of IVIG can resolve inflammation in ICM and has proven to be successful as interferon therapy in adenoviral and enteroviral myocarditis. Immunosuppressive and Immunomodulating treatment has been proven to be active, particularly in a single-center trial (TIMIC study), for virus negative ICM. Contrast media-enhanced MRI also helps in visualizing the activity, localization, the extent of the inflammation and the disease transition as it also serves as a powerful noninvasive diagnostic tool in acute myocarditis.

The Dallas criteria remain the gold standard for diagnosis, but a new clinicopathological staging system has however been proposed. EMB's should be considered for highly selected group (5%) of patients, particularly those with increased myocardial enhancement on cardiac MRI, unexplained ventricular dysfunction in the presence of an autoimmune disease known to affect the myocardium and rapidly progressive cardiomyopathy. Randomized large-scale clinical trials to evaluate treatment strategies and establish diagnosis have been limited due to the relatively low incidence. Although the magnitude of spontaneous improvement in infective ICM and acute myocarditis with an average of five years survival rate as reported in experienced centers provides some optimism and hope for the future. However, ongoing clinical trials should be channeled in clarifying whether immune-modulating strategies can also improve this prognosis. The recognition in the overlap of virus-mediated damage, inflammation, and autoimmune dysregulation is pivotal in the understanding of this complex disease.

Prospective randomized placebo-controlled trials should be based on etiological diagnosis (viral *vs.* autoimmune patients) to provide new treatment options and possibly a better prognosis. Future research should be focused on the related immune responses and understanding underlying genetic susceptibility that explains why some patients are susceptible to developing clinical symptoms of myocarditis following viral infection, whereas others spontaneously improve afterward or progress to an idiopathic dilated cardiomyopathy later.

LIST OF ABBREVIATIONS

ACC American College of Cardiology

AHA American Heart Association

ACE Angiotensin Converting Enzyme

ARBS Angiotensin- II- receptor

aabs Autoantibodies

CMR Cardiovascular Magnetic Resonance Imaging

CT Computer Tomography

DCM Dilated Cardiomyopathy

EMB Endomyocardial Biopsy

ESC European Society of Cardiology

EF Ejection Fraction

ECG Electrocardiography

IVIG Intravenous Immunoglobulin

IC Infective Cardiomyopathy>

ICM Inflammatory Cardiomyopathy

LV Left Ventricular

LGE Late Gadolinium Enhancement

MRI Magnetic Resonance Imaging

NYHA New York Heart Association

PCR Polymerase Chain Reaction

CONSENT FOR PUBLICATION

Not applicable.

CONFLICT OF INTEREST

The authors confirm that this chapter contents have no conflict of interest.

ACKNOWLEDGEMENTS

Declared none.

REFERENCE

[1] Schölmerich P. Myocarditis — Cardiomyopathy Historic Survey and Definition. International Boehringer Mannheim Symposia 1983; 1: 5.

[2] Joseph Friedrich Sobernheim. Praktische Diagnostik der inneren Krankheiten mit vorzueglicher Ruecksicht auf pathologische Anatomic. Berlin: Hirschwald 1837; p. 117.

[3] Jared W, Magnani G, William Dec. Myocarditis Archived 2013-12-16 at the Wayback Machine, Circulation 2006; 113: 876-90.

[4] Basso C, Calabrese F, Corrado D, Thiene G. Postmortem diagnosis in sudden cardiac death victims: macroscopic, microscopic and molecular findings. Cardiovasc Res 2001; 50(2): 290-300. [http://dx.doi.org/10.1016/S0008-6363(01)00261-9] [PMID: 11334833]

[5] Towbin JA, Lowe AM, Colan SD, *et al.* Incidence, causes, and outcomes of dilated cardiomyopathy in children. JAMA 2006; 296(15): 1867-76. [http://dx.doi.org/10.1001/jama.296.15.1867] [PMID: 17047217]

[6] Caforio AL, Calabrese F, Angelini A, *et al.* A prospective study of biopsy-proven myocarditis: prognostic relevance of clinical and aetiopathogenetic features at diagnosis. Eur Heart J 2007; 28(11): 1326-33. [http://dx.doi.org/10.1093/eurheartj/ehm076] [PMID: 17493945]

[7] Stuehr DJ, Marletta MA. Induction of nitrite/nitrate synthesis in murine macrophages by BCG infection, lymphokines, or interferon-γ. J Immunol 1987; 139(2): 518-25. [PMID: 3110273]

[8] Adams V, Nehrhoff B, Späte U, *et al.* Induction of iNOS expression in skeletal muscle by IL-1beta and NFkappaB activation: an *in vitro* and *in vivo* study. Cardiovasc Res 2002; 54(1): 95-104. [http://dx.doi.org/10.1016/S0008-6363(02)00228-6] [PMID: 12062366]

[9] Song W, Lu X, Feng Q. Tumor necrosis factor-alpha induces apoptosis *via* inducible nitric oxide synthase in neonatal mouse cardiomyocytes. Cardiovasc Res 2000; 45(3): 595-602. [http://dx.doi.org/10.1016/S0008-6363(99)00395-8] [PMID: 10728381]

[10] Mungrue IN, Gros R, You X, *et al.* Cardiomyocyte overexpression of iNOS in mice results in peroxynitrite generation, heart block, and sudden death. J Clin Invest 2002; 109(6): 735-43. [http://dx.doi.org/10.1172/JCI0213265] [PMID: 11901182]

[11] Aretz HT. Myocarditis: The Dallas criteria. Hum Pathol 1987; 18(6): 619-24. [http://dx.doi.org/10.1016/S0046-8177(87)80363-5] [PMID: 3297992]

[12] Leone O, Veinot JP, Angelini A, *et al.* 2011 consensus statement on endomyocardial biopsy from the Association for European Cardiovascular Pathology and the Society for Cardiovascular Pathology. Cardiovasc Pathol 2012; 21(4): 245-74. [http://dx.doi.org/10.1016/j.carpath.2011.10.001] [PMID: 22137237]

[13] Kindermann I, Barth C, Mahfoud F, *et al.* Update on myocarditis. J Am Coll Cardiol 2012; 59(9): 779-92. [http://dx.doi.org/10.1016/j.jacc.2011.09.074] [PMID: 22361396]

[14] Schultz JC, Hilliard AA, Cooper LT Jr, Rihal CS. Diagnosis and treatment of viral myocarditis. Mayo Clin Proc 2009; 84(11): 1001-9. [http://dx.doi.org/10.1016/S0025-6196(11)60670-8] [PMID: 19880690]

[15] Baughman KL. Diagnosis of myocarditis: death of Dallas criteria. Circulation 2006; 113(4): 593-5. [http://dx.doi.org/10.1161/CIRCULATIONAHA.105.589663] [PMID: 16449736]

[16] Kearney MT, Cotton JM, Richardson PJ, Shah AM. Viral myocarditis and dilated cardiomyopathy: Mechanisms, manifestations, and management. Postgrad Med J 2001; 77(903): 4-10. [http://dx.doi.org/10.1136/pmj.77.903.4] [PMID: 11123385]

[17] Caforio AL, *et al.* Current state of knowledge on aetiology, diagnosis, management, therapy of myocarditis: a position statement of the European Society of Cardiology Working Group on Myocardial and Pericardial Diseases. Eur Heart J 2013; 34(33): 2636-48. [http://dx.doi.org/10.1093/eurheartj/eht210]

[18] Dec GW Jr, Palacios IF, Fallon JT, *et al.* Active myocarditis in the spectrum of acute dilated cardiomyopathies. Clinical features, histologic correlates, and clinical outcome. N Engl J Med 1985; 312(14): 885-90. [http://dx.doi.org/10.1056/NEJM198504043121404] [PMID: 3974674]

[19] Yamada T, Matsumori A, Tamaki N, Nohara R, Konishi J, Sasayama S. Indium-111 antimyosin antibody imaging and thallium-201 imaging-a comparative myocardial scintigraphic study using single-photon emission computed tomography in patients with myocarditis and dilated cardiomyopathy. Jpn Circ J 1997; 61(10): 827-35. [http://dx.doi.org/10.1253/jcj.61.827] [PMID: 9387064]

[20] Theleman KP, Kuiper JJ, Roberts WC. Acute myocarditis sudden death without heart failure. Am J Cardiol 2001; 88: 1078-83. [http://dx.doi.org/10.1016/S0002-9149(01)02000-8] [PMID: 11704019]

[21] Choudhury L, Mahrholdt H, Wagner A, *et al.* Myocardial scarring in asymptomatic or mildly symptomatic patients with hypertrophic cardiomyopathy. J Am Coll Cardiol 2002; 40(12): 2156-64. [http://dx.doi.org/10.1016/S0735-1097(02)02602-5] [PMID: 12505229]

[22] Lieberman EB, Hutchins GM, Herskowitz A, Rose NR, Baughman KL. Clinicopathologic description of myocarditis. J Am Coll Cardiol 1991; 18(7): 1617-26. [http://dx.doi.org/10.1016/0735-1097(91)90493-S] [PMID: 1960305]

[23] McCarthy RE III, Boehmer JP, Hruban RH, *et al.* Long-term outcome of fulminant myocarditis as compared with acute (nonfulminant) myocarditis. N Engl J Med 2000; 342(10): 690-5. [http://dx.doi.org/10.1056/NEJM200003093421003] [PMID: 10706898]

[24] Heart Failure Society of America. HFSA guidelines for the management of patients with heart failure due to left ventricular systolic dysfunction-pharmacological approaches. Congest Heart Fail 2000; 6(1): 11-39.
[PMID: 12029200]

[25] Hauck AJ, Kearney DL, Edwards WD. Evaluation of postmortem endomyocardial biopsy specimens from 38 patients with lymphocytic myocarditis: implications for role of sampling error. Mayo Clin Proc 1989; 64(10): 1235-45.
[http://dx.doi.org/10.1016/S0025-6196(12)61286-5] [PMID: 2593714]

[26] Felker GM, Hu W, Hare JM, Hruban RH, Baughman KL, Kasper EK. The spectrum of dilated cardiomyopathy. The Johns Hopkins experience with 1,278 patients. Medicine (Baltimore) 1999; 78(4): 270-83.
[http://dx.doi.org/10.1097/00005792-199907000-00005] [PMID: 10424207]

[27] Parrillo JE. Inflammatory cardiomyopathy (myocarditis): which patients should be treated with anti-inflammatory therapy? Circulation 2001; 104(1): 4-6.
[http://dx.doi.org/10.1161/hc2601.092124] [PMID: 11435327]

[28] Wojnicz R, Nowalany-Kozielska E, Wodniecki J, *et al.* Immunohistological diagnosis of myocarditis. Potential role of sarcolemmal induction of the MHC and ICAM-1 in the detection of autoimmune mediated myocyte injury. Eur Heart J 1998; 19(10): 1564-72.
[http://dx.doi.org/10.1053/euhj.1998.1085] [PMID: 9820996]

[29] D'Ambrosio A, Patti G, Manzoli A, *et al.* The fate of acute myocarditis between spontaneous improvement and evolution to dilated cardiomyopathy: a review. Heart 2001; 85(5): 499-504.
[http://dx.doi.org/10.1136/heart.85.5.499] [PMID: 11302994]

[30] Grogan M, Redfield MM, Bailey KR, *et al.* Long-term outcome of patients with biopsy-proved myocarditis: Comparison with idiopathic dilated cardiomyopathy. J Am Coll Cardiol 1995; 26(1): 80-4.
[http://dx.doi.org/10.1016/0735-1097(95)00148-S] [PMID: 7797779]

[31] Kühl U, Pauschinger M, Noutsias M, *et al.* High prevalence of viral genomes and multiple viral infections in the myocardium of adults with "idiopathic" left ventricular dysfunction. Circulation 2005; 111(7): 887-93.
[http://dx.doi.org/10.1161/01.CIR.0000155616.07901.35] [PMID: 15699250]

[32] Dec GW Jr, Waldman H, Southern J, Fallon JT, Hutter AM Jr, Palacios I. Viral myocarditis mimicking acute myocardial infarction. J Am Coll Cardiol 1992; 20(1): 85-9.
[http://dx.doi.org/10.1016/0735-1097(92)90141-9] [PMID: 1607543]

[33] Dec GW. Introduction to clinical myocarditis. Myocarditis: From Bench to Bedside. Totowa, NJ: Humana Press 2003; pp. 257-81.

[34] Fabre A, Sheppard MN. Sudden adult death syndrome and other non-ischaemic causes of sudden cardiac death. Heart 2006; 92(3): 316-20.
[http://dx.doi.org/10.1136/hrt.2004.045518] [PMID: 15923280]

[35] Doolan A, Langlois N, Semsarian C. Causes of sudden cardiac death in young Australians. Med J Aust 2004; 180(3): 110-2.
[http://dx.doi.org/10.5694/j.1326-5377.2004.tb05830.x] [PMID: 14748671]

[36] Puranik R, Chow CK, Duflou JA, Kilborn MJ, McGuire MA. Sudden death in the young. Heart Rhythm 2005; 2(12): 1277-82.
[http://dx.doi.org/10.1016/j.hrthm.2005.09.008] [PMID: 16360077]

[37] Virmani R, Burke AP, Farb A. Sudden cardiac death. Cardiovasc Pathol 2001; 10(5): 211-8.
[http://dx.doi.org/10.1016/S1054-8807(01)00091-6] [PMID: 11673058]

[38] Kawai C. From myocarditis to cardiomyopathy: mechanisms of inflammation and cell death: learning from the past for the future. Circulation 1999; 99(8): 1091-100.

[http://dx.doi.org/10.1161/01.CIR.99.8.1091] [PMID: 10051305]

[39] Calabrese F, Basso C, Carturan E, Valente M, Thiene G. Arrhythmogenic right ventricular cardiomyopathy/dysplasia: is there a role for viruses? Cardiovasc Pathol 2006; 15(1): 11-7. [http://dx.doi.org/10.1016/j.carpath.2005.10.004] [PMID: 16414451]

[40] Archard LC, Khan MA, Soteriou BA, *et al.* Characterization of Coxsackie B virus RNA in myocardium from patients with dilated cardiomyopathy by nucleotide sequencing of reverse transcription-nested polymerase chain reaction products. Hum Pathol 1998; 29(6): 578-84. [http://dx.doi.org/10.1016/S0046-8177(98)80006-3] [PMID: 9635677]

[41] Schultheiss H-P, Kühl U, Cooper LT. The management of myocarditis. Eur Heart J 2011; 32(21): 2616-25. [http://dx.doi.org/10.1093/eurheartj/ehr165] [PMID: 21705357]

[42] Richardson P, McKenna W, Bristow M, *et al.* Report of the 1995 World Health Organization/International Society and Federation of Cardiology Task Force on the Definition and Classification of cardiomyopathies. Circulation 1996; 93(5): 841-2. [http://dx.doi.org/10.1161/01.CIR.93.5.841] [PMID: 8598070]

[43] Cooper LT Jr. Myocarditis. N Engl J Med 2009; 360(15): 1526-38. [http://dx.doi.org/10.1056/NEJMra0800028] [PMID: 19357408]

[44] Kindermann I, Barth C, Mahfoud F, *et al.* Update on myocarditis. J Am Coll Cardiol 2012; 59(9): 779-92. [http://dx.doi.org/10.1016/j.jacc.2011.09.074] [PMID: 22361396]

[45] Dennert R, Crijns HJ, Heymans S. Acute viral myocarditis. Eur Heart J 2008; 29(17): 2073-82. [http://dx.doi.org/10.1093/eurheartj/ehn296] [PMID: 18617482]

[46] Noutsias M, Pauschinger M, Poller W-C, Schultheiss H-P, Kühl U. Current insights into the pathogenesis, diagnosis and therapy of inflammatory cardiomyopathy. Heart Fail Monit 2003; 3(4): 127-35. [PMID: 12709733]

[47] Maisch B, Pankuweit S. Current treatment options in (peri)myocarditis and inflammatory cardiomyopathy. Herz 2012; 37(6): 644-56. [http://dx.doi.org/10.1007/s00059-012-3679-9] [PMID: 22996288]

[48] Caforio ALP, Bottaro S, Iliceto S. Dilated cardiomyopathy (DCM) and myocarditis: classification, clinical and autoimmune features. Appl Cardiopulm Pathophysiol 2012; 16(1): 82-95.

[49] Wehlou C, Delanghe JR. Detection of antibodies in cardiac autoimmunity. Clin Chim Acta 2009; 408(1-2): 114-22. [http://dx.doi.org/10.1016/j.cca.2009.08.002] [PMID: 19682445]

[50] Caforio ALP, Mahon NJ, Tona F, McKenna WJ. Circulating cardiac autoantibodies in dilated cardiomyopathy and myocarditis: pathogenetic and clinical significance. Eur J Heart Fail 2002; 4(4): 411-7. [http://dx.doi.org/10.1016/S1388-9842(02)00010-7] [PMID: 12167378]

[51] Rose NR. Myocarditis: infection versus autoimmunity. J Clin Immunol 2009; 29(6): 730-7. [http://dx.doi.org/10.1007/s10875-009-9339-z] [PMID: 19826933]

[52] Caforio ALP, Marcolongo R, Basso C, Iliceto S. Clinical presentation and diagnosis of myocarditis. Heart 2015; 101(16): 1332-44. [http://dx.doi.org/10.1136/heartjnl-2014-306363] [PMID: 26109587]

[53] Frustaci A, Chimenti C, Calabrese F, Pieroni M, Thiene G, Maseri A. Immunosuppressive therapy for active lymphocytic myocarditis: virological and immunologic profile of responders versus nonresponders. Circulation 2003; 107(6): 857-63. [http://dx.doi.org/10.1161/01.CIR.0000048147.15962.31] [PMID: 12591756]

[54] Wojnicz R, Nowalany-Kozielska E, Wojciechowska C, *et al.* Randomized, placebo-controlled study for immunosuppressive treatment of inflammatory dilated cardiomyopathy: two-year follow-up results. Circulation 2001; 104(1): 39-45.
[http://dx.doi.org/10.1161/01.CIR.104.1.39] [PMID: 11435335]

[55] Stanton C, Mookadam F, Cha S, *et al.* Greater symptom duration predicts response to immunomodulatory therapy in dilated cardiomyopathy. Int J Cardiol 2008; 128(1): 38-41.
[http://dx.doi.org/10.1016/j.ijcard.2007.05.016] [PMID: 17707091]

[56] Frustaci A, Russo MA, Chimenti C. Randomized study on the efficacy of immunosuppressive therapy in patients with virus-negative inflammatory cardiomyopathy: the TIMIC study. Eur Heart J 2009; 30(16): 1995-2002.
[http://dx.doi.org/10.1093/eurheartj/ehp249] [PMID: 19556262]

[57] Maisch B, Richter A, Sandmöller A, Portig I, Pankuweit S. Inflammatory dilated cardiomyopathy (DCMI). Herz 2005; 30(6): 535-44.
[http://dx.doi.org/10.1007/s00059-005-2730-5] [PMID: 16170686]

[58] Kindermann I, Kindermann M, Kandolf R, *et al.* Predictors of outcome in patients with suspected myocarditis. Circulation 2008; 118(6): 639-48.
[http://dx.doi.org/10.1161/CIRCULATIONAHA.108.769489] [PMID: 18645053]

[59] McManus BM, Chow LH, Wilson JE, *et al.* Direct myocardial injury by enterovirus: a central role in the evolution of murine myocarditis. Clin Immunol Immunopathol 1993; 68(2): 159-69.
[http://dx.doi.org/10.1006/clin.1993.1113] [PMID: 7689428]

[60] Maekawa Y, Ouzounian M, Opavsky MA, Liu PP. Connecting the missing link between dilated cardiomyopathy and viral myocarditis: virus, cytoskeleton, and innate immunity. Circulation 2007; 115(1): 5-8.
[http://dx.doi.org/10.1161/CIRCULATIONAHA.106.670554] [PMID: 17200452]

[61] Lawson CM. Evidence for mimicry by viral antigens in animal models of autoimmune disease including myocarditis. Cell Mol Life Sci 2000; 57(4): 552-60.
[http://dx.doi.org/10.1007/PL00000717] [PMID: 11130455]

[62] Badorff C, Knowlton KU. Dystrophin disruption in enterovirus-induced myocarditis and dilated cardiomyopathy: From bench to bedside. Med Microbiol Immunol (Berl) 2004; 193(2-3): 121-6.
[http://dx.doi.org/10.1007/s00430-003-0189-7] [PMID: 12920582]

[63] Mason JW. Myocarditis and dilated cardiomyopathy: An inflammatory link. Cardiovasc Res 2003; 60(1): 5-10.
[http://dx.doi.org/10.1016/S0008-6363(03)00437-1] [PMID: 14522402]

[64] Liu PP, Schultheiss HP. Myocarditis Baunwald (ed):, Heart Disease 8 ed Philadelphia: W B Saunders co. 2008; pp. 1775-92.

[65] Mahrholdt H, Wagner A, Judd RM, Sechtem U. Assessment of myocardial viability by cardiovascular magnetic resonance imaging. Eur Heart J 2002; 23(8): 602-19.
[http://dx.doi.org/10.1053/euhj.2001.3038] [PMID: 11969275]

[66] Friedrich MG, Sechtem U, Schulz-Menger J, *et al.* Cardiovascular magnetic resonance in myocarditis: A JACC White Paper. J Am Coll Cardiol 2009; 53(17): 1475-87.
[http://dx.doi.org/10.1016/j.jacc.2009.02.007] [PMID: 19389557]

[67] Felker GM, Thompson RE, Hare JM, *et al.* Underlying causes and long-term survival in patients with initially unexplained cardiomyopathy. N Engl J Med 2000; 342: 1077-84.

[68] Cooper LT, Baughman KL, Feldman AM, *et al.* The role of endomyocardial biopsy in the management of cardiovascular disease: a scientific statement from the American Heart Association, the American College of Cardiology, and the European Society of Cardiology. Endorsed by the Heart Failure Society of America and the Heart Failure Association of the European Society of Cardiology. J Am Coll Cardiol 2007; 50: 1914-31.

[69] Sarda L, Colin P, Boccara F, *et al.* Myocarditis in patients with clinical presentation of myocardial infarction and normal coronary angiograms. J Am Coll Cardiol 2001; 37(3): 786-92. [http://dx.doi.org/10.1016/S0735-1097(00)01201-8] [PMID: 11693753]

[70] Liu PP, Yan AT. Cardiovascular magnetic resonance for the diagnosis of acute myocarditis: Prospects for detecting myocardial inflammation. J Am Coll Cardiol 2005; 45(11): 1823-5. [http://dx.doi.org/10.1016/j.jacc.2005.03.002] [PMID: 15936613]

[71] Bültmann BD, Klingel K, Näbauer M, Wallwiener D, Kandolf R. High prevalence of viral genomes and inflammation in peripartum cardiomyopathy. Am J Obstet Gynecol 2005; 193(2): 363-5. [http://dx.doi.org/10.1016/j.ajog.2005.01.022] [PMID: 16098856]

[72] Ukena C, Mahfoud F, Kindermann I, Kandolf R, Kindermann M, Böhm M. Prognostic electrocardiographic parameters in patients with suspected myocarditis. Eur J Heart Fail 2011; 13(4): 398-405. [http://dx.doi.org/10.1093/eurjhf/hfq229] [PMID: 21239404]

[73] Wu LA, Lapeyre AC III, Cooper LT. Current role of endomyocardial biopsy in the management of dilated cardiomyopathy and myocarditis. Mayo Clin Proc 2001; 76(10): 1030-8. [http://dx.doi.org/10.4065/76.10.1030] [PMID: 11605687]

[74] Hunt SA, Baker DW, Chin MH, *et al.* American College of Cardiology/American Heart Association Task Force on Practice Guidelines (Committee to Revise the 1995 Guidelines for the Evaluation and Management of Heart Failure); International Society for Heart and Lung Transplantation; Heart Failure Society of America. ACC/AHA Guidelines for the Evaluation and Management of Chronic Heart Failure in the Adult: Executive Summary A Report of the American College of Cardiology/American Heart Association Task Force on Practice Guidelines (Committee to Revise the 1995 Guidelines for the Evaluation and Management of Heart Failure): Developed in Collaboration With the International Society for Heart and Lung Transplantation; Endorsed by the Heart Failure Society of America. Circulation 2001; 104(24): 2996-3007. [http://dx.doi.org/10.1161/hc4901.102568] [PMID: 11739319]

[75] Kühl U, Pauschinger M, Seeberg B, *et al.* Viral persistence in the myocardium is associated with progressive cardiac dysfunction. Circulation 2005; 112(13): 1965-70. [http://dx.doi.org/10.1161/CIRCULATIONAHA.105.548156] [PMID: 16172268]

[76] Mahrholdt H, Goedecke C, Wagner A, *et al.* Cardiovascular magnetic resonance assessment of human myocarditis: a comparison to histology and molecular pathology. Circulation 2004; 109(10): 1250-8. [http://dx.doi.org/10.1161/01.CIR.0000118493.13323.81] [PMID: 14993139]

[77] Mahrholdt H, Wagner A, Deluigi CC, *et al.* Presentation, patterns of myocardial damage, and clinical course of viral myocarditis. Circulation 2006; 114(15): 1581-90. [http://dx.doi.org/10.1161/CIRCULATIONAHA.105.606509] [PMID: 17015795]

[78] Noutsias M, Pauschinger M, Schultheiss H, K hl U. Phenotypic characterization of infiltrates in dilated cardiomyopathy - diagnostic significance of T-lymphocytes and macrophages in inflammatory cardiomyopathy. Med Sci Monit 2002; 8(7): CR478-87. [PMID: 12118194]

[79] Maisch B, Portig I, Ristic A, Hufnagel G, Pankuweit S. Definition of inflammatory cardiomyopathy (myocarditis): on the way to consensus. A status report. Herz 2000; 25(3): 200-9. [http://dx.doi.org/10.1007/s000590050007] [PMID: 10904839]

[80] Karjalainen J, Heikkilä J. "Acute pericarditis": myocardial enzyme release as evidence for myocarditis. Am Heart J 1986; 111(3): 546-52. [http://dx.doi.org/10.1016/0002-8703(86)90062-1] [PMID: 3953365]

[81] Lauer B, Niederau C, Kühl U, *et al.* Cardiac troponin T in patients with clinically suspected myocarditis. J Am Coll Cardiol 1997; 30(5): 1354-9. [http://dx.doi.org/10.1016/S0735-1097(97)00317-3] [PMID: 9350939]

[82] Takeda N. Cardiomyopathy: molecular and immunological aspects (review). Int J Mol Med 2003; 11(1): 13-6.
[PMID: 12469210]

[83] Afanasyeva M, Georgakopoulos D, Rose NR. Autoimmune myocarditis: Cellular mediators of cardiac dysfunction. Autoimmun Rev 2004; 3(7-8): 476-86.
[http://dx.doi.org/10.1016/j.autrev.2004.08.009] [PMID: 15546794]

[84] Schwimmbeck PL, Badorff C, Schultheiss HP, Strauer BE. Transfer of human myocarditis into severe combined immunodeficiency mice. Circ Res 1994; 75(1): 156-64.
[http://dx.doi.org/10.1161/01.RES.75.1.156] [PMID: 8013075]

[85] Okazaki T, Tanaka Y, Nishio R, *et al.* Autoantibodies against cardiac troponin I are responsible for dilated cardiomyopathy in PD-1-deficient mice. Nat Med 2003; 9(12): 1477-83.
[http://dx.doi.org/10.1038/nm955] [PMID: 14595408]

[86] O'Donoghue HL, Lawson CM, Reed WD. Autoantibodies to cardiac myosin in mouse cytomegalovirus myocarditis. Immunology 1990; 71(1): 20-8.
[PMID: 2170269]

[87] Felker GM, Boehmer JP, Hruban RH, *et al.* Echocardiographic findings in fulminant and acute myocarditis. J Am Coll Cardiol 2000; 36(1): 227-32.
[http://dx.doi.org/10.1016/S0735-1097(00)00690-2] [PMID: 10898439]

[88] Dec GW, Palacios I, Yasuda T, *et al.* Antimyosin antibody cardiac imaging: Its role in the diagnosis of myocarditis. J Am Coll Cardiol 1990; 16(1): 97-104.
[http://dx.doi.org/10.1016/0735-1097(90)90463-Y] [PMID: 2358612]

[89] Baccouche H, Mahrholdt H, Meinhardt G, *et al.* Diagnostic synergy of non-invasive cardiovascular magnetic resonance and invasive endomyocardial biopsy in troponin-positive patients without coronary artery disease. Eur Heart J 2009; 30(23): 2869-79.
[http://dx.doi.org/10.1093/eurheartj/ehp328] [PMID: 19696191]

[90] Yilmaz A, Kindermann I, Kindermann M, *et al.* Comparative evaluation of left and right ventricular endomyocardial biopsy: Differences in complication rate and diagnostic performance. Circulation 2010; 122(9): 900-9.
[http://dx.doi.org/10.1161/CIRCULATIONAHA.109.924167] [PMID: 20713901]

[91] Laissy JP, Messin B, Varenne O, *et al.* MRI of acute myocarditis: A comprehensive approach based on various imaging sequences. Chest 2002; 122(5): 1638-48.
[http://dx.doi.org/10.1378/chest.122.5.1638] [PMID: 12426265]

[92] Cerqueira MD, Weissman NJ, Dilsizian V, *et al.* American Heart Association Writing Group on Myocardial Segmentation and Registration for Cardiac Imaging. Standardized myocardial segmentation and nomenclature for tomographic imaging of the heart. A statement for healthcare professionals from the Cardiac Imaging Committee of the Council on Clinical Cardiology of the American Heart Association. Circulation 2002; 105(4): 539-42.
[http://dx.doi.org/10.1161/hc0402.102975] [PMID: 11815441]

[93] Hiramitsu S, Morimoto S, Kato S, *et al.* Transient ventricular wall thickening in acute myocarditis: A serial echocardiographic and histopathologic study. Jpn Circ J 2001; 65(10): 863-6.
[http://dx.doi.org/10.1253/jcj.65.863] [PMID: 11665789]

[94] Zagrosek A, Wassmuth R, Abdel-Aty H, Rudolph A, Dietz R, Schulz-Menger J. Relation between myocardial edema and myocardial mass during the acute and convalescent phase of myocarditis--a CMR study. J Cardiovasc Magn Reson 2008; 10: 19.
[http://dx.doi.org/10.1186/1532-429X-10-19] [PMID: 18447954]

[95] Kim RJ, Choi KM, Judd RM, *et al.* Assessment of myocardial viability by contrast-enhancement.Cardiovascular MRI and MRA. Philadelphia, PA: Lippincott-Williams & Wilkins 2003; pp. 209-36.

[96] Aretz HT, Billingham ME, Edwards WD, *et al.* Myocarditis. A histopathologic definition and classification. Am J Cardiovasc Pathol 1987; 1(1): 3-14. [PMID: 3455232]

[97] Simonetti OP, Kim RJ, Fieno DS, *et al.* An improved MR imaging technique for the visualization of myocardial infarction. Radiology 2001; 218(1): 215-23. [http://dx.doi.org/10.1148/radiology.218.1.r01ja50215] [PMID: 11152805]

[98] Abdel-Aty H, Zagrosek A, Schulz-Menger J, *et al.* Delayed enhancement and T2-weighted cardiovascular magnetic resonance imaging differentiate acute from chronic myocardial infarction. Circulation 2004; 109(20): 2411-6. [http://dx.doi.org/10.1161/01.CIR.0000127428.10985.C6] [PMID: 15123531]

[99] Abdel-Aty H, Boyé P, Zagrosek A, *et al.* Diagnostic performance of cardiovascular magnetic resonance in patients with suspected acute myocarditis: comparison of different approaches. J Am Coll Cardiol 2005; 45(11): 1815-22. [http://dx.doi.org/10.1016/j.jacc.2004.11.069] [PMID: 15936612]

[100] Gutberlet M, Spors B, Thoma T, *et al.* Suspected chronic myocarditis at cardiac MR: diagnostic accuracy and association with immunohistologically detected inflammation and viral persistence. Radiology 2008; 246(2): 401-9. [http://dx.doi.org/10.1148/radiol.2461062179] [PMID: 18180335]

[101] McMurray JJ, Adamopoulos S, Anker SD, *et al.* ESC committee for practice guidelines. ESC guidelines for the diagnosis and treatment of acute and chronic heart failure 2012: the Task Force for the diagnosis and treatment of acute and chronic heart failure 2012 of the European Society of Cardiology. Developed in collaboration with the Heart Failure Association of the ESC (HFA). Eur Heart J 2012; 33: 1787-847. [http://dx.doi.org/10.1093/eurheartj/ehs104] [PMID: 22611136]

[102] Hsu KH, Chi NH, Yu HY. Wang CH, Huang SC,Wang SS, Ko WJ, Chen YS. Extracorporeal membranous oxygenation support for acute fulminant myocarditis: analysis of a single center's experience. Eur J Cardiothorac Surg 2011; 12-050.

[103] Zipes DP, Camm AJ, Borggrefe M, *et al.* American College of Cardiology/American Heart Association Task Force; European Society of Cardiology Committee for Practice Guidelines; European Heart Rhythm Association and the Heart Rhythm Society. ACC/AHA/ESC 2006 guidelines for management of patients with ventricular arrhythmias and the prevention of sudden cardiac death--executive summary: A report of the American College of Cardiology/American Heart Association Task Force and the European Society of Cardiology Committee for Practice Guidelines (Writing Committee to Develop Guidelines for Management of Patients with Ventricular Arrhythmias and the Prevention of Sudden Cardiac Death) Developed in collaboration with the European Heart Rhythm Association and the Heart Rhythm Society. Eur Heart J 2006; 27(17): 2099-140. [http://dx.doi.org/10.1093/eurheartj/ehl199] [PMID: 16923744]

[104] Vardas PE, Auricchio A, Blanc JJ, *et al.* European Society of Cardiology; European Heart Rhythm Association. Guidelines for cardiac pacing and cardiac resynchronization therapy: The Task Force for Cardiac Pacing and Cardiac Resynchronization Therapy of the European Society of Cardiology. Developed in collaboration with the European Heart Rhythm Association. Eur Heart J 2007; 28(18): 2256-95. [http://dx.doi.org/10.1093/eurheartj/ehm305] [PMID: 17726042]

[105] Dickstein K, Vardas PE, Auricchio A, *et al.* ESC Committee for Practice Guidelines (CPG). 2010 Focused Update of ESC Guidelines on device therapy in heart failure: an update of the 2008 ESC Guidelines for the diagnosis and treatment of acute and chronic heart failure and the 2007 ESC guidelines for cardiac and resynchronization therapy. Developed with the special contribution of the Heart Failure Association and the European Heart Rhythm Association. Eur Heart J 2010; 31(21): 2677-87. [http://dx.doi.org/10.1093/eurheartj/ehq337] [PMID: 20801924]

[106] Camm AJ, Lip GY, De Caterina R, *et al.* ESC Committee for Practice Guidelines (CPG). 2012 focused update of the ESC Guidelines for the management of atrial fibrillation: an update of the 2010 ESC Guidelines for the management of atrial fibrillation. Developed with the special contribution of the European Heart Rhythm Association. Eur Heart J 2012; 33(21): 2719-47.
[http://dx.doi.org/10.1093/eurheartj/ehs253] [PMID: 22922413]

[107] European Heart Rhythm Association. European Association for Cardio-Thoracic Surgery, Camm AJ, Kirchhof P, Lip GY, *et al.* Guidelines for the management of atrial fibrillation: the Task Force for the Management of Atrial Fibrillation of the European Society of Cardiology (ESC). Eur Heart J 2010; 31: 2369-429.

[108] Basso C, Carturan E, Corrado D, Thiene G. Myocarditis and dilated cardiomyopathy in athletes: diagnosis, management, and recommendations for sport activity. Cardiol Clin 2007; 25(3): 423-429, vi.
[http://dx.doi.org/10.1016/j.ccl.2007.08.008] [PMID: 17961796]

[109] Pelliccia A, Fagard R, Bjørnstad HH, *et al.* Study Group of Sports Cardiology of the Working Group of Cardiac Rehabilitation and Exercise Physiology; Working Group of Myocardial and Pericardial Diseases of the European Society of Cardiology. Recommendations for competitive sports participation in athletes with cardiovascular disease: A consensus document from the Study Group of Sports Cardiology of the Working Group of Cardiac Rehabilitation and Exercise Physiology and the Working Group of Myocardial and Pericardial Diseases of the European Society of Cardiology. Eur Heart J 2005; 26(14): 1422-45.
[http://dx.doi.org/10.1093/eurheartj/ehi325] [PMID: 15923204]

[110] Krueger GR, Ablashi DV. Human herpesvirus-6: A short review of its biological behavior. Intervirology 2003; 46(5): 257-69.
[http://dx.doi.org/10.1159/000073205] [PMID: 14555846]

[111] Kühl U, Pauschinger M, Schwimmbeck PL, *et al.* Interferon-beta treatment eliminates cardiotropic viruses and improves left ventricular function in patients with myocardial persistence of viral genomes and left ventricular dysfunction. Circulation 2003; 107(22): 2793-8.
[http://dx.doi.org/10.1161/01.CIR.0000072766.67150.51] [PMID: 12771005]

[112] Kühl U, Lassner D, von Schlippenbach J, Poller W, Schultheiss HP. Interferon-Beta improves survival in enterovirus-associated cardiomyopathy. J Am Coll Cardiol 2012; 60(14): 1295-6.
[http://dx.doi.org/10.1016/j.jacc.2012.06.026] [PMID: 23017536]

[113] Orange JS, Hossny EM, Weiler CR, *et al.* Primary Immunodeficiency Committee of the American Academy of Allergy, Asthma and Immunology. Use of intravenous immunoglobulin in human disease: A review of evidence by members of the Primary Immunodeficiency Committee of the American Academy of Allergy, Asthma and Immunology. J Allergy Clin Immunol 2006; 117(4) (Suppl.): S525-53.
[http://dx.doi.org/10.1016/j.jaci.2006.01.015] [PMID: 16580469]

[114] Tzartos SJ, Bitzopoulou K, Gavra I, *et al.* Antigen-specific apheresis of pathogenic autoantibodies from myasthenia gravis sera. Ann N Y Acad Sci 2008; 1132: 291-9.
[http://dx.doi.org/10.1196/annals.1405.017] [PMID: 18567880]

[115] Dickstein K, Cohen-Solal A, Filippatos G, *et al.* ESC Committee for Practice Guidelines (CPG). ESC Guidelines for the diagnosis and treatment of acute and chronic heart failure 2008: The Task Force for the Diagnosis and Treatment of Acute and Chronic Heart Failure 2008 of the European Society of Cardiology. Developed in collaboration with the Heart Failure Association of the ESC (HFA) and endorsed by the European Society of Intensive Care Medicine (ESICM). Eur Heart J 2008; 29(19): 2388-442.
[http://dx.doi.org/10.1093/eurheartj/ehn309] [PMID: 18799522]

CHAPTER 3

Familiar Dilated Cardiomyopathy: A Comprehensive Overview

Iroegbu Chukwuemeka Daniel[1], **Wangping Chen**[1], **Luo Cheng**[1], **Zhou Zhongxin**[2] and **Jinfu Yang**[1,*]

[1] *Department of Cardiovascular Surgery, The Second Xiangya Hospital, Central South University, Middle Renmin Road 139, 410011 Changsha, China*

[2] *Department of Thoracic and Cardiovascular Surgery, Affiliated Hospital of Xuzhou Medical University, Xuzhou, 99 Huaihai Road West Xuzhou, Jiangsu Province 221000, China*

Abstract: Genetic testing over the years has grown to be a crucial aspect in medical practice for inheritable forms of cardiomyopathies. However, though a great deal of progress in understanding the genetic basis of dilated cardiomyopathy has been made, issues of rare variants, prevalence, penetrance, mismatch, noncausal options, the burden of heart failure, and the more-complex genomics that underlie dilated cardiomyopathy still exist in cardiovascular genetics today. The challenging aspect of identifying common and rare genetic variants contributing to systolic heart failure is made difficult due to its diverse and multiple etiology. Improving our understanding of the genetic basis of both systolic heart failure and dilated cardiomyopathies, would lead to the discovery of rare novel variant(s), identify malignant phenotypes, help optimize treatment and clarify the diagnosis. Hence, this chapter aims to provide a detailed and concise overview of dilated cardiomyopathy genetic etiology, discuss the latest phenomic and genomic available data which are vital to understanding the emerging complexity of familial dilated cardiomyopathy as well as the clinical utilities and limitations of genetic testing. The chapter will also, examine the genetic underpinnings of heart failure syndromes, advances in the common and rare variant discovery and the interpretation in dilated cardiomyopathy and systolic heart failure. With this in mind, this chapter will further aim to define the diagnostic criteria(s) of familial dilated cardiomyopathy, current clinical management options/strategies and the implications, these findings hold for patient care and future research.

Keywords: Arrhythmias, Beta-Myosin Heavy Chain, Cardiomyopathy, Cardiac Troponin-I, dilated cardiomyopathy, Diagnosis, Genes, Genetic testing, Genetic counselling, Human genetics, Heart failure, left ventricular dysfunction, Left ventricular function normalization, Myosin, Molecular biology, Mutation, Next-

* **Corresponding author Jinfu Yang:** Department of Cardiovascular Surgery, The Second Xiangya Hospital, Central South University, Middle Renmin Road 139, 410011 Changsha, China; E-mails: yjf19682005@csu.edu.cn, Dr.iroegbu_daniel@yahoo.com, Dr.iroegbu_daniel@csu.edu.cn

Jinfu Yang & Iroegbu Chukwuemeka Daniel (Eds.)

generation sequencing technology, Patients, Sudden cardiac death, Troponin T, Tropomyosin, Therapeutics.

INTRODUCTION

Dilated cardiomyopathy (DCM) is a cardiac muscle disorder (primary myocardial disease and genetically heterogeneous disorder) defined by the presence of a dilated/enlarged cardiac chamber(s), inadequate left ventricle (LV) function, and progressive systolic dysfunction/impaired systolic function (almost always diastolic). DCM can also, be clinically defined as cardiac chamber dilatation and inefficient myocardial contractility in the absence of ischemic heart disease more than enough to cause global systolic impairment or abnormal loading conditions (valve disease, hypertension). DCM is often associated with arrhythmias and conduction system diseases, progressive/congestive/refractory heart failure (HF), thromboembolic disease and sudden cardiac death (SCD) which could also, but all be asymptomatic. DCM is a multigenic disorder and over the past decade, various genes (more than 30) have been identified to be associated with DCM, coding a variety of proteins and contributing to development of the disease such as: sarcoplasmic reticulum, cardiac sarcomeric units, desmosomal proteins, nuclear envelope, ion channels, transcription factors, intermediary filament, and dystrophin-associated cytoskeletal complex [1]. Furthermore, DCM can, however, sporadically appear in a family member (single) which is then called idiopathic DCM (IDC). DCM may also be inherited (autosomal-dominant pattern) hence termed familial DCM (FDC) (been discussed here in the chapter), contributing 20-48% of DCMs. However, FCM can also be seen as an autosomal recessive or X-linked recessive trait. The principal causes of FDC are genetic mutations affecting cardiac myocytes. Accordingly, based on molecular and clinical genetic data, different forms can be distinguished:

I. The autosomal dominant pure FDC with three known chromosomal loci mapped on chromosome 1q32 [2], 9q13-22 [3], and 10q21-23 [4].
II. The autosomal dominant form in which DCM appears after conduction defects, with two disease loci mapped on chromosome 3p22-p25 [5] and 1p1-1q1 [6].
III. The autosomal dominant form associated with myopathy [7].
IV. The autosomal recessive form.
V. The X-linked DCM due to dystrophin gene mutations/deletions both in the critical region of the 5' end [8, 9] and the region of exons 48-49 [10].
VI. Mitochondrial DCM, characterized by a matrilineal transmission and
VII. Right ventricular cardiomyopathy which can mimic DCM, and other unclassifiable forms of cardiomyopathies.

Consequently, DCM accounts for 30-50% of all HF cases in large clinical trials posing the leading cause for heart transplantation [11]. It is important to note that, DCM does not equate with systolic HF as DCM is predominantly an imaging diagnosis, whereas HF is a clinical and imaging diagnosis. Also, of equal importance, the small size of contemporary families in clinical trials and registries can conceal the genetic nature of the disease [12]. HF represents the final common phenotypic pathway in most cases in response to genetic insults, which affect approximately 40 million people with FDC globally [13]. Great efforts towards the understanding of the genetic basis of FDC have currently been made with the use of genome-wide association studies (GWAS), and candidate gene sequencing as well as linkage gene analyses in families [14, 15] to help in the identification of risk variants and genes causing mutations. However, the main issue in cardiovascular genetic medicine is determining if a putative mutation in a gene known to be associated with DCM is indeed causative of disease. Although a molecular genetic diagnosis may not help guide the treatment and impact the outcome of a proband with the disease advanced, however, clinical surveillance, medical and antiarrhythmic device therapy for an at-risk pre-symptomatic relative who carries the disease-causing mutation may prevent disease progression and life-threatening complications. Novel sequencing approaches in the practice of cardiovascular genetic medicine [16 - 19] have empowered and transformed clinical genetic testing. Hence, the knowledge of FDC is highly essential for cardiovascular genetic medicine clinic staffs, and for geneticists in general, including a primary and clinical geneticist, and genetic counselors. By contrast, the genetic basis of DCM is highly diverse (involving various genetic pathways leading to an increased propensity to SCD) with genetic and phenotypic overlap between arrhythmogenic right ventricular cardiomyopathy (ARVC) and hypertrophic cardiomyopathy (HCM) [20 - 29].

Finally, despite the adequate tremendous progress made in the field so far, ongoing and lingering questions remain such as:

I. How the familiar type of the disease apart from its genetic basis differs from the others, *e.g.*, IDC?
II. Which genetic pathways or specific genes are most relevant? and
III. Whether other genetic mechanisms (*e.g.*, mitochondrial mutations, DNA structural variants, and others) are operative in DCM?

The chapter aims to provide a detailed and concise overview of DCM genetic etiology, discuss the latest phenomic and genomic available data which are crucial to understanding the emerging complexity of FDC as well as the clinical utilities and limitations of genetic testing. The chapter will also examine the genetic underpinnings of HF syndromes, advances in the common and rare variant discovery and the interpretation in DCM and systolic HF. With this in mind, this chapter will further aim to define the diagnostic criteria of FDC, current clinical management options/strategies, and what the implications these findings hold for patient care and future research.

DEFINITION AND NOMENCLATURE

DCM is characterized by LV enlargement and systolic dysfunction with an ejection fraction (EF) of 50% [30] or, more stringently, 45% [31]. "DCM" as a name is most at times confusing as it is a term commonly used mostly in clinical trial literature which is on the morphological basis (ischemic or nonischemic) [32] of the LV (systolic dysfunction, dilatation) irrespective of the etiology. In that note, both European Consortium consensus and the American Heart Association (AHA) documents exclude DCM from ischemic heart disease (IHD). However, other secondary causes of DCM are recognized [33, 34]. The continuous confusion of the term "DCM" in cardiovascular genetic literature in one case arise where it is used to refer to IDC (where the genetic cause is inferred and/or suspected) and in another case to indicated specifically "a genetic-caused" form of DCM. Although, the term "familiar"-DCM is strongly used to imply a genetic cause as its classification is assigned according to pedigree assessments and phenotype and not molecular genetic data (Table **1**).

Table 1. Causes of dilated cardiomyopathy.

Young
Myocarditis (infective/toxic/immune)
Carnitine deficiency
Selenium deficiency
Anomalous coronary arteries
Arteriovenous malformations
Kawasaki disease
Endocardial fibroelastosis
Non-compacted myocardium
Calcium deficiency
Familial IDC
Barth syndrome
Adolescent/Adults
Familial IDC
X linked

(Table 1) cont.....

Alcohol
Myocarditis (infective/toxic/immune)
Tachycardiomyopathy
Mitochondrial
Arrhythmogenic right ventricular cardiomyopathy
Eosinophilic (Churg Strauss syndrome)
Drugs—anthracyclines
Peripartum
Endocrine
Nutritional—thiamine, carnitine deficiency, hypophosphatemia, hypocalcemia

EPIDEMIOLOGICAL PREVALENCE

In general, DCM prevalence varies vastly, likely reflecting ethnic and geographical differences, as well as the methodologies, used [35, 36]. Although much common in African-Americans than in Caucasians (three times more frequent in blacks and males than whites and females), it may occur in any patient population. In the current guidelines and clinical practice, the prevalence of FDC is assumed to be approximately 30% to 50% [37 - 40] with about 30% of them having an identifiable genetic cause [40]. Studies from Japan (14/100 000) [35], England (8.3/100 000) [41], and Italy (7.0/100 000) [42] identifies the remarkable geographical and ethnic diversity of the disease. Although, the prevalence of DCM is still very much underestimated or overestimated [43] as the case may be.

CLINICAL SIGNS AND SYMPTOMS OF DILATED CARDIOMYOPATHY

DCM can appear along a spectrum of absent to mild or severe symptoms with cases of congestive HF (CHF). When only subtle signs exist, infants and younger children are most times diagnosed with recurrent pneumonia or an upper respiratory tract infection (viral) with the physician not realizing that a fundamental genetic heart problem is the basis for presenting symptoms in the infant or child. However, unlike in younger children and infants, the early presenting symptoms include fatigue and a decreased exercise tolerance rate making clinicians less likely to diagnose older children and adolescents with viral syndromes. Although, with signs and symptoms of CHF, infants and younger children will usually present with noticeable clinical changes such as failure to thrive, irritability, facial paleness, wheezing, and increased sweating especially with activities. Not until DCM diagnosis is made, the wheezing and chronic cough would be misinterpreted as asthma. Symptoms such as arrhythmias can also be either the first symptom or appearing after the diagnosis of DCM has been made. Other rhythmic symptoms include syncope, seizure, palpitations, and possible SCD. It is also imperative to note that, even if other severe symptoms of CHF are yet to appear, these symptoms can, however, occur at any age and stage of cardiomyopathy.

MOLECULAR GENETICS OF DILATED CARDIOMYOPATHY AND ITS GENOMIC ARCHITECTURE

Identified "genetic" diseases can typically be classified into two categories: Monogenic (Mendelian) diseases which are rare with only one mutation in a given gene responsible for its inheritance in a given family and multifactorial diseases which are often complex due to the addictive effect or the interaction of multiple genes, more common, and often recognized as "running in the family". DCM in cardiovascular genetics can, however, be sub-classified as monogenic diseases, caused by mutations in key genes that lead to either an abnormality or the absence of myocardial proteins [44]. Mutations in more than 30 genes of diverse ontology are reported causing DCM, which is by stark contrast, more than the mutations causing ARVC and HCM. Notably, a number of these genes encode proteins of the sarcomere, including those relevant to HCM. Also, well-represented are genes encoding Z-disk proteins. Others include genes encoding proteins related to potassium or calcium channels, mitochondria, nuclear envelope, and heat-shock chaperones.

Furthermore, allelic heterogeneities are also hallmarks for DCMs. Consequently, it often complicates the prediction of a phenotype and establishes a clear relationship between genotype and phenotype. Also, issues of a single mutation manifesting as DCM in one individual and HCM in another only expands the cardiomyopathic complexity. In addition to the disease complexity, most DCM-associated mutations are sometimes "private" (unique to a family or an individual) [45]. Although rarity does not automatically equate to pathogenicity, some variants are as well significant myocardial protein defects and are more likely to be pathogenic. Thus, as already stated previously, pathological mechanisms leading to DCM are different such as mutations in genes encoding sarcomeric, desmosomal, cytoskeletal, mitochondrial, nuclear membrane, and RNA-binding proteins have all been linked to DCM (Fig. **1** & Table **2**). Listed below are the most commonly implicated genes, and also in order of their frequency and contribution to DCM.

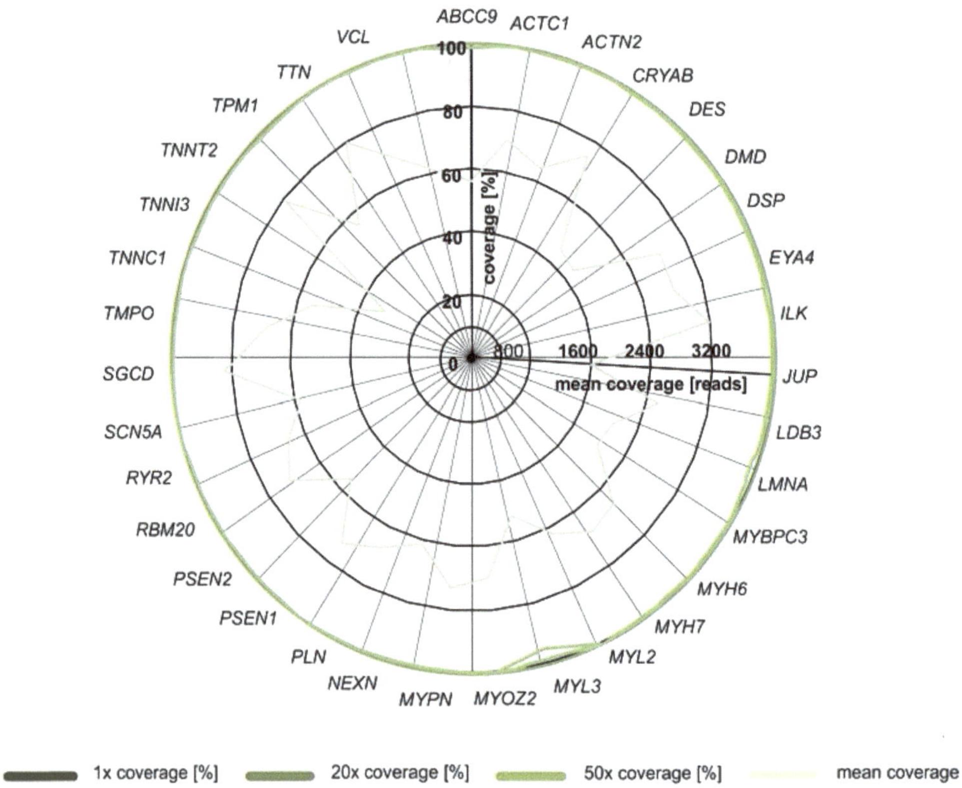

Fig. (1). Figure representing the known list and sequence coverage of dilated cardiomyopathy genes (both definitive and putative DCM Genes). The vertical axis is showing the target coverage for every gene; color codes give the read depth of coverage. The horizontal axis is providing the mean coverage in reads per gene (pale green line).

Table 2. Genes associated with dilated cardiomyopathy.

Gene	Encoded Protein	Function
Major Genetic Factors		
LMNA	lamins A/C	building blocks of the nuclear lamina
TNNT2	cardiac troponin T (cTnT)	regulation of muscle contraction
β-MYH7	β -myosin heavy chain	conversion of chemical energy into mechanical force
Other Genetic Factors		
SCN5A	the alpha subunit of type V voltage-gated sodium channel	controlling sodium ion flow into cardiac muscle cells
TCAP	titin-cap (telethonin)	regulation of sarcomere assembly

(Table 2) cont.....

Gene	Encoded Protein	Function
HBEGF	heparin-binding epidermal growth factor	regulation of cell growth and differentiation
SRA1	steroid receptor RNA activator 1	stimulation of proliferation and apoptosis
IK	cytokine	down-regulation of expression of HLA class II antigens
TPM1	α-tropomyosin	regulation of actin-myosin interaction
PSEN 1/2	presenilin 1 / 2	multi-pass transmembrane proteins
Dnm1l	dynamin-1-like	establishing mitochondrial morphology
LDB3	LIM domain binding 3	interaction with α-actinin-2 and protein kinase C

TTN

The most significant known protein expressed in the heart and the discovery of the role of TTN-truncating variants is one of the significant advances made in cardiovascular genetics [46]. It functions as a spring regulating sarcomere contraction and signaling by providing passive force [47] with domains accommodating passive stiffness [48]. The I band of the TTN gene is encoded by 220 of TTN's 360 exons which includes proline-glutamate-valine-lysine repetitive region which regulates its passive force/tension. The extensive alternative splicing of TTN, repetitive nature, and size makes it challenging for genetic analysis. Throughout the heart's early development, TTN is notably differentially spliced and adaptive to distinct physiological states, including HF [49]. However, there is also, the tendency for TTN truncations to distribute to A bands, rather than the I band [50]. Overall, in the general population, caution needs to be applied in interpreting (familial segregation analysis) the presence of TTN-truncating variants.

LMNA

LMNA mutations are inherited just like TTN in an autosomal dominant manner. LMNA mutations linked to autosomal dominant DCM are both frameshifting and missense in nature, and occurring throughout the entire length of the coding region (Fig. **2**). The missense and truncating mutations of LMNA account for 5% to 9% of genetic DCM [51, 52]. Mutations in lamin A leads to accumulation of prelamin A (progerin), and a constellation of diseases from premature aging syndrome (Hutchinson-Gilford progeria) [53], to myopathies and DCM [54]. The single LMNA gene encodes lamins A and C, and differential splicing at the 3′ end results in two proteins that are identical across their first 566 amino acids. LMNA loss leads to a defect in mechano-signaling [55, 56] as Lamins A and C are both implicated in many different cellular processes from DNA replication, to mechano-sensing, a gene regulating expression, and nuclear to cytoplasmic transport.

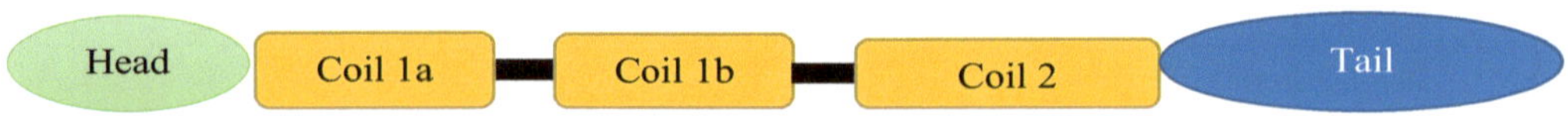

Fig. (2). Human lamin structure.

PLN

The un-phosphorylation of PLN gene which encodes a 52 amino acid residue transmembrane protein (phospholamban) typically inhibits sarcoplasmic reticulum Ca2+-ATPase. The phenotype with PLN mutations is variable. However, several dominant mutations in PLN have been associated with DCM, including the R14del severe phenotype (Germany and Netherlands) [57] although, the much milder phenotype can also be seen [58, 59]. Early onset DCM with lethal ventricular arrhythmias are also known [60, 61].

RBM20

A 1227 amino acid in length highly found in both atria and ventricles, and contains an RNA recognition motif domain between residues 525 and 600 amino acid. Dominant mutations in the RBM20 gene were first described in DCM, where they contribute to 1% to 5% of DCM [62, 63]. A second conserved domain can also be found between 650 and 725 amino acids. More recently, RBM20 have been identified in a third conserved region (glutamate-rich area) [64]. RBM20, as an RNA-binding protein is involved in tissue-specific splicing relevant to adaptation and the development of the diseases state. RBM20 modulates cardiac splicing, including the splicing of TTN in the heart [65 - 67] hence, mutations with RBM20 may share similarities to those occurring from TTN-truncating variants.

SCN5A

SCN5A encodes the primary sodium channel expressed in the heart (Fig. **3**). SCN5A missense mutations have also been described in FDC, and these mutations carry a higher risk for arrhythmias (the long QT and Brugada syndromes) [68, 69] due to the distinct roles of SCN5A plays in the myocardium and the conduction system. However, it is quite challenging to interpret rare variation in the SCN5A gene due to is considerable genetic heterogeneity in the general population [70]. Although genotype-phenotype association studies can help guide genotype-based therapies.

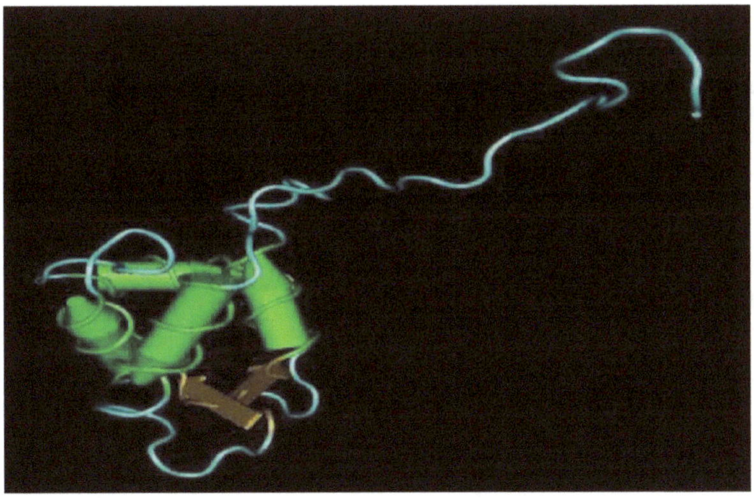

Fig. (3). Structure of the C-terminal Ef-hand domain of human cardiac sodium channel.

Cytoskeletal Genes

Genes encoding cardiac cytoskeletal proteins have been implicated in DCM such as dystrophin mutations link to cardiomyopathy in Duchenne muscular dystrophy, X-linked DCM [71], and sarcoglycan genes mutations [72]. Thus, the absence of these genes leads to heart dysfunctions and cardiomyocyte lose as these gene products play crucial roles in sarcolemmal stability.

Mitochondrial Mutations

Mitochondrial genomes mutations are challenging to interpret and identify given the role of heteroplasmy also coupled with the fact that most genetic testing relies on peripheral blood DNA, which may or may not match what occurs in the heart. Both mitochondrial-encoded and nuclear-encoded mitochondrial genes lead to cardiomyopathy [1, 73]. However, mitochondrial-encoded genes show maternal inheritance, whereas Nuclear-encoded mitochondrial genes follow either autosomal dominant or recessive inheritance.

Other Major Genetic Causes of Dilated Cardiomyopathy

Cardiac Troponin T (TNNT2): Troponin T located on the thin filament of the contractile apparatus is the tropomyosin-binding protein in the troponin regulatory complex (Fig. **4**). There are three isotype forms of troponin T: cardiac troponin T, slow and fast skeletal muscle isotypic forms. Cardiac troponin T is encoded by the TNNT2 gene; which alterations significantly contribute to DCM [74]. K210 (deletion of lysine in residue 210) mutation is one of the most common variants observed in patients suffering DCM [75].

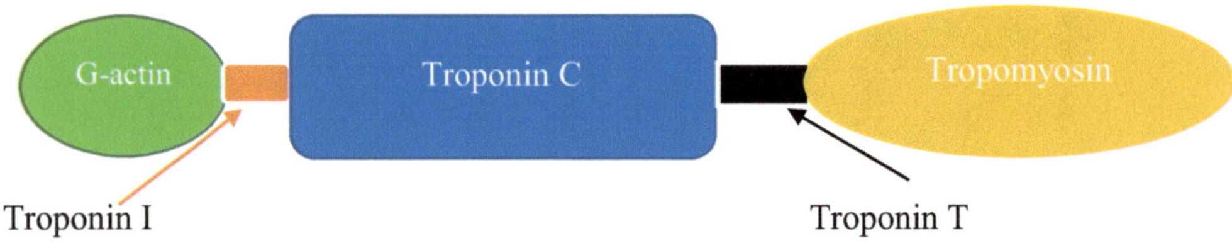

Fig. (4). Location of troponin T in the troponin regulatory complex.

β-myosin Heavy Chain (MYH7): Myosin within the cell, it is organized as two pairs of light chains and a pair of heavy chains which is a highly asymmetric molecule with a rod-like tail and a globular head (Figs. **5** & **6**). The globular head contains a catalytic domain with actin and ATP-binding sites and a light chain-binding domain [76]. Myosin is a protein that converts chemical energy into mechanical force through hydrolysis of ATP. Currently, more than 50 different mutations have been identified in MYH7 gene in association with DCM [77] with 4.2% of cases reported [78]. Disease-causing dominant mutations of MYH7 (S532P and F764L) located at chromosome 14q11.2-13 results in a diminished contractile function and ventricular dilatation [79, 80].

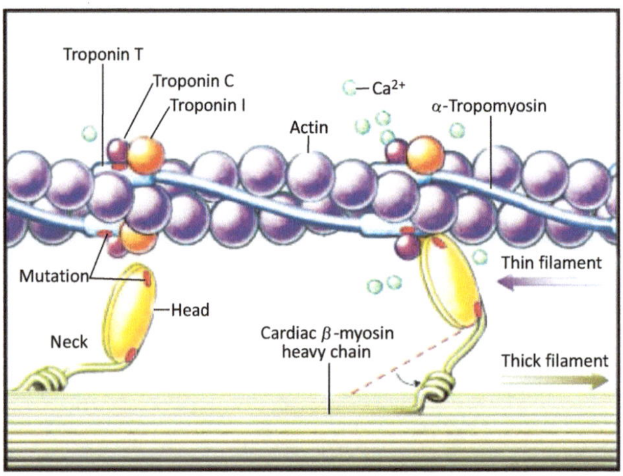

Fig. (5). Generation of a Power Stroke by Myosin and Actin in Sarcomere Filaments.

Additional Genetic Mutations in Dilated Cardiomyopathy

DCM best considered as a cardiomyopathy of mixed origin, there are other known genetic mutations though not as frequently identified as others described above. TPM1, BAG3 [81], Presenilin genes (PSEN1 and PSEN2) [82], and heparin-binding epidermal growth factor (HBEGF), steroid receptor RNA activator 1 (SRA1) and IK cytokine (Fig. 7).

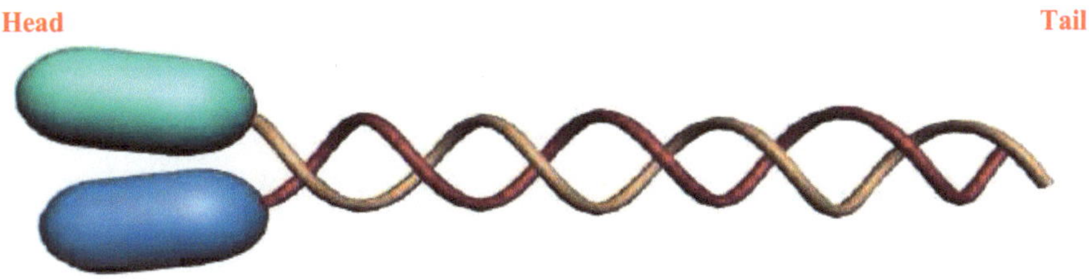

Fig (6). A pair of myosin heavy chains.

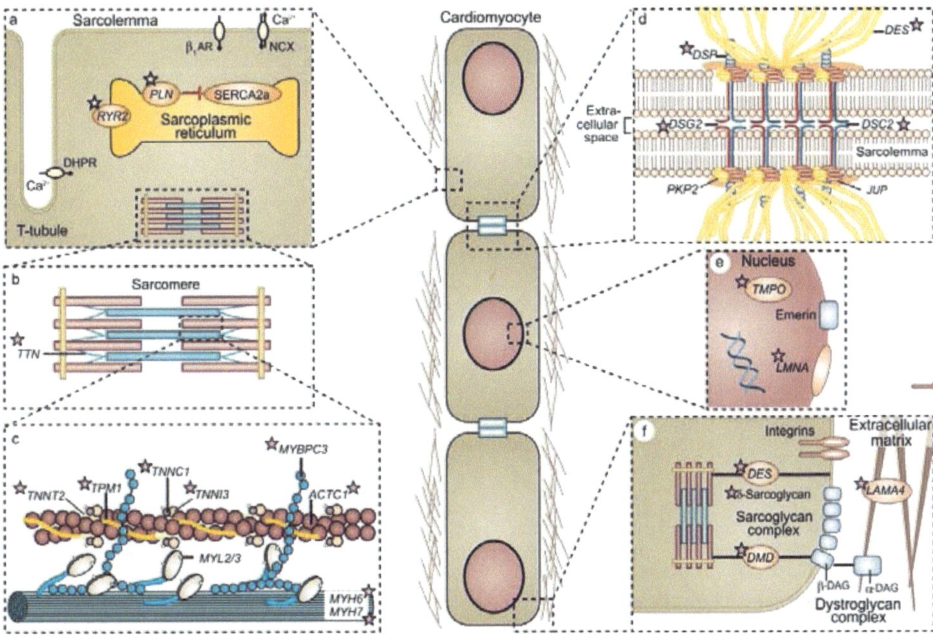

Fig. (7). Heterogeneous set of rare genetic variants. **(A)** The cardiomyocyte membrane (sarcolemma), transverse (T)-tubule, and sarcoplasmic reticulum. **(B, C)** The sarcomere: the force-generating structure in cardiomyocytes. **(D)** Desmosomal junctions, which assist in force transmission during muscle contraction. **(E)** The cardiomyocyte nucleus. **(F)** Cardiomyocyte membrane and extracellular matrix proteins.

COMPLEX GENETIC ARCHITECTURE OF HEART FAILURE SYNDROMES AND THE CHALLENGES IN THE INTERPRETATION OF GENETIC VARIANTS

DCM known as a multigenic disorder or cardiomyopathy of mixed origin carries several early and late clinical presentations. Systolic HF a “catch-all phenotypic diagnosis” and can be caused by a variety of insults ranging from myocardial ischemia to cardiomyopathy (Fig. **8**).

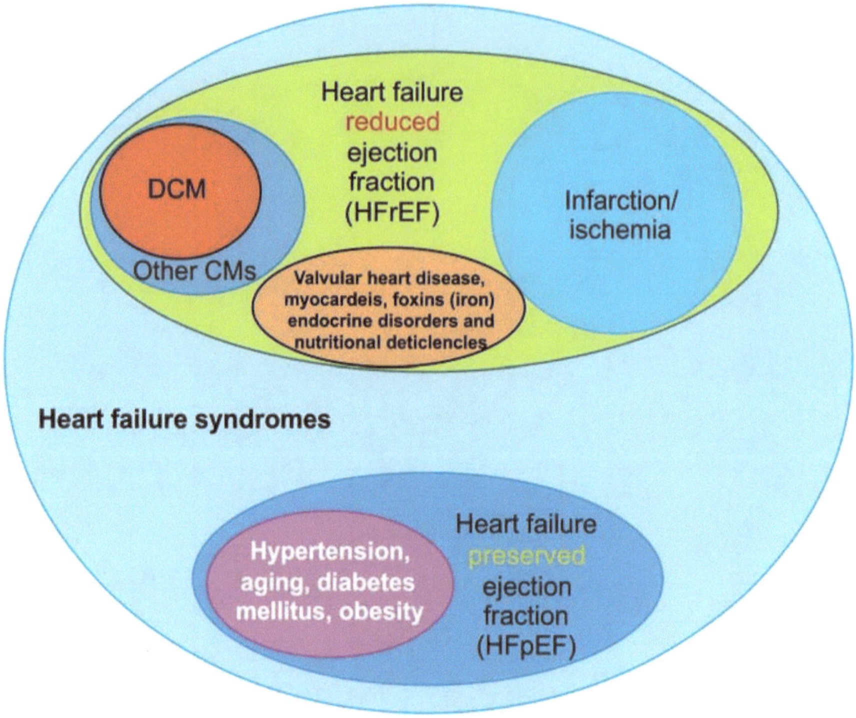

Fig. (8). An overview of heart failure syndromes showing where dilated cardiomyopathy (DCM) and systolic heart failure fit about all heart failure syndromes.

However, this lack of specificity limits our knowledge and understanding of genetic variants the contributing to systolic HF. Rare variants are typically defined as "unique" having a minor allele frequency of <1%, though varies on reported cases [83]. Understanding rare variants, a disease-specific cut-off informed by disease penetrance, prevalence, and allelic contribution to disease [84, 85] is crucial. Identification approaches can be carried out as traditional Sanger capillary-based sequencing, whole-genome or whole-exome sequencing, or panel-based sequencing. Furthermore, common variants should be identified by genotyping on chips containing hundreds of thousands of single-nucleotide polymorphisms (SNPs) or genotyping of SNPs on candidate gene studies. These approaches form the basis of GWAS. DCM known as a multigenic disorder or cardiomyopathy of mixed origin carries several early and late clinical presentations. Systolic HF a "catch-all phenotypic diagnosis" and can be caused by a variety of insults ranging from myocardial ischemia to cardiomyopathy. However, this lack of specificity limits our knowledge and understanding of genetic variants the contributing to systolic HF. Excluding contributions of monogenic cardiomyopathies that are novel alleles, private or rare, to the risk of systolic HF are limited due to the complex etiology of systolic HF as each associated condition might have its genetic basis (for example, diabetes, and hypertension) making it difficult to distinguish primary from secondary effects [83]. Also, HF has an inheritable component estimated at 18% based on analyses of the Framingham data-set [86]. Although, primary cardiomyopathies might play little or no role in common HF, but can highlight more molecular pathways that are important for HF syndromes more generically [87].

Translational Implications

Although no clear emerging novel drug targets or new mechanistic pathways yet, as discussed above, many recent genetic studies of systolic HF have suggested the involvement of novel genes and loci. However, among emerging studies, the most striking findings have been that, among those genes linked to systolic HF, not all are expressed exclusively within the heart such as the CLCKNA gene encoding chloride channels in the kidney.

CLINICAL GENETICS OF DILATED CARDIOMYOPATHY

Family History and Pedigree Analysis

The importance of this step cannot be overemphasized as it is a critical aspect of evaluating a patient with DCM before considering a genetic cause. It is essential for clinicians to obtain a proper family history from patients and relatives and also, patients seeking information by themselves from relatives. This history should include three-to-four generations following up on subtle hints of FDC [88]. Although, the time required to obtain a complete family history in outpatient's clinical settings is prohibitive. Therefore, it is imperative that questionnaires either internet based or paper-based are provided or recommended to them before a clinic visit which would change history taking from a one-time event to a process where before and after a clinic visit, a patient carefully investigate their family history. Also, medical records should be requested and reviewed whenever possible. Nevertheless, even detailed family history can be negative in a patient with FDC, because the asymptomatic period of the DCM-causal pathway can extend for years hence, clinical screening (discussed further in the chapter) is an essential complement to family history. Care should also be taken not to presume inheritance patterns based on preliminary data.

Reduced and Age-Dependent Penetrance

In its strictest definition, penetrance is an 'all-or-nothing' phenomenon, where an individual must reach old age without the disease before a reduced penetrance can be established. Therefore, a reduced penetrance can be seen practically as where an individual who has both an affected parent and affected children is unaffected with absolutely no sign of LV enlargement or systolic dysfunction despite harboring a pathogenic DCM mutation after reaching and/ or surpassing the mean age, *i.e.* from neonates to adulthood ≥60 years old [89].

Variable Expressivity

Evidence of a phenotypic penetrance is determined by whether phenotypic expressions can be observed, whereas variable expression accounts for variability, severity, or degree of a phenotype. For example, in large kindred harboring the same DCM mutation, some siblings can have only a mild LV systolic dysfunction with no evidence of HF whereas, others might have a profound decrease in LV systolic function accompanied by an overt HF.

CLINICAL DIAGNOSIS OF DILATED CARDIOMYOPATHY

Clinical Presentation: FDC most times are diagnosed incidentally in asymptomatic individuals during routine medical screening or family evaluation of patients with an established diagnosis. However, first clinical presentations can be the development of arrhythmia, in particular, atrial fibrillation (AF), low cardiac output, pulmonary congestion, systemic embolism an even SCD.

Electrocardiography (ECG): ECG in patients with FDC are sometimes remarkably normal, but abnormalities ranging from prolongation of atrioventricular (AV) conduction, isolated T wave changes to septal Q waves in patients with extensive LV fibrosis, and bundle branch block, sinus tachycardia and supraventricular arrhythmias may be observed.

Echocardiography: LV measurements are essential to diagnose DCM. Systolic and diastolic LV dimensions can be determined by M-mode and 2-dimensional echocardiography. Hence, the state of LV enlargement is recognized as a prodrome to DCM [90]. Echocardiography also helps detect strain and strain rate differences in first-degree relatives of those with newly diagnosed nonischemic DCM.

Cardiac Magnetic Resonance (CMR): Strain measurements and LV chamber dimensions can also be accurately determined by CMR imaging. Contrast agents, main gadolinium, can be used with CMR to evaluate fibrosis, providing additional information on myocardial tissue quality. The degree of fibrosis in DCM is a predictor of all-cause mortality, which is detected by the delayed gadolinium contrast enhancement, identifying the need for future hospitalization [91].

Exercise Testing: Symptom-limited upright exercise testing and respiratory gas analysis are valuable when assessing functional limitation, especially when combined with metabolic exercise testing (MET). MET facilitates the assessment of disease progression, gives an objective measure of exercise capacity, provide diagnostic information about LV impairment, helps assess prognosis, and is useful in patient's selection for a heart transplant.

Endomyocardial Biopsy (EMB): EMB can be used to confirm the diagnosis. However, with improved cardiac imaging, EMB is less frequently used. Although, despite technically enhanced imaging techniques, EMBs can be the preferred choice in some settings such as amyloid, iron overload, and other infiltrative processes [92]. EMBs can further be used to evaluate myocarditis and in the background of unexplained HF [93, 94]. Be it as it may, the complication rates such as tamponades and perforation further limit its use, and the non-uniform nature of infiltrative diseases also limits its sensitivity [95].

Noninvasive Arrhythmia Monitoring: Generally, DCMs are associated with an increased risk for cardiac arrhythmias and SCD [96], and some specific genetic DCM subtypes are especially prone to arrhythmias. Therefore, due to the increased risk of SCD with DCM and the susceptibility of some subtypes to arrhythmias, there is hence the need for arrhythmic surveillance to be able to properly deploy device management such as implantable cardioverter defibrillators (ICDs) and peacemakers. For its ease, Holter monitoring remains a mainstay enabling a two to three days sampling and regulation. However, for long-term information and real-time transmitted data, implantable loop recorders offer long-term information which would also, provide more findings ventricular tachycardia (VT) and ventricular ectopy [97].

CRITERIA FOR THE DIAGNOSIS OF FAMILIAR DILATED CARDIOMYOPATHY

The diagnosis of familial dilated cardiomyopathy is made (Fig. **9**):

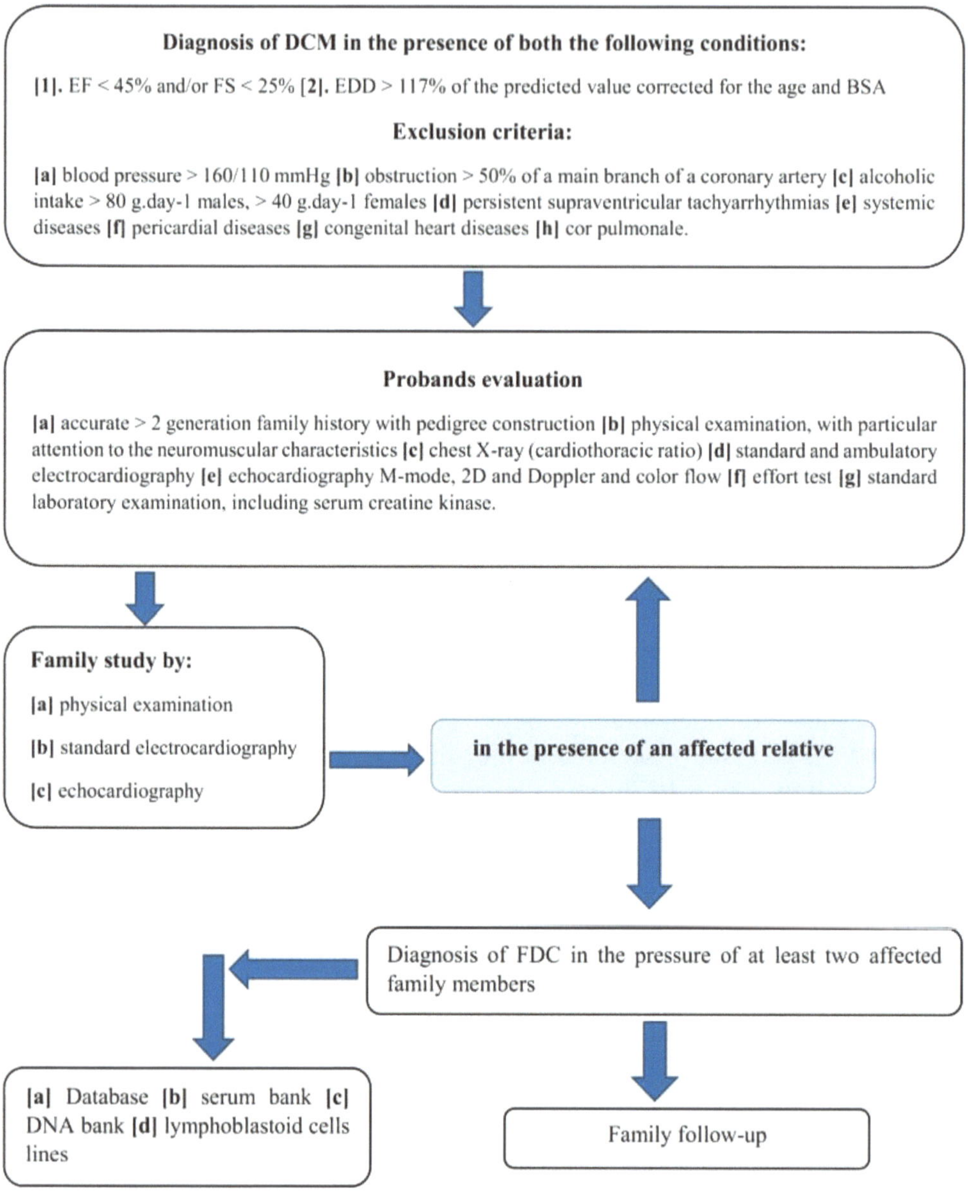

Fig. (9). Protocol for the clinical and molecular genetic studies of familial dilated cardiomyopathy (DC). EF=ejection fraction; FS=fractional shortening; EDD=end diastolic diameter; BSA=body surface area.

I. In the presence of two or more affected individuals in a single family or
II. In the presence of a first-degree relative of a DCM patient, with a well-documented unexplained sudden death at <35 years of age.

DEFINITION OF THE CLINICAL STATUS OF FAMILIES WITH FAMILIAR DILATED CARDIOMYOPATHY

Major Criteria

I. Defined criteria for DCM (as stated above).

Minor Criteria

I. LV dilatation >112% of the predicted value.
II. LV dysfunction: EF <50% or fractional shortening <28%.
III. Unexplained sudden death or stroke before 50 years of age.
IV. Segmental wall motion abnormalities (<1 segment, or 1 if not previously present) in the absence of intraventricular conduction defect or ischemic heart disease.
V. Unexplained ventricular (>1000. 24 h”1) or supraventricular (sustained arrhythmias or AF) arrhythmias, frequent or repetitive (three or more beats with >120 beats. min”1) before the age of 50. Stroke before 50 years of age or sudden unexplained death.
VI. Unexplained conduction disease: nodal sinus dysfunction, II or III atrioventricular conduction defects, and left-ventricular bundle branch block.

Assessment of Clinical Status

I. Affected
- Systolic dysfunction and LV dilatation (major criteria) and
- one minor criterion + LV dilatation (>117%) and/ or
- Three minor criteria's (as stated above).

II. Unaffected
- Individuals with normal hearts.
- Presence of other causes of myocardial disease.

III. Unknown
- Presence of one or two minor criteria.

CURRENT MEDICAL TREATMENTS AND MANAGEMENT STRATEGIES FOR DILATED CARDIOMYOPATHY

Currently, there are no existing therapies that can “cure” DCM; however, treatments are available, which can improve symptoms and decrease risk in patients with DCM (Fig. **10**). Therefore, the therapeutic management of DCM is focused on (i) LV dimension and function, (ii) arrhythmia surveillance and treatment, (iii) reducing congestive symptoms if present, and (iv) preventing the disease progression and complications such as progressive HF, SCD, and thromboembolism. The specific therapy depends on the clinical condition of the patient, ability of the patient to tolerate the treatment, and the risk of dangerous events.

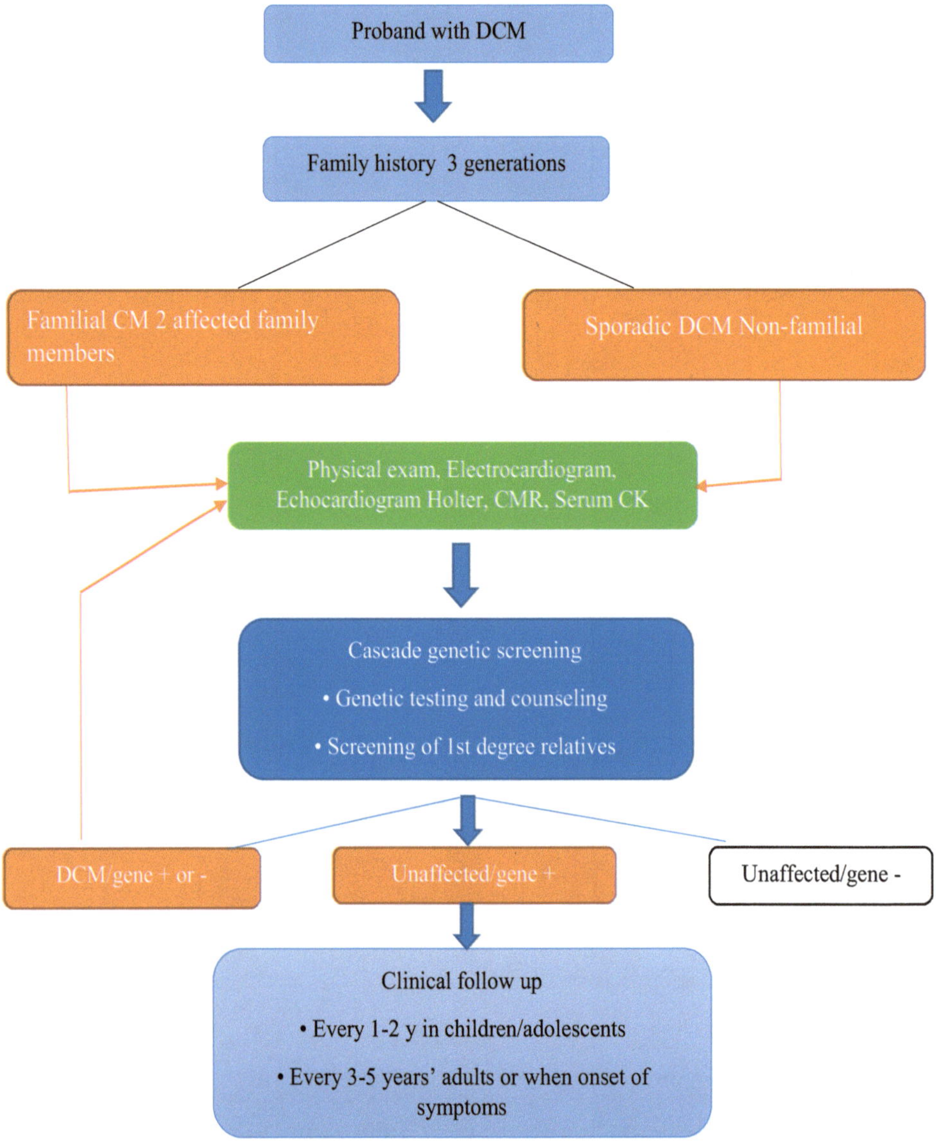

Fig. (10). Algorithm for the management of a patient with dilated cardiomyopathy.

Anti-arrhythmia Medications

The use of amiodarone and procainamide can help prevent or control abnormal rhythm (VTs or supraventricular tachycardias). General side effects include headache, nausea/constipation, slower heart rate, lower blood pressure, depressed mood, dizziness, skin rash, and difficulties concentrating, among others.

Angiotensin II Receptor Blockers (ARBs)

ARBs are essential and an essential armory to have for the treatment of HF. Though ARBs have similar hemodynamic effects as angiotensin-converting enzyme (ACE) inhibitors, they are somewhat better tolerated and pharmacologically clinically overcome the "escape" of ARBs system blockade seen in some patients on ACE inhibitors. However, unlike ACE inhibitors, ARBs do not inhibit bradykinin metabolism and thus lack a potentially beneficial vasodilatory effect.

Angiotensin Converting Enzyme Inhibitors (ACE)

Renin-angiotensin-aldosterone system (RAAS) activation is central to the pathophysiology of HF of whatever underlying etiology. For this reason, ACE inhibitors are the mainstays of treatment in patients with FDC, irrespective of the severity of HF [98]. Therapy with ACE inhibitors improve exercise intolerance, dyspnea, and reduce both hospitalization rates and cardiovascular mortality. They further also prevent or slow disease progression in asymptomatic patients.

β Blockers

Despite progress with the use of ACE inhibitors, death continues to be high in patients with HF. It however, not come as a surprise given that ACE inhibitors act on only one aspect of the RAAS that contributes to progressive LV dysfunction. Patients should not be started on B blockers if they have signs or symptoms of decompensated HF, and initial doses should be low (bisoprolol 1.25 mg once daily, carvedilol 3.125 mg twice daily, metoprolol SR 12.5 mg once daily). Doses should be increased gradually every 3-6 weeks, monitoring carefully for hypotension, bradycardia or worsening HF until sides effects occur or the target dose is achieved.

Diuretics (Spironolactone)

ACE inhibition usually results in only a transient decrease in aldosterone concentrations, which is as a result of aldosterone reduced hepatic clearance rather than angiotensin dependent adrenal secretion. High plasma concentrations of aldosterone are frequent in patients with moderate to severe HF and contribute to potassium loss, sodium retention, myocardial fibrosis, baroreceptor dysfunction, and sympathetic activation. Spironolactone should, however, be considered in all patients presenting with moderate to severe HF symptoms.

Inotropes

Inotropic agents such as Vasopressin, milrinone, dobutamine, dopamine, epinephrine, norepinephrine (intravenous) and digoxin (oral) are used to help the heart contract more effectively and to support children who have severe HF and are not stable enough to be home.

Anticoagulation Medications

Although the risk for thromboembolism is relatively low, there is a risk of blood clots formation high, especially in a patient with a heart that does not contract properly. The reasonable likelihood of blood clot forming will determine the choice of anticoagulants used. The use of lesser anticoagulants, such as aspirin and dipyridamole, is recommended to prevent fetal outcomes. Stronger anticoagulants like warfarin should be administered in patients with a history of thromboembolism or evidence of intracardiac thrombus with regular blood testing and monitoring.

Pacing Therapies

Pacemakers: Small, battery-operated devices usually placed under the skin of the abdomen or chest attached to electrical leads which are threaded to the heart. The help monitors heartbeats and maintains a regular rhythm in patients who are prone to having abnormal heartbeats either "too slow" due to slow conduction of impulses through the heart or as a side effect of medications or "extremely fast" life-threatening arrhythmias (VT and fibrillation). In adults with end-stage HF, bi-ventricular pacing system can also be employed although not yet recommended for use in children.

Implantable Cardioverter Defibrillator (ICD): ICDs are designed and used to prevent SCD from a severe arrhythmia as it's used to monitor heart rates, and when VT or VF are detected, shocks are delivered to the heart restoring the rhythm. We (authors) recommended its use for both adults and children with DCM. Current average five-year survival rates for children and adults with DCM are 40-50% and 30-40%, respectively.

NON-PHARMACOLOGICAL TREATMENT OF ADVANCED HEART FAILURE

Though heart transplant remains the cornerstone for advanced HF management in patients with refractory HF and end-stage cardiac diseases, however, transplantation remains limited by the scarcity of suitable organs and the development of graft vasculopathy. Therefore, in response to this dilemma, the use of left ventricular assist device (LVAD) and a novel approach, "the BATISTA procedure" are been employed. Though the later not in routine use especially in in-experienced centers managing advanced HF.

Left Ventricular Assist Devices (LVADs): LVADs have recently received approval from the US Food and Drug Administration for use in patients with end-stage heart failure as a bridge to cardiac transplantation. However, technical advances and LVAD designs serve as an alternative to transplantation in patients who are not transplanted, candidates. We (authors) recommended its use for adults with DCM.

BATISTA Procedure (Partial Left Ventriculectomy): This procedure is based on Laplace's law hence, reducing the LV size by removing part of its circumference should minimize wall stress and improve ventricular hemodynamics. Though the method is based on hypothesis, in experienced centers, this procedure has proven to be excellent given the nature of the surgical procedure. However, its downside is its strict patient selection, and patients can only survive with a combination of LAVD therapy [99].

POTENTIAL PHARMACOLOGICAL NOVEL TREATMENTS

Natriuretic Peptides

Released in response to stretch from atrial myocytes, suppresses the renin-angiotensin system and induces vasodilatation, natures, and diuresis. The circulating concentrations of atrial natriuretic peptides (ANP) are increased in congestive HF and correspond with the prognosis and functional class of NYHA. Both brain natriuretic peptide and ANP are potent diuretics, and vasodilators but clinical trials have shown tolerance developing during i.v administration. It can be overcome by producing an enzyme responsible for the breakdown of natriuretic peptides and drugs that inhibit neutral endopeptidase.

Cytokine Antagonist

Cachectin or Tumor necrosis factor á (TNFá) is a proinflammatory cytokine released from failing myocardium, T cells, and activated macrophages. It circulates at high concentrations in patients with congestive HF. Cytokines are increasingly thought to promote HF progression as other proinflammatory cytokines and raised plasma concentrations of TNFá have been interpreted as epiphenomena of HF.

MANAGEMENT OF GENOTYPE-POSITIVE PHENOTYPE NEGATIVE PATIENTS

Genotype-positive/phenotype negative family members can be identified through genetic testing, which would prove useful for lifestyle recommendation, adjustments (restriction from competitive sports) [100], and preventive strategies. Current guidelines recommend observation in asymptomatic at-risk relatives with the yearly clinical assessment [101] and control of risk factors at this stage, such as hypertension [102]. Although, less consensus exists on timing, management, and intervention in this patient.

GENETIC TESTING, SCREENING, TESTING APPROACHES, AND COUNSELLING

Clinical Genetic Testing and Guidelines

DCM clinical genetic testing has been rapidly evolving over the years which have seen the previously published guidelines [101] outdated from testing one or two genes, on a gene-by-gene basis, to panels containing 12-30 genes. According to the American Heart Association (AHA) 2016 Scientific Statement on DCM [37], genetic testing is recommended (with moderate level of consensus) in patients with familial (Level of Evidence A) although there is a healthy level of agreement (nonfamiliar) in approving mutation-specific genetic testing for family members after the identification of a DCM-causative mutation in the proband (Level of Evidence B). Showing lack of a complete consensus in the field, the European Society of Cardiology (ESC) 2016 Position Statement [103] is slightly different and recommends genetic testing in all familial DCM or nonfamiliar with clinical clues (such as creatine kinase elevation or atrioventricular block). Of note, the ESC Position Statement recommends that genetic testing should be oriented by clinical diagnostic clues and restricted to genes known to cause DCM although considering large panels of genes only when the family structure is large enough to permit segregation analysis.

Testing Approaches Within a Family

According to standard family-based genetic testing principles, testing should begin with the available and the most severely affected family member. Emphasis should be placed on a careful physical examination and family history to rule out syndromic disease. Also, a thorough discussion and the reasonable likelihood of finding a variant of unknown significance should be born in mind. In situations where an affected family member is unavailable, investigations should be conducted to identify stored tissue suitable for DNA analysis from an affected, deceased family member. In the absence of this, expert counseling and communication of the limitations of this testing approach with a cardiovascular geneticist are advised.

Family Screening

DCM genetic evaluations should begin with a very accurate and extensive accurate assessment of the patient's family history, involving at least three generations and including the history of cardiomyopathy and history of SCD (unexpected) death at a young age (<30-40 years) [37, 101]. Information gotten from these would go a long way in providing excellent care to family members, identify at-risk relatives, guiding testing, and aid interpretation of the results.

Clinical Cardiovascular Screening of Relatives

Screening for first-degree relatives of probands is mandatory. Standards for cardiac testing includes careful medical and family history taking, a thorough and proper physical examination, ECG, and an echocardiogram. If any cardiovascular abnormalities are detected, a full cardiovascular evaluation by a cardiovascular specialist is indicated as this is particularly relevant when signs and symptoms of DCM are identified in those whose coronary disease risk is increasing. CMR imaging is also useful in questions or suspicion of overlap.

Screening Asymptomatic Relatives and Screening Intervals

It is important to understand that genetic DCM can occur in individuals who are entirely asymptomatic. Therefore, a pre-symptomatic diagnosis gives room for early intervention and may result in the prevention or delayed onset of HF or SCD [101]. Regardless of an already established mutation, genetic testing that has shown a variant of unknown significance, negative or no genetic testing, asymptomatic relatives with any evidence suggestive of DCM on cardiac screening studies should be rescreened regularly [101]. A follow-up plan/schedule is also advised. Also, for families where mutations have not been identified yet in a proband, relatives with negative clinical cardiac screening should be rescreened every 3-5 years beginning from childhood [14].

Genetic Counselling

With the growing and ever-increasing twist and current state of cardiomyopathic genetic testing, the need for genetic counselors to provide both pre and post-test counseling and communicate with specialized cardiovascular genetic specialist and clinics cannot be overemphasized (Fig. **11**).

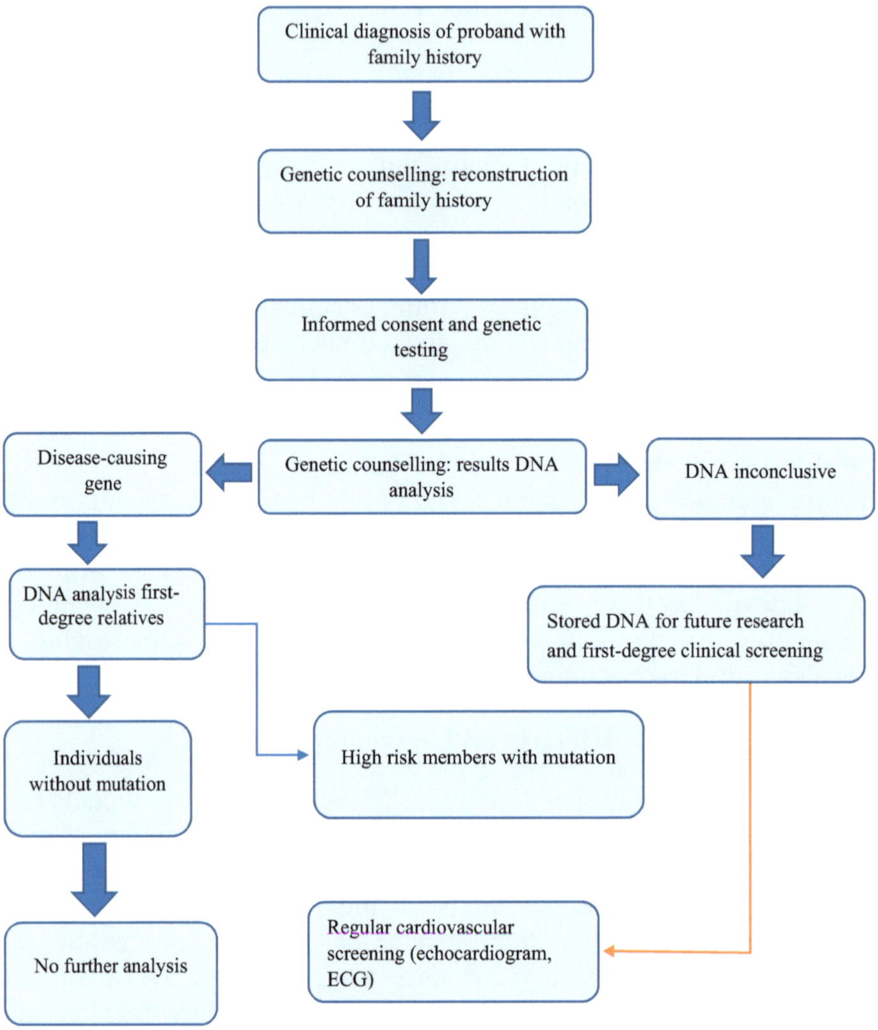

Fig. (11). Flow chart showing the clinical management and genetic counseling of heritable cardiomyopathies.

Pre-test counseling should discuss genetic results of (i) benign genetic variants, (ii) variants of uncertain significance, and (iii) benign genetic variants. The post-test counseling should, however, focus on (i) family testing (ii) interpretation/possible reinterpretation, and (iii) reproductive risks to offspring. If and once a genetic mutation is identified, genetic cascade screening (evaluates the specific family mutation rather than a gene panel) can be conducted with family members.

METHODS OF INVESTIGATION

Protocol for Probands Evaluation

I. Basic evaluation
- Family history with pedigree construction
- Physical examination, with particular attention to neuromuscular characteristics
- Ambulatory electrocardiography
- Chest X-ray (cardiothoracic ratio)
- Echocardiography: M-mode, 2D and Doppler and color flow
- Effort test: bicycle maximal or treadmill, symptom-limited, with increments of 10 Watt. min"1
- Standard laboratory examination.

II. Suggested studies
- Signal-averaged ECG
- Enzyme dosage (troponin T)
- Serum analyses of cardiac organ-specific autoantibodies
- VO2 max
- CT scan for muscular involvement
- Ventriculographic, a hemodynamic and coronary angiographic study
- Non-invasive evaluation of myocardial ischemia
- Right and left endomyocardial biopsy
- Clinical assessment by a neuromuscular specialist
- Study of viral persistence

Family Study

I. Evaluation of the proband's relatives
- Physical examination
- Blood sampling
- Standard ECG, signal-averaged ECG (optional)
- Echocardiography (M-mode and 2D; color flow optional)

II. Evaluation of the affected relatives
- Review of previous hospital records
- Non-invasive examinations and, when indicated, invasive investigations
- The pedigree extension (the study of first-degree relatives of new affected family members)
- Genetic counseling.

III. Analysis of retrospective cases
- Review of hospital records
- Interview of family physicians

  - Discussion of multiple informants among close relatives

IV. Material sampling
  - Clinical database
  - Serum bank, according to standard procedures, stored at 20°C
  - DNA: extracted from 10-40 ml of peripheral blood according to standard procedures
  - Isolated lymphocytes extracted from 10-20 ml of peripheral blood in heparin or acetate-citrate-dextrose
  - EMB, skeletal muscle biopsies (if available)

V. Family follow-up studies (should be performed every 2-3 years)
  - Physical examination
  - ECG
  - Echocardiography

CONCLUSION AND FUTURE DIRECTIONS

Although, it is always challenging to find the genetic cause of multigenic disorders, especially if it is considered that mutations in the genome are only one of the contributing factors of disease. However, a great deal of progress has been made over the years in understanding the genetic basis of DCM. Nevertheless, a deep basic and clinical understanding of the genetic basis underlying DCM would prove very useful in the diagnoses, treatment, and management of the disease hence, giving a chance to early diagnosis thereby, increasing the prognostic and therapeutic outcomes.

Future research should be directed towards understanding DCM phenome better, medical management of specific types of genetic DCM, and improving next-generation sequencing technology (NGST). In addition to sequencing technology, the efficient use and improvement in NGST would provide an accurate diagnostic and cost-effective method to yield biomarkers that indicate disease risk, especially within families. With this improvement, further re-evaluation of the molecular diagnosis over time would be required with more and more stringent criteria. It is also lingering questions in the field such as (i) the correct asymptomatic DCM pre-clinical treatment of gene carriers (ii) genetic testing interpretations, and (iii) development of gene- and mechanism-specific therapies need to be tackled as soon as possible.

LIST OF ABBREVIATIONS

ARVC Arrhythmogenic right ventricular cardiomyopathy

AF Atrial fibrillation

ARB Angiotensin II receptor blocker

AHA American Heart Association

ANP	Atrial natriuretic peptide
CMR	Cardiac magnetic resonance
CHF	Congestive heart failure
DCM	Dilated cardiomyopathy
ESC	European Society of Cardiology
EF	Ejection fraction
ECG	Electrocardiography
EMB	Endomyocardial biopsy
FDC	Familiar dilated cardiomyopathy
GWAS	Genome-wide association study
HF	Heart failure
HCM	Hypertrophic cardiomyopathy
IDC	Idiopathic dilated cardiomyopathy
IHD	Ischemic heart disease
ICD	Implantable cardioverter defibrillator
LVAD	Left ventricular assist device
LV	Left ventricle
LVEF	Left ventricular ejection fraction
MET	Metabolic exercise testing
NGST	Next-generation sequencing technology
SNPs	Single nucleotide polymorphisms
SCD	Sudden cardiac death
RAAS	Renin-angiotensin system
VT	Ventricular tachycardia

CONSENT FOR PUBLICATION

Not applicable.

CONFLICT OF INTEREST

The authors confirm that this chapter contents have no conflict of interest.

ACKNOWLEDGEMENTS

Declared none.

REFERENCES

[1] Ashrafian H, Docherty L, Leo V, *et al.* A mutation in the mitochondrial fission gene Dnml1 leads to cardiomyopathy. PLoS Genet 2010; 6(6): e1001000.
[http://dx.doi.org/10.1371/journal.pgen.1001000] [PMID: 20585624]

[2] Durand J-B, Bachinski LL, Bieling LC, *et al.* Localization of a gene responsible for familial dilated cardiomyopathy to chromosome 1q32. Circulation 1995; 92(12): 3387-9.
[http://dx.doi.org/10.1161/01.CIR.92.12.3387] [PMID: 8521556]

[3] Krajinovic M, Pinamonti B, Sinagra G, *et al.* Linkage of familial dilated cardiomyopathy to chromosome 9. Am J Hum Genet 1995; 57(4): 846-52.
[PMID: 7573045]

[4] Bowles KR, Gajarski R, Porter P, *et al.* Gene mapping of familial autosomal dominant dilated cardiomyopathy to chromosome 10q21-23. J Clin Invest 1996; 98(6): 1355-60.
[http://dx.doi.org/10.1172/JCI118922] [PMID: 8823300]

[5] Olson TM, Keating MT. Mapping a cardiomyopathy locus to chromosome 3p22-p25. J Clin Invest 1996; 97(2): 528-32.
[http://dx.doi.org/10.1172/JCI118445] [PMID: 8567977]

[6] Kass S, MacRae C, Graber HL, *et al.* A gene defect that causes conduction system disease and dilated cardiomyopathy maps to chromosome 1p1-1q1. Nat Genet 1994; 7(4): 546-51.
[http://dx.doi.org/10.1038/ng0894-546] [PMID: 7951328]

[7] Messina DN, Speer MC, Pericak-Vance MA, McNally EM. Linkage of familial dilated cardiomyopathy with conduction defect and muscular dystrophy to chromosome 6q23. Am J Hum Genet 1997; 61(4): 909-17.
[http://dx.doi.org/10.1086/514896] [PMID: 9382102]

[8] Milasin J, Muntoni F, Severini GM, *et al.* A point mutation in the 5′ splice site of the dystrophin gene first intron responsible for X-linked dilated cardiomyopathy. Hum Mol Genet 1996; 5(1): 73-9.
[http://dx.doi.org/10.1093/hmg/5.1.73] [PMID: 8789442]

[9] Ortiz-Lopez R, Li H, Su J, Goytia V, Towbin JA. Evidence for a dystrophin missense mutation as a cause of X-linked dilated cardiomyopathy. Circulation 1997; 95(10): 2434-40.
[http://dx.doi.org/10.1161/01.CIR.95.10.2434] [PMID: 9170407]

[10] Muntoni F, Di Lenarda A, Porcu M, *et al.* Dystrophin gene abnormalities in two patients with idiopathic dilated cardiomyopathy. Heart 1997; 78(6): 608-12.
[http://dx.doi.org/10.1136/hrt.78.6.608] [PMID: 9470882]

[11] International Society of Heart and Lung Transplantation Quarterly Report 2015.

[12] McNally EM, Golbus JR, Puckelwartz MJ. Genetic mutations and mechanisms in dilated cardiomyopathy. J Clin Invest 2013; 123(1): 19-26.
[http://dx.doi.org/10.1172/JCI62862] [PMID: 23281406]

[13] Ziaeian B, Fonarow GC. Epidemiology and aetiology of heart failure. Nat Rev Cardiol 2016; 13(6): 368-78.
[http://dx.doi.org/10.1038/nrcardio.2016.25] [PMID: 26935038]

[14] Meder B, Ruhle F, Weis T, *et al.* A genome-wide association study identifies 6p21 as novel risk locus for dilated cardiomyopathy. Eur Heart J 2013; 35(16): 1069-77.

[15] Meder B, Haas J, Keller A, *et al.* Targeted next-generation sequencing for the molecular genetic diagnostics of cardiomyopathies. Circ Cardiovasc Genet 2011; 4(2): 110-22.
[http://dx.doi.org/10.1161/CIRCGENETICS.110.958322] [PMID: 21252143]

[16] Lakdawala NK, Funke BH, Baxter S, *et al.* Genetic testing for dilated cardiomyopathy in clinical practice. J Card Fail 2012; 18(4): 296-303.
[http://dx.doi.org/10.1016/j.cardfail.2012.01.013] [PMID: 22464770]

[17] Teekakirikul P, Kelly MA, Rehm HL, Lakdawala NK, Funke BH. Inherited cardiomyopathies: molecular genetics and clinical genetic testing in the postgenomic era. J Mol Diagn 2013; 15(2): 158-70.
[http://dx.doi.org/10.1016/j.jmoldx.2012.09.002] [PMID: 23274168]

[18] MacRae CA. Action and the actionability in exome variation. Circ Cardiovasc Genet 2012; 5(6): 597-8.
[http://dx.doi.org/10.1161/CIRCGENETICS.112.965152] [PMID: 23250897]

[19] Sturm AC, Hershberger RE. Genetic testing in cardiovascular medicine: current landscape and future horizons. Curr Opin Cardiol 2013; 28(3): 317-25.
[http://dx.doi.org/10.1097/HCO.0b013e32835fb728] [PMID: 23571470]

[20] Hershberger RE, Morales A, Siegfried JD. Clinical and genetic issues in dilated cardiomyopathy: a review for genetics professionals. Genet Med 2010; 12(11): 655-67.
[http://dx.doi.org/10.1097/GIM.0b013e3181f2481f] [PMID: 20864896]

[21] Fatkin D, Otway R, Richmond Z. Genetics of dilated cardiomyopathy. Heart Fail Clin 2010; 6(2): 129-40.
[http://dx.doi.org/10.1016/j.hfc.2009.11.003] [PMID: 20347783]

[22] Jefferies JL, Towbin JA. Dilated cardiomyopathy. Lancet 2010; 375(9716): 752-62.
[http://dx.doi.org/10.1016/S0140-6736(09)62023-7] [PMID: 20189027]

[23] Dellefave L, McNally EM. The genetics of dilated cardiomyopathy. Curr Opin Cardiol 2010; 25(3): 198-204.
[http://dx.doi.org/10.1097/HCO.0b013e328337ba52] [PMID: 20186049]

[24] Jacoby D, McKenna WJ. Genetics of inherited cardiomyopathy. Eur Heart J 2012; 33(3): 296-304.
[http://dx.doi.org/10.1093/eurheartj/ehr260] [PMID: 21810862]

[25] Piran S, Liu P, Morales A, Hershberger RE. Where genome meets phenome: rationale for integrating genetic and protein biomarkers in the diagnosis and management of dilated cardiomyopathy and heart failure. J Am Coll Cardiol 2012; 60(4): 283-9.
[http://dx.doi.org/10.1016/j.jacc.2012.05.005] [PMID: 22813604]

[26] Posafalvi A, Herkert JC, Sinke RJ, *et al.* Clinical utility gene card for: dilated cardiomyopathy (CMD). Eur J Hum Genet 2013; 21: 10.
[http://dx.doi.org/10.1038/ejhg.2012.276] [PMID: 23249954]

[27] Houle D, Govindaraju DR, Omholt S. Phenomics: the next challenge. Nat Rev Genet 2010; 11(12): 855-66.
[http://dx.doi.org/10.1038/nrg2897] [PMID: 21085204]

[28] Evans JP, Berg JS. Next-generation DNA sequencing, regulation, and the limits of paternalism: the next challenge. JAMA 2011; 306(21): 2376-7.
[http://dx.doi.org/10.1001/jama.2011.1788] [PMID: 22147382]

[29] Bagnall RD, Ingles J, Semsarian C. Molecular diagnostics of cardiomyopathies: the future is here. Circ Cardiovasc Genet 2011; 4(2): 103-4.
[http://dx.doi.org/10.1161/CIRCGENETICS.110.959247] [PMID: 21505198]

[30] Burkett EL, Hershberger RE. Clinical and genetic issues in familial dilated cardiomyopathy. J Am Coll Cardiol 2005; 45(7): 969-81.
[http://dx.doi.org/10.1016/j.jacc.2004.11.066] [PMID: 15808750]

[31] Mestroni L, Maisch B, McKenna WJ, *et al.* Guidelines for the study of familial dilated cardiomyopathies. Eur Heart J 1999; 20(2): 93-102.
[http://dx.doi.org/10.1053/euhj.1998.1145] [PMID: 10099905]

[32] Yancy CW. ACCF/AHA guideline for the management of heart failure: a report of the American College of Cardiology Foundation/American Heart Association Task Force on Practice Guidelines.

Circulation 2013.

[33] Elliott P, Andersson B, Arbustini E, *et al.* Classification of the cardiomyopathies: a position statement from the European Society Of Cardiology Working Group on Myocardial and Pericardial Diseases. Eur Heart J 2008; 29(2): 270-6. [http://dx.doi.org/10.1093/eurheartj/ehm342] [PMID: 17916581]

[34] Maron BJ, Towbin JA, Thiene G, *et al.* Contemporary definitions and classification of the cardiomyopathies: an American Heart Association Scientific Statement from the Council on Clinical Cardiology, Heart Failure and Transplantation Committee; Quality of Care and Outcomes Research and Functional Genomics and Translational Biology Interdisciplinary Working Groups; and Council on Epidemiology and Prevention. Circulation 2006; 113(14): 1807-16. [http://dx.doi.org/10.1161/CIRCULATIONAHA.106.174287] [PMID: 16567565]

[35] Miura K, Nakagawa H, Morikawa Y, *et al.* Epidemiology of idiopathic cardiomyopathy in Japan: results from a nationwide survey. Heart 2002; 87(2): 126-30. [http://dx.doi.org/10.1136/heart.87.2.126] [PMID: 11796547]

[36] Amoah AG, Kallen C. Aetiology of heart failure as seen from a National Cardiac Referral Centre in Africa 2000. [http://dx.doi.org/10.1159/000006996]

[37] Bozkurt B, Colvin M, Cook J, *et al.* Current diagnostic and treatment strategies for specific dilated cardiomyopathies: a scientific statement from the american heart association. Circulation 2016; 134(23): e579-646. [http://dx.doi.org/10.1161/CIR.0000000000000455] [PMID: 27832612]

[38] Sweet M, Taylor MR, Mestroni L. Diagnosis, prevalence, and screening of familial dilated cardiomyopathy. Expert Opin Orphan Drugs 2015; 3(8): 869-76. [http://dx.doi.org/10.1517/21678707.2015.1057498] [PMID: 27547593]

[39] Petretta M, Pirozzi F, Sasso L, Paglia A, Bonaduce D. Review and metaanalysis of the frequency of familial dilated cardiomyopathy. Am J Cardiol 2011; 108(8): 1171-6. [http://dx.doi.org/10.1016/j.amjcard.2011.06.022] [PMID: 21798502]

[40] Ganesh SK, Arnett DK, Assimes TL, *et al.* Genetics and genomics for the prevention and treatment of cardiovascular disease: update: a scientific statement from the American Heart Association. Circulation 2013; 128(25): 2813-51. [http://dx.doi.org/10.1161/01.cir.0000437913.98912.1d] [PMID: 24297835]

[41] Williams DG, Olsen EG. Prevalence of overt dilated cardiomyopathy in two regions of England. Br Heart J 1985; 54(2): 153-5. [http://dx.doi.org/10.1136/hrt.54.2.153] [PMID: 4015924]

[42] Rakar S, Sinagra G, Di Lenarda A, *et al.* Epidemiology of dilated cardiomyopathy. A prospective post-mortem study of 5252 necropsies. Eur Heart J 1997; 18(1): 117-23. [http://dx.doi.org/10.1093/oxfordjournals.eurheartj.a015092] [PMID: 9049523]

[43] Hershberger RE, Hedges DJ, Morales A. Dilated cardiomyopathy: the complexity of a diverse genetic architecture. Nat Rev Cardiol 2013; 10(9): 531-47. [http://dx.doi.org/10.1038/nrcardio.2013.105] [PMID: 23900355]

[44] Robin NH, Tabereaux PB, Benza R, Korf BR. Genetic testing in cardiovascular disease. J Am Coll Cardiol 2007; 50(8): 727-37. [http://dx.doi.org/10.1016/j.jacc.2007.05.015] [PMID: 17707176]

[45] Norton N, Robertson PD, Rieder MJ, *et al.* Evaluating pathogenicity of rare variants from dilated cardiomyopathy in the exome era. Circ Cardiovasc Genet 2012; 5(2): 167-74. [http://dx.doi.org/10.1161/CIRCGENETICS.111.961805] [PMID: 22337857]

[46] Herman DS, Lam L, Taylor MR, *et al.* Truncations of titin causing dilated cardiomyopathy. N Engl J Med 2012; 366(7): 619-28.

[http://dx.doi.org/10.1056/NEJMoa1110186] [PMID: 22335739]

[47] LeWinter MM, Granzier HL. Cardiac titin and heart disease. J Cardiovasc Pharmacol 2014; 63(3): 207-12.
[http://dx.doi.org/10.1097/FJC.0000000000000007] [PMID: 24072177]

[48] Anderson BR, Granzier HL. Titin-based tension in the cardiac sarcomere: molecular origin and physiological adaptations. Prog Biophys Mol Biol 2012; 110(2-3): 204-17.
[http://dx.doi.org/10.1016/j.pbiomolbio.2012.08.003] [PMID: 22910434]

[49] Nagueh SF, Shah G, Wu Y, *et al.* Altered titin expression, myocardial stiffness, and left ventricular function in patients with dilated cardiomyopathy. Circulation 2004; 110: 155-60.
[http://dx.doi.org/10.1161/01.CIR.0000135591.37759.AF]

[50] Roberts AM, Ware JS, Herman DS, *et al.* Integrated allelic, transcriptional, and phenomic dissection of the cardiac effects of titin truncations in health and disease. Sci Transl Med 2015; 7(270): 270ra6.
[http://dx.doi.org/10.1126/scitranslmed.3010134] [PMID: 25589632]

[51] van Tintelen JP, Hofstra RM, Katerberg H, *et al.* High yield of LMNA mutations in patients with dilated cardiomyopathy and/or conduction disease referred to cardiogenetics outpatient clinics. Am Heart J 2007; 154(6): 1130-9.
[http://dx.doi.org/10.1016/j.ahj.2007.07.038] [PMID: 18035086]

[52] Parks SB, Kushner JD, Nauman D, *et al.* Lamin A/C mutation analysis in a cohort of 324 unrelated patients with idiopathic or familial dilated cardiomyopathy. Am Heart J 2008; 156(1): 161-9.
[http://dx.doi.org/10.1016/j.ahj.2008.01.026] [PMID: 18585512]

[53] Young SG, Meta M, Yang SH, Fong LG. Prelamin A farnesylation and progeroid syndromes. J Biol Chem 2006; 281(52): 39741-5.
[http://dx.doi.org/10.1074/jbc.R600033200] [PMID: 17090536]

[54] Lu JT, Muchir A, Nagy PL, Worman HJ. LMNA cardiomyopathy: cell biology and genetics meet clinical medicine. Dis Model Mech 2011; 4(5): 562-8.
[http://dx.doi.org/10.1242/dmm.006346] [PMID: 21810905]

[55] Nikolova V, Leimena C, McMahon AC, *et al.* Defects in nuclear structure and function promote dilated cardiomyopathy in lamin A/C-deficient mice. J Clin Invest 2004; 113(3): 357-69.
[http://dx.doi.org/10.1172/JCI200419448] [PMID: 14755333]

[56] Lammerding J, Schulze PC, Takahashi T, *et al.* Lamin A/C deficiency causes defective nuclear mechanics and mechanotransduction. J Clin Invest 2004; 113(3): 370-8.
[http://dx.doi.org/10.1172/JCI200419670] [PMID: 14755334]

[57] van der Zwaag PA, van Rijsingen IA, Asimaki A, *et al.* Phospholamban R14del mutation in patients diagnosed with dilated cardiomyopathy or arrhythmogenic right ventricular cardiomyopathy: evidence supporting the concept of arrhythmogenic cardiomyopathy. Eur J Heart Fail 2012; 14(11): 1199-207.
[http://dx.doi.org/10.1093/eurjhf/hfs119] [PMID: 22820313]

[58] DeWitt MM, MacLeod HM, Soliven B, McNally EM. Phospholamban R14 deletion results in late-onset, mild, hereditary dilated cardiomyopathy. J Am Coll Cardiol 2006; 48: 1396-8.

[59] Truszkowska GT, Bilińska ZT, Kosińska J, *et al.* A study in Polish patients with cardiomyopathy emphasizes pathogenicity of phospholamban (PLN) mutations at amino acid position 9 and low penetrance of heterozygous null PLN mutations. BMC Med Genet 2015; 16: 21.
[http://dx.doi.org/10.1186/s12881-015-0167-0] [PMID: 25928149]

[60] Haghighi K, Kolokathis F, Gramolini AO, *et al.* A mutation in the human phospholamban gene, deleting arginine 14, results in lethal, hereditary cardiomyopathy. Proc Natl Acad Sci USA 2006; 103(5): 1388-93.
[http://dx.doi.org/10.1073/pnas.0510519103] [PMID: 16432188]

[61] Liu GS, Morales A, Vafiadaki E, *et al.* A novel human R25C-phospholamban mutation is associated with super-inhibition of calcium cycling and ventricular arrhythmia. Cardiovasc Res 2015; 107(1):

164-74.
[http://dx.doi.org/10.1093/cvr/cvv127] [PMID: 25852082]

[62] Brauch KM, Karst ML, Herron KJ, *et al.* Mutations in ribonucleic acid binding protein gene cause familial dilated cardiomyopathy. J Am Coll Cardiol 2009; 54(10): 930-41.
[http://dx.doi.org/10.1016/j.jacc.2009.05.038] [PMID: 19712804]

[63] Li D, Morales A, Gonzalez-Quintana J, *et al.* Identification of novel mutations in RBM20 in patients with dilated cardiomyopathy. Clin Transl Sci 2010; 3(3): 90-7.
[http://dx.doi.org/10.1111/j.1752-8062.2010.00198.x] [PMID: 20590677]

[64] Beqqali A, Bollen IA, Rasmussen TB, *et al.* A mutation in the glutamate-rich region of RNA-binding motif protein 20 causes dilated cardiomyopathy through missplicing of titin and impaired Frank-Starling mechanism. Cardiovasc Res 2016; 112(1): 452-63.
[http://dx.doi.org/10.1093/cvr/cvw192] [PMID: 27496873]

[65] Guo W, Schafer S, Greaser ML, *et al.* RBM20, a gene for hereditary cardiomyopathy, regulates titin splicing. Nat Med 2012; 18(5): 766-73.
[http://dx.doi.org/10.1038/nm.2693] [PMID: 22466703]

[66] Li S, Guo W, Dewey CN, Greaser ML. Rbm20 regulates titin alternative splicing as a splicing repressor. Nucleic Acids Res 2013; 41(4): 2659-72.
[http://dx.doi.org/10.1093/nar/gks1362] [PMID: 23307558]

[67] Maatz H, Jens M, Liss M, *et al.* RNA-binding protein RBM20 represses splicing to orchestrate cardiac pre-mRNA processing. J Clin Invest 2014; 124(8): 3419-30.
[http://dx.doi.org/10.1172/JCI74523] [PMID: 24960161]

[68] McNair WP, Sinagra G, Taylor MR, *et al.* Familial Cardiomyopathy Registry Research Group. SCN5A mutations associate with arrhythmic dilated cardiomyopathy and commonly localize to the voltage-sensing mechanism. J Am Coll Cardiol 2011; 57: 2160-8.

[69] Mann SA, Castro ML, Ohanian M, *et al.* R222Q SCN5A mutation is associated with reversible ventricular ectopy and dilated cardiomyopathy. J Am Coll Cardiol 2012; 60(16): 1566-73.
[http://dx.doi.org/10.1016/j.jacc.2012.05.050] [PMID: 22999724]

[70] Walsh R, Thomson KL, Ware JS, *et al.* Reassessment of Mendelian gene pathogenicity using 7,855 cardiomyopathy cases and 60,706 reference samples. Genet Med 2017; 19(2): 192-203.
[http://dx.doi.org/10.1038/gim.2016.90] [PMID: 27532257]

[71] Feng J, Yan J, Buzin CH, Towbin JA, Sommer SS. Mutations in the dystrophin gene are associated with sporadic dilated cardiomyopathy. Mol Genet Metab 2002; 77(1-2): 119-26.
[http://dx.doi.org/10.1016/S1096-7192(02)00153-1] [PMID: 12359139]

[72] McNally EM. New approaches in the therapy of cardiomyopathy in muscular dystrophy. Annu Rev Med 2007; 58: 75-88.
[http://dx.doi.org/10.1146/annurev.med.58.011706.144703]

[73] Sibbing D, Pfeufer A, Perisic T, *et al.* Mutations in the mitochondrial thioredoxin reductase gene TXNRD2 cause dilated cardiomyopathy. Eur Heart J 2011; 32(9): 1121-33.
[http://dx.doi.org/10.1093/eurheartj/ehq507] [PMID: 21247928]

[74] Kamisago M, Sharma SD, DePalma SR, *et al.* Mutations in sarcomere protein genes as a cause of dilated cardiomyopathy. N Engl J Med 2000; 343(23): 1688-96.
[http://dx.doi.org/10.1056/NEJM200012073432304] [PMID: 11106718]

[75] Otten E, Lekanne Dit Deprez RH, Weiss MM, *et al.* Recurrent and founder mutations in the Netherlands: mutation p.K217del in troponin T2, causing dilated cardiomyopathy. Neth Heart J 2010; 18(10): 478-85.
[http://dx.doi.org/10.1007/BF03091819] [PMID: 20978592]

[76] Khabaeva Z. Genetic analysis in hypertrophic cardiomyopathy: missense mutations in the ventricular myosin regulatory light chain gene. Humboldt University, 2002.

[77] Tanjore R, RangaRaju A, Vadapalli S, *et al.* Genetic variations of MYH7 in hypertrophic cardiomyopathy and dilated cardiomyopathy. Indian J Hum Genet 2010; 16: 67-71. [http://dx.doi.org/10.4103/0971-6866.69348] [PMID: 21031054]

[78] Hershberger RE, Parks SB, Kushner JD, *et al.* Coding sequence mutations identified in MYH7, TNNT2, SCN5A, CSRP3, LBD3, and TCAP from 313 patients with familial or idiopathic dilated cardiomyopathy. Clin Transl Sci 2008; 1(1): 21-6. [http://dx.doi.org/10.1111/j.1752-8062.2008.00017.x] [PMID: 19412328]

[79] Kärkkäinen S, Heliö T, Jääskeläinen P, *et al.* Two novel mutations in the beta-myosin heavy chain gene associated with dilated cardiomyopathy. Eur J Heart Fail 2004; 6(7): 861-8. [http://dx.doi.org/10.1016/j.ejheart.2004.04.017] [PMID: 15556047]

[80] Villard E, Duboscq-Bidot L, Charron P, *et al.* Mutation screening in dilated cardiomyopathy: prominent role of the beta myosin heavy chain gene. Eur Heart J 2005; 26(8): 794-803. [http://dx.doi.org/10.1093/eurheartj/ehi193] [PMID: 15769782]

[81] Norton N, Li D, Rieder MJ, *et al.* Genome-wide studies of copy number variation and exome sequencing identify rare variants in BAG3 as a cause of dilated cardiomyopathy. Am J Hum Genet 2011; 88(3): 273-82. [http://dx.doi.org/10.1016/j.ajhg.2011.01.016] [PMID: 21353195]

[82] Li D, Parks SB, Kushner JD, *et al.* Mutations of presenilin genes in dilated cardiomyopathy and heart failure. Am J Hum Genet 2006; 79(6): 1030-9. [http://dx.doi.org/10.1086/509900] [PMID: 17186461]

[83] Dorn GW II. Genetics of common forms of heart failure. Curr Opin Cardiol 2011; 26(3): 204-8. [http://dx.doi.org/10.1097/HCO.0b013e328345d336] [PMID: 21464711]

[84] Gibson G. Rare and common variants: twenty arguments. Nat Rev Genet 2012; 13(2): 135-45. [http://dx.doi.org/10.1038/nrg3118] [PMID: 22251874]

[85] Whiffin N, Minikel E, Walsh R, *et al.* Using high-resolution variant frequencies to empower clinical genome interpretation. Genet Med 2017; 19(10): 1151-8. [http://dx.doi.org/10.1038/gim.2017.26]

[86] Velagaleti RS, O'Donnell CJ. Genomics of heart failure. Heart Fail Clin 2010; 6(1): 115-24. [http://dx.doi.org/10.1016/j.hfc.2009.08.002]

[87] MacRae CA. The genetics of congestive heart failure. Heart Fail Clin 2010; 6(2): 223-30. [http://dx.doi.org/10.1016/j.hfc.2009.11.004] [PMID: 20347790]

[88] Ruiter JS, Berkenbosch-Nieuwhof K, van den Berg MP, van Dijk R, Middel B, van Tintelen JP. The importance of the family history in caring for families with long QT syndrome and dilated cardiomyopathy. Am J Med Genet A 2010; 152A(3): 607-12. [http://dx.doi.org/10.1002/ajmg.a.33270] [PMID: 20186837]

[89] Brodt C, Siegfried JD, Hofmeyer M, *et al.* Temporal relationship of conduction system disease and ventricular dysfunction in LMNA cardiomyopathy. J Card Fail 2013; 19(4): 233-9. [http://dx.doi.org/10.1016/j.cardfail.2013.03.001] [PMID: 23582089]

[90] Fatkin D. Guidelines for the diagnosis and management of familial dilated cardiomyopathy. Heart Lung Circ 2011; 20(11): 691-3. [http://dx.doi.org/10.1016/j.hlc.2011.07.008] [PMID: 21885340]

[91] Assomull RG, Prasad SK, Lyne J, *et al.* Cardiovascular magnetic resonance, fibrosis, and prognosis in dilated cardiomyopathy. J Am Coll Cardiol 2006; 48(10): 1977-85. [http://dx.doi.org/10.1016/j.jacc.2006.07.049] [PMID: 17112987]

[92] Gil KE, Pawlak A, Gil RJ, Frontczak-Baniewicz M, Bil J. The role of invasive diagnostics and its impact on the treatment of dilated cardiomyopathy: a systematic review 2016. [http://dx.doi.org/10.1016/j.advms.2016.07.001]

[93] Caforio AL, Pankuweit S, Arbustini E, *et al.* Current state of knowledge on aetiology, diagnosis, management, and therapy of myocarditis: a position statement of the European Society of Cardiology Working Group on Myocardial and Pericardial Diseases 2013. [http://dx.doi.org/10.1093/eurheartj/eht210]

[94] Cooper LT, Baughman KL, Feldman AM, *et al.* The role of endomyocardial biopsy in the management of cardiovascular disease: a scientific statement from the American Heart Association, the American College of Cardiology, and the European Society of Cardiology. Circulation 2007; 116(19): 2216-33. [http://dx.doi.org/10.1161/CIRCULATIONAHA.107.186093] [PMID: 17959655]

[95] Cooper LT, Baughman KL, Feldman AM, *et al.* The role of endomyocardial biopsy in the management of cardiovascular disease: a scientific statement from the American Heart Association, the American College of Cardiology, and the European Society of Cardiology Endorsed by the Heart Failure Society of America and the Heart Failure Association of the European Society of Cardiology. Eur Heart J 2007; 28(24): 3076-93. [http://dx.doi.org/10.1093/eurheartj/ehm456] [PMID: 17959624]

[96] Felker GM, Thompson RE, Hare JM, *et al.* Underlying causes and long-term survival in patients with initially unexplained cardiomyopathy. N Engl J Med 2000; 342(15): 1077-84. [http://dx.doi.org/10.1056/NEJM200004133421502] [PMID: 10760308]

[97] Spezzacatene A, Sinagra G, Merlo M, *et al.* Familial Cardiomyopathy Registry. Arrhythmogenic phenotype in dilated cardiomyopathy: natural history and predictors of life-threatening arrhythmias. J Am Heart Assoc 2015; 4(10)e002149 [http://dx.doi.org/10.1161/JAHA.115.002149] [PMID: 26475296]

[98] The treatment of heart failure. Task Force of the Working Group on Heart Failure of the European Society of Cardiology. Eur Heart J 1997; 18(5): 736-53. [http://dx.doi.org/10.1093/oxfordjournals.eurheartj.a015339] [PMID: 9152644]

[99] McCarthy JF, McCarthy PM, Starling RC, *et al.* Partial left ventriculectomy and mitral valve repair for end-stage congestive heart failure. Eur J Cardiothorac Surg 1998; 13(4): 337-43. [http://dx.doi.org/10.1016/S1010-7940(98)00013-X] [PMID: 9641329]

[100] Saberi S, Day SM. Exercise prescription for the athlete with cardiomyopathy. Cardiol Clin 2016; 34(4): 591-601. [http://dx.doi.org/10.1016/j.ccl.2016.06.008] [PMID: 27692227]

[101] Hershberger RE, Lindenfeld J, Mestroni L, Seidman CE, Taylor MR, Towbin JA. Genetic evaluation of cardiomyopathy-a Heart Failure Society of America practice guideline. J Card Fail 2009; 15(2): 83-97. [http://dx.doi.org/10.1016/j.cardfail.2009.01.006] [PMID: 19254666]

[102] Yancy CW, Jessup M, Bozkurt B, *et al.* 2013 ACCF/AHA guideline for the management of heart failure: a report of the American College of Cardiology Foundation/American Heart Association Task Force on Practice Guidelines. J Am Coll Cardiol 2013; 62(16): e147-239. [http://dx.doi.org/10.1016/j.jacc.2013.05.019] [PMID: 23747642]

[103] Pinto YM, Elliott PM, Arbustini E, *et al.* Proposal for a revised definition of dilated cardiomyopathy, hypokinetic non-dilated cardiomyopathy, and its implications for clinical practice: a position statement of the ESC working group on myocardial and pericardial diseases. Eur Heart J 2016; 37(23): 1850-8. [http://dx.doi.org/10.1093/eurheartj/ehv727] [PMID: 26792875]

CHAPTER 4

Current Perspectives in Hypertrophic Cardiomyopathy: Novel Therapeutic Medical Approaches, Misconceptions, and The Present Prevalent Issues

Iroegbu Chukwuemeka Daniel[1], **Chengming Fan**[1], **Shiyuan Tang**[1], **Xin Chen**[2] and **Jinfu Yang**[1,*]

[1] *Department of Cardiovascular Surgery, The Second Xiangya Hospital, Central South University, Middle Renmin Road 139, 410011 Changsha, China*

[2] *Department of Cardiovascular Surgery, The First Affiliated Hospital of Nanjing Medical University, Jiangsu, PR, China*

Abstract: One of Cardiology's "great masqueraders" and the most common heritable cardiovascular disease with a heterogeneous clinical presentation, hypertrophic cardiomyopathy (HCM) has been investigated extensively over the past two decades affecting approximately 1 in 500 individuals. HCM is one of the primary causes of sudden death in young people and a significant cause of heart failure at any age. Once considered deadly, untreatable, and relentless as delays and mistakes in diagnosis abound, it has become a highly treatable disease, though contemporary with the help of genomic medicine. The continuous research and discovery of new HCM susceptibility genes, recent advances in the diagnosis and treatment of HCM, a growing amount of data from genotype-phenotype correlation studies, and the introduction of commercially available genetic tests for HCM have been crucial in decreasing the frequency of adverse clinical events. However, complete elimination of sudden cardiac death remains an elusive gain. Therefore, it is essential that a modern-day basic or clinical physician, cardiologist, cardiac surgeons, and cardiovascular geneticist understand the diagnostic, prognostic, and therapeutic implications of HCM. This chapter aims to evaluate the new development and the novel achievements made compared to previous eras of the disease across published European registries. It also analyses the prevalent issues and misconceptions regarding HCM that persist among practicing physicians today. The chapter further focuses on the risk assessment, the various diagnosis and treatment therapies in children, adolescent, adults, and athletes in contrast to the current European set guidelines for the diagnosis and management of HCM patients.

* **Corresponding author Jinfu Yang:** Department of Cardiovascular Surgery, The Second Xiangya Hospital, Central South University, Middle Renmin Road 139, 410011 Changsha, China;
E-mails: yjf19682005@csu.edu.cn, dr.iroegbu_daniel@yahoo.com, dr.iroegbu_daniel@csu.edu.cn

Jinfu Yang & Iroegbu Chukwuemeka Daniel (Eds.)

Keywords: Atrial fibrillation, Athletes, Alcohol septal ablation, Cardiomyopathy, Cardiovascular pathology, Complications, Cardiac transplant, Children, Dual chamber pacing, Echocardiography, Genomics, Guidelines for eligibility and disqualification, Hypertrophic cardiomyopathy, Heart failure, Implantable cardioverter defibrillator, Inappropriate shock, Mortality, Reverse remodeling, Risk stratifications, Sudden cardiac death, Septal reduction therapy, Ventricular Arrhythmias.

INTRODUCTION

Initial contemporary morphological description of hypertrophic cardiomyopathy (HCM) was reported first in 1958 by Teare [1]. HCM is an inherited autosomal dominant disease characterized by more or less unexplained hypertrophy of the myocardium that is not explained solely by abnormal loading conditions [2] in the absence of other possible systemic or cardiac disease that itself would be capable of producing the magnitude of hypertrophy [3]. HCM was regarded as "asymmetrical hypertrophy of the heart in young adults" and since then, it has been referred to by an array of names namely; hypertrophic obstructive cardiomyopathy [4], idiopathic hypertrophic subaortic stenosis [5], and muscular subaortic stenosis [6] which portrays its relatively rare clinical occurrence in our daily cardiologic practice. A comprehensive clinical description of HCM was made by the Braunwald group at the National Institutes of Health fifty-five years ago [7], and since then, the spectrum of HCM has measurably evolved over the years and markedly different from the diseases of previous eras. Presently as a common monogenic cardiovascular disorder in clinical practice, the natural history, and its different presentation are frequently misunderstood and also often underrecognized and diagnosed [8 - 10]. HCM is the most common cardiomyopathy [11, 12] a disease marked by genotypic and phenotypic heterogeneity with a prevalence rate of 1 in every 500 individuals in the general population [12]. HCM can manifest from a negligible to extreme hypertrophy, absent to severe left ventricular outflow tract obstruction (LVOT), minimal to extensive fibrosis and myocyte disarray on microscopy and distinct septal morphologies such as sigmoidal, apical, and reverse curve HCM. Its clinical course varies as well, ranging from an asymptomatic lifelong course to dyspnea and angina refractory to pharmacotherapy to sudden death. HCM is the most common medical cause of sudden death in young athletes [13] and older children [14]. The differential diagnosis includes infiltrative storage disorders or metabolic diseases [14], causing physiologic remodeling associated with athletic training and hypertensive heart disease [15, 16]. It is also difficult to differentiate nonobstructive HCM from hypertensive left ventricular (LV) hypertrophy in some patients [15] because the phenotypes of each condition can overlap [17, 18].

However, a subset of patients with HCM has hypertrophic obstructive cardiomyopathy (HOCM). Malposition of the anterior papillary muscle, hyperdynamic LV contraction (drag forces through a Venturi effect) with an enlarged posterior mitral leaflet and systolic septal bulging into the LVOT provoke systolic anterior motion of the anterior leaflet of the mitral valve contributing to the creation of the LVOT gradient. LVOT obstruction is generally variable to a degree with only a few patients presenting with any significant sign of LVOT gradient at rest. Obstructions seen are only latent or provokable by stimuli such as drugs (amyl nitrate), Valsalva maneuvers, and other exercises [19]. Before the introduction of ICDs, the most common causes of death in the HCM population were heart failure, sudden cardiac death (SCD), and stroke. Identification of patients with HCM at high risk of SCD has been made possible due to the better risk stratification models borne out of multi-center registries which provide more accurate identification of patients who are suitable for an implantable cardioverter defibrillator (ICD) as a form of primary prevention of SCD [20, 21]. Rhythm disturbances in a patient with HCM are virtually common but unpredictable [22]. Ventricular fibrillation or ventricular tachycardia may cause SCD without prompt resuscitation, whereas, atrial fibrillation contributes to worsening heart failure or thromboembolism. Therefore, ICD's effectively terminates ventricular fibrillation or ventricular tachycardia and also used to treat HCM patients who are at increased risk for these potentially life-threatening arrhythmias [22, 23 - 27]. Patients who are unresponsive to medical therapy and have developed refractory heart failure and fatal arrhythmia, heart transplantation is a treatment option apart from the known myectomy (septal reduction therapy) and alcohol septal ablation (ASA) [28, 29].

This chapter aims to evaluate the new development and the novel achievements made compared to previous eras of the disease across published European registries. It also analyses the prevalent issues and misconceptions regarding HCM that persist among practicing physicians today. The chapter further focuses on the risk assessment, the various diagnosis and treatment therapies in children, adolescent, adults, and athletes in contrast to the current European set guidelines for the diagnosis and management of HCM patients.

NATURAL HISTORY, EPIDEMIOLOGIC FEATURES, CLINICAL COURSE, AND GLOBAL BURDEN

Since the initial description of a hypertrophied heart and the various clinical descriptions used [1, 2], HOCM is frequently used mostly to stress the fact that the patient is symptomatic due to obstructions after clinical investigations. The recently published European guidelines recommend the usage of HCM and avoiding former nomenclature even though the guidelines provide recommendations for establishing the degree of obstruction using pharmacological and physiological provocations of obstructiveness. Echocardiography-based epidemiologic studies in the USA have shown a disease prevalence of 1:500 persons in the general population who have been confirmed in other geographical parts of the world with highly available resources of diagnostic tools (Fig. **1**) [30]. However, patients with mutations associated with HCM (genotype) without hypertrophy [phenotype], the prevalence is 1:350 [31], making HCM the most prevalent inherited myocardial disease. The clinical spectrum of HCM is however diverse, ranging from an utterly asymptomatic state to symptoms related to progressive heart failure, diastolic dysfunction, outflow tract obstruction, various tachyarrhythmias, and sudden cardiac death [32]. HCM has been identified in over a hundred countries (representing approximately 90% of the world population), with spontaneous mutations describing the extent of the disease burden affecting nearly 20 million people globally [33].

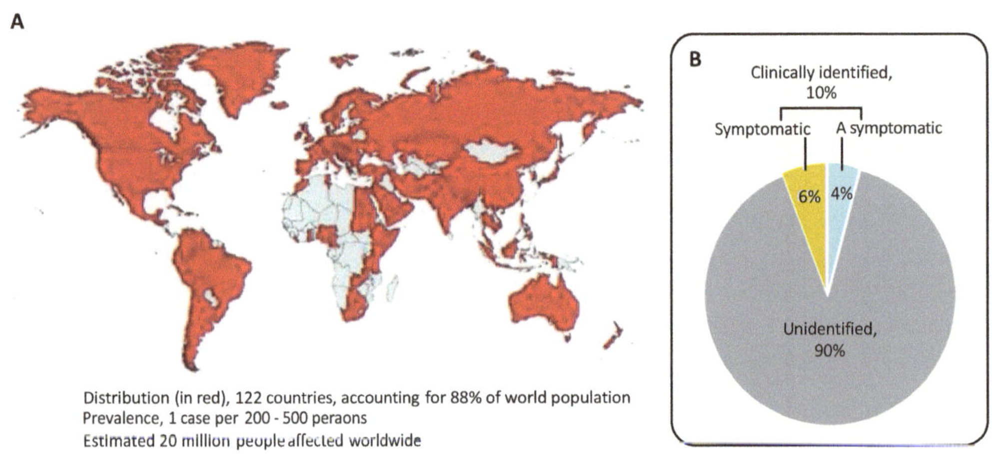

Fig. (1). Epidemiologic Features of Hypertrophic Cardiomyopathy. Panel A shows the worldwide distribution of the disease (in red). Panel B shows the proportions of clinically identified and unidentified cases.

SIGNS AND SYMPTOMS

Dyspnea is the initial predominant symptom which leads to an echocardiographic evaluation. Complaints of shortness of breath are highly pronounced at exertion due to relaxation disturbances of the left ventricle during diastole and outflow tract obstruction [34]. The obstructions produced is dynamic with regards to heart rate, filling pressure, body position and can also be affected by medications that have any effect to the cardiovascular system with patients having an adopted lifestyle to decrease physical stamina and constant tiredness. Other symptoms include chest pain (without coronary disease) [35], palpitations, tachyarrhythmias, syncope, microvascular dysfunction, and fibrosis, which shows the disease progression [36].

FAMILY HISTORY AND INHERITANCE

Due to the increased research activities and the widened new genetic panels, the cause of HCM can be explained, and its outcome partly predicted [37, 38]. The vast majority of mutations associated with HCM affects myosin proteins; myosin-binding protein (MYBPC3) and beta-myosin heavy chain (MYH7) (Fig. **2**), (Tables **1** & **2**).

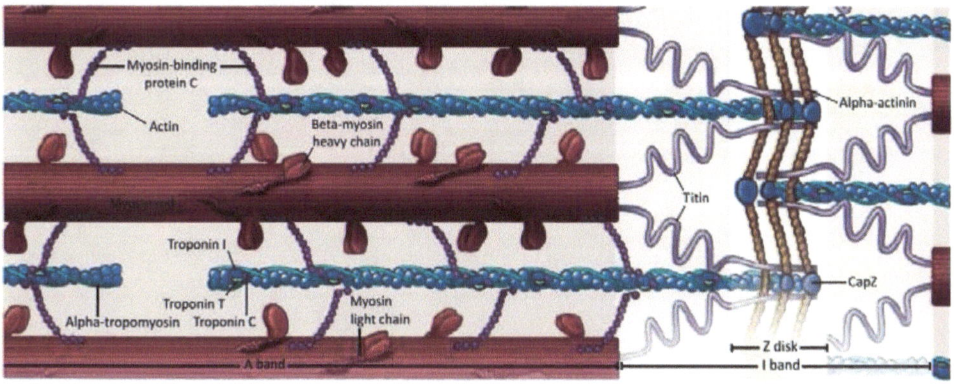

Fig. (2). Pathophysiological Substrate of Hypertrophic Cardiomyopathy (HCM) showing eleven HCM sarcomere genes.

HCM mutations patterns are autosomal dominant except the X-linked Danon disease due to lysosome-associated membrane protein 2 [39]. Hypertrophy of the heart in children is part of a syndrome, and the most common metabolic disease-causing hypertrophy of the heart is Anderson-Fabry, which is a storage dysfunction of the lysosomes. Constellations of malformations may lead suspicion towards Noonan's disease, LEOPARD, or even more rare diseases. Amyloidosis in adults should be part of the differential diagnosis. Family-history taking is mandatory for the initial evaluation of a patient with a suspected or confirmed hypertrophy. The clinician should systematically document the patients' report on family members who died suddenly or suffered from unexplained syncope or other symptoms suggesting an inheritance. The history taken should go beyond first and second-degree relatives for past medical records, and military service test if applicable to the individual patient.

Table 1. Hypertrophic cardiomyopathy susceptibility genes summary.

Gene	Locus	Protein	Frequency (%)
Myofilament HCM			
TTN	2q24.3	Titin	<1
MYH7	14q11.2–q12	β-myosin heavy chain	15–25
MYH6	14q11.2–q12	α-myosin heavy chain	<1
MYL2	12q23–q24.3	Ventr. Reg. myo. Lht. cha.	<2
MYL3	3p21.2–p21.3	Ventr. Esst. myo. Lht. cha.	<1
MYBPC3	11p11.2	Card. myo. Bin. prot. C	15–25
TNNT2	1q32	Cardiac troponin T	<4
TNNI3	19p13.4	Cardiac troponin I	<4
TPM1	15q22.1	α -tropomyosin	<4
ACTC	15q14	α-cardiac actin	<2
TNNC1	3p21.3–p14.3	Cardiac troponin C	<2
Z-disc HCM			
LBD3	10q22.2–q23.3	LIM binding domain 3	1-5
CSRP3	11p15.1	Muscle LIM protein	<1
TCAP	17q12–q21.1	Telethonin	<1
VCL	10q22.1–q23	Vinculin/metavinculin	<1
ACTN2	1q42–q43	Alpha-actinin 2	<1
MYOZ2	4q26–q27	Myozenin 2	<1
Calcium-handling HCM			
JPH2	20q12	Junctophilin-2	<1
PLN	6q22.1	Phospholamban	<1

Ventr-ventricular, Reg-Regulatory, Myo-myosin, Lht-Light, Cha-chain, Bin-binding, Prot-Protein

WALL THICKNESS AND ESTABLISHED RISK FACTORS OF LEFT VENTRICULAR HYPERTROPHY (ECHOCARDIOGRAPHIC BASED)

Patients with a ≥30 mm maximal wall thickness have a three-fold increased strong risk factor for HCM, although, between 25-29 mm thickness would probably be enough for most clinicians. Practically, hypertrophy is more or less unevenly distributed as this can influence the echocardiographic risk factor in practice. However, echocardiography also plays a crucial part in affecting the risk factor as it does not always provide accurate estimations in certain parts notably the apex of the heart although, other imaging techniques can resolve this problem in individuals. Extreme hypertrophy (defined as a maximum wall thickness >30 mm measured in diastole) frequently occurs in younger patients and 0.5% in patients over 50 years [40]. LV hypertrophy and a wall thickness >30 mm is an established marker of increased risk for SCD in HCM patients. However, this does not imply that risk is necessarily low when the wall thickness is <30 mm as other risk factors may be present as the majority of documented cases of patients who suddenly die are found to have a wall thickness <30 mm [41, 42].

Table 2. HCM phenocopies.

Gene	Locus	Protein	Syndrome
TAZ	Xq28	Tafazzin (G4.5)	Barth syndrome/LVNC
DTNA	18q12	Alpha-dystrobrevin	Barth syndrome/LVNC
PRKAG2	7q35–q36.36	AMP-activated protein kinase	WPW/HCM
LAMP2	Xq24	Lysosome-associated membrane protein 2	Danon's syndrome/WPW
GAA	17q25.2–q25.3	Alpha-1,4-glucosidase deficiency	Pompe's disease
GLA	Xq22	Alpha-galactosidase A	Fabry's disease
AGL	1p21	Amylo-1,6-glucosidase	Forbes disease
FXN	9q13	Frataxin	Friedrich's ataxia
PTPN11	12q24.1	Protein tyrosine phosphatase, nonreceptor type 11, SHP-2	Noonan's syndrome, LEOPARD syndrome
RAF1	3p25	V-RAF-1 murine leukemia viral oncogene homolog 1	Noonan's syndrome, LEOPARD syndrome
KRAS	12p12.1	v-Ki-ras2 Kirsten rat sarcoma viral oncogene homolog	Noonan's syndrome
SOS1	2p22-p21	Son of seven less homolog 1	Noonan's syndrome

AMP - adenosine monophosphate; HCM- hypertrophic cardiomyopathy; LEOPARD- mnemonic for syndrome with clinical characteristics of lentigines, electrocardiographic conduction abnormalities, ocular hypertelorism, pulmonary hypertension, abnormal genitalia, retarded growth, deafness; LVNC - left ventricular noncompaction; WPW - Wolff-Parkinson-White syndrome.

LEFT VENTRICULAR OUT-FLOW TRACT OBSTRUCTION AND REVERSE REMODELING

The outflow gradient of the left chamber varies tremendously among individual patients and also changes with exercise or can be provoked by drugs. Available data on the effect of LVOT obstruction on clinical outcome is mainly derived from large consecutive series and observational studies. Based on available data, LVOT obstruction of >30 mmHg should be regarded as only a minor risk factor for SCD and not the sole or even predominant deciding clinical marker for the implantation of an ICD (discussed in detail elsewhere in the chapter) [43, 44].

Reverse remodeling (LV mass reduction) is enhanced by a progressive and significant reduction in LVOT gradient [45]. The ongoing thinning that occurs is seen on the interventricular septum [45, 46]. Although, studies show it can be evident in the posterior wall of the LV [45] which is not coming as a surprise considering LV hypertrophy in young patients with HOCM is partially secondary to LVOT obstruction and that myectomies induce LV to reverse remodeling with wall thinning in areas distant from the interventricular septum [47].

IMPLANTABLE CARDIO-DEFIBRILLATOR THERAPY

ICD is an effective way to prevent SCD in HCM as several studies have confirmed its usefulness in HCM patients [24]. It protects from bradycardia and is indicated in high degree AV-block, tachy-brady, and occasionally to reduce outflow gradients in a patient where options are not suitable [2, 48]. Ventricular pacing from the right apical part may relieve obstruction electrical dyssynchrony between the lateral and septal segments of the LV. However, in any case, for an indication to implant an ICD in a patient with obstruction, a dual chamber system should be considered.

Implant Procedure

The procedure to implant an ICD is essentially the same as in other indication for HCM patient. Typical vascular access is from the left side either through punctures of the subclavian or axillary vein or a cephalic cut-down. If R-waves and thresholds can be favorably obtained at the apical region, the ventricular lead can thus, be implanted at the apical-right ventricular position. It is essential to check for T-wave oversensing before deciding the final place of the lead. In obstructive HCM, it is of particular importance to implant the lead in apex as this could facilitate a reduction in outflow gradient if AV-pacing is tried. The device could be subcutaneously or intramuscularly implanted. Patients can be discharged the same day as the typical procedure time is less than an hour. Modern ICDs batteries can last for 8-10 years, depending on amount pacing and, in a few cases, the demand for therapies.

Inappropriate Shocks and Triggers

There are varied differences in the reported incidence of shocks, which can be explained by the different definitions of inappropriate shock and the differences in follow-up time. Although, new devices with more competent algorithms have reduced the risk as an inappropriate shock is indeed a catastrophic event. Atrial arrhythmias mainly Atrial fibrillation and T-wave oversensing is the most common culprit for an inappropriate shock.

Indications and Safety of ICD Implantation in Adults, Adolescents, and Children

The implantation of an ICD is strongly warranted for secondary prevention in those patients who have experienced spontaneous or sustained ventricular tachycardia VT (class I indication based on the American College of Cardiology/ American Heart Association/National Association for Sport and Physical Education [ACC/AHA/NASPE] guidelines 2002) [49]. However, the decision to implant an ICD for primary prevention is more complicated. If a patient is felt to be at an unacceptably high risk owing to the presence of two or more established risk factors [explained in details further in the chapter], then an ICD warrants strong consideration after a discussion with the patient regarding the benefits and risks of device therapy (class IIb indication based on the ACC/AHA/NASPE guidelines 2002) [49]. For those in whom only a single risk factor is present, an assessment of risk needs to be made on an individual basis, as the presence of a particularly malignant pedigree despite the absence of other risk factors may still pose an unacceptably high risk to the patient and physician.

Nevertheless, the criteria for the placement of ICDs in pediatric patients remains somewhat controversial. Although, a revised consensus statement from the ACC and AHA does not provide any specific categorization for pediatric patients and adolescents, but suggests that indications are similar to those in adults [50]. The complication rates associated with the implantation of ICDs in children are relatively low and are comparable to those seen in adults [51, 52]. Lead-related complications (dislodgements and lead failures) and infections are commonly seen in both groups but at a higher frequency in the pediatric population.

ICD Placement in Children and Adolescents

There are significant setbacks in the pediatric aspect of patients with ICD placement and considerations that need to be looked into. However, this is more or less likely to increase as the need for an ICD implant expands in this group of patients.

Setbacks

I. No defibrillators have explicitly been produced or developed for children and to some considerable extent, adolescents as they only make up a small percentage of ICDs in the market.
II. New generation set of devices in the market weigh more ranging from 60/70 to 100g with volumes of 30 to 60/65ml which is considerably thicker than peacemakers, generally having a volume of about 8 to 11/12 ml.

III. High-energy capacitors and battery life are a constant limiting factor to ICDs, which contributes largely to its increased weight and volume.

Considerations

I. Although weight and volume are pressing issues in selecting an appropriate device for an individual patient, battery life should be considered as this is critical in a child who receives an ICD implant early in his/her life and would so require multiple generator changes during their lifetime.
II. Implant site for the pulse generator should be adequately taken into consideration most especially in thin children preferably deep pectoralis major muscle as it provides an improved cosmetic appearance in children with thin chest walls and a lack of adipose tissue [53, 54].

TYPE OF PLACEMENT SYSTEMS IN PEDIATRIC AND ADULT POPULATION

Epicardial *vs.* Transvenous Lead System

Epicardial placement system is gradually fading away as the preferable choice of lead system for pacing and defibrillating in both pediatric and adult patients. Epicardial systems require pace-sensing electrodes, and its hardware's to either be sewn or screwed to the epicardial surface of the heart to complete the defibrillation circuit. This particular system is associated with a high morbidity and mortality rate as its placement requires a thoracotomy whereas, transvenous lead systems have the advantage of avoiding a surgical thoracotomy and a surgical recovery time. Although transvenous lead systems implant methods was associated with an increased rate of crush damage to the leads. However, modifications to its initial approach (subclavian vein) resulted to new access routes such as axillary, cephalic and extra-thoracic subclavian vein which significantly decreased the high rate of lead crush and its complications [55]. Transvenous ICD leads can be secured to the myocardium either through active or passive fixation mechanism. Active-fixation leads have a helical screw that is deployed into the myocardium at the time of placement while passive-fixation leads have tines that are designed to anchor into ventricular trabeculae which are prone to been caught in the heavily trabeculated right ventricle especially in children forming strong adhesions. Transvenous defibrillation leads are comprised of one or two high-voltage coils that deliver a high energy shock to the myocardium. Single-coil leads have a coil located near the distal right ventricular lead tip as the defibrillator vector is created between the distal coil and the pulse generator itself. Dual-coil leads have both distal right ventricular apical coil and a proximal coil located a few centimeters from the lead tip. When placed in a healthy sized adult, this proximal coil lies within the superior vena cava.

However, in children, the fixed location of the proximal lead may not lie in a position to produce an optimal defibrillation vector, diminishing the value of the new coil.

NOVEL EPICARDIAL LEAD SYSTEMS

A subcutaneous approach is a unique approach which was developed initially as an adjunct to transvenous defibrillator leads as a means of improving higher defibrillation thresholds. This new approach involves several finger-like unipolar coil leads that are tunneled within the subcutaneous fascia around the lateral ribcage providing a wavefront discharge that covered a vast area of the myocardium, resulting in successful defibrillation hence utilizing lesser energy [56]. Also, unique leadless ICDs are currently in development as such devices would sense ventricular activity and deliver a defibrillation charge to the heart when necessary through the pulse generator itself. As it would highly obviate the technical limitations that both epicardial and transvenous defibrillation leads impose on the growing child and also be of significant benefit to adults as well. For example, patients who had previously undergone surgery under cardiopulmonary bypass will typically have the right atrial appendage amputated during cannulation. It would further, limit the ability to place an atrial lead in the usual right atrial appendage location and require the use of active fixation atrial points for attachment. However, same difficulties would be faced in a patient who has just undergone a Cavo pulmonary anastomosis such as the Fontan or Glenn procedures and venous anomalies of the upper extremities such as persistent left superior vena cava without a bridging vein.

DEATH DESPITE IMPLANTABLE CARDIO-DEFIBRILLATOR

Death despite ICD is mostly attributed to progressive heart failure (discussed in detail elsewhere in the chapter). Compared to the general population, the mortality rate despite ICD therapies is 3.4 (95% confidence interval 2.4–4.5) [57] (**See Appendix**). It, however, implies that, for successful treatment with or after an ICD implantation, heart failure needs to be addressed and taking seriously if an improved survival rate is to be expected.

UNDERLYING PATHOPHYSIOLOGY AND RISK ASSESSMENT

The pathophysiology of SCD is complex and is believed to require the interaction between an underlying substrate and a transient event. This process induces electric instability and lethal ventricular arrhythmias followed by hemodynamic collapse. Although the challenge remains to predict when such interactions prove harmful, a variety of risk factors have been proposed. SCD generally refers to unexpected death from a cardiovascular cause in a person with or without preexisting heart disease. The specificity of this definition varies depending on whether the event was witnessed. However, most cases presented are either a witnessed collapse, an unexpected death that occurred within the past twenty -four hours and/or deaths occurring within an hour of an acute change in clinical status of the individual [58]. The risk of SCD during infancy is low and also varies both with age and clinical features. After that, the risk is too small between 2 and 8 years of age, but it peaks in the 9 to 17-year-old age group. SCD events are attributable to ventricular tachyarrhythmias – ventricular tachycardia/ ventricular fibrillation – and usually occur in the presence of ≥ 1 of the major risk markers. In adult and teenagers, the generally accepted major risk factors for SCD are massive LV hypertrophy ≥ 3 cm, unexplained syncope, previous cardiac arrest, first-degree family history of sudden premature death, blunted systolic blood pressure response to exercise, and Nonsustained VT (repetitive and >120 bpm) (Fig. **3**). In children, massive LV hypertrophy can be quantified as either maximal wall thickness >2 cm or either maximal wall thickness >190% of an upper limit for age, (z score >3.72) [59]. However, only some of these risk factors for SCD have been verified in pediatrics HCM patients [60]. Apart from previous cardiac arrest, these individual risk factors have low predictive accuracy in the pediatric population except electrocardiogram (ECG) risk score a newer candidate risk assessment strategy. Other notable risk factors include; structural heart disease [61] (*e.g.*, Coronary heart disease or congestive heart failure), congenital heart disease, nutritional or dietary patterns [62 - 65], and various dysregulation in metabolic, inflammatory and neurohumoral pathways.

PRECIPITANTS

SCD risk in the population is not only a function of the underlying substrate and its vulnerability to arrhythmias but also the frequency of exposure to acute precipitants which in turn, precipitates to arrhythmias and SCD (Fig. **4**).

I. Physical Activity [66].
II. Genetic Predisposition to SCD [67].
III. Psychosocial Determinants [68].
IV. Diurnal/Seasonal Variation [69].

SYNCOPE

When it comes to interviewing patients with HCM, syncope deserves special attention. This, however, includes observations gotten from witnesses about signs and durations which can most times be overestimated. The body position and activity may aid essential clues. Carotid sinus mechanism for syncope can sometimes be reproduced. Prompt evaluation is highly needed in exercise-induced syncope as a malignant cause is probably likely. Also, tiredness and seizures experienced indicate epilepsy, but cardiac causes should be ruled out.

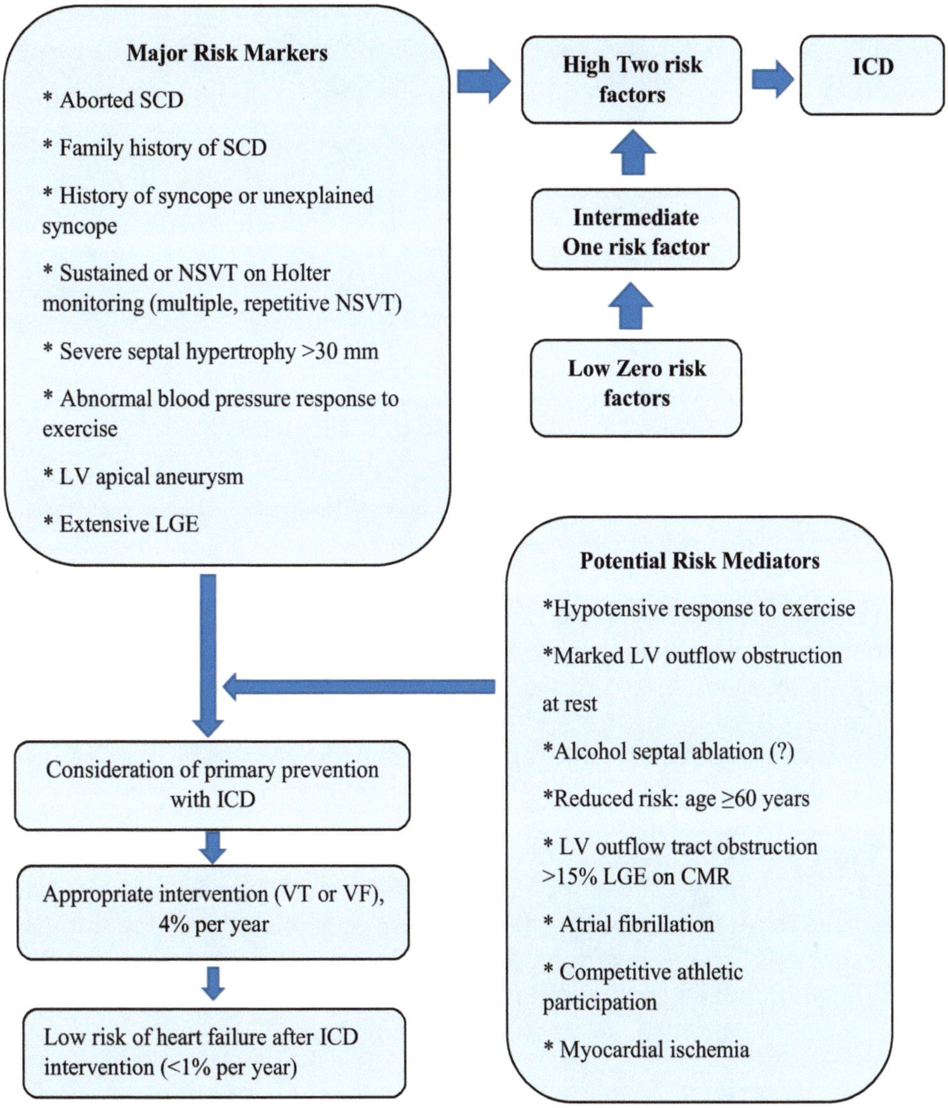

Fig. (3). Risk stratification and Primary Prevention of Sudden Death with ICDs in Patients with hypertrophic cardiomyopathy. ICD: Implantable cardioverter–defibrillator; NSVT: Nonsustained ventricular tachycardia; SCD: Sudden cardiac death.

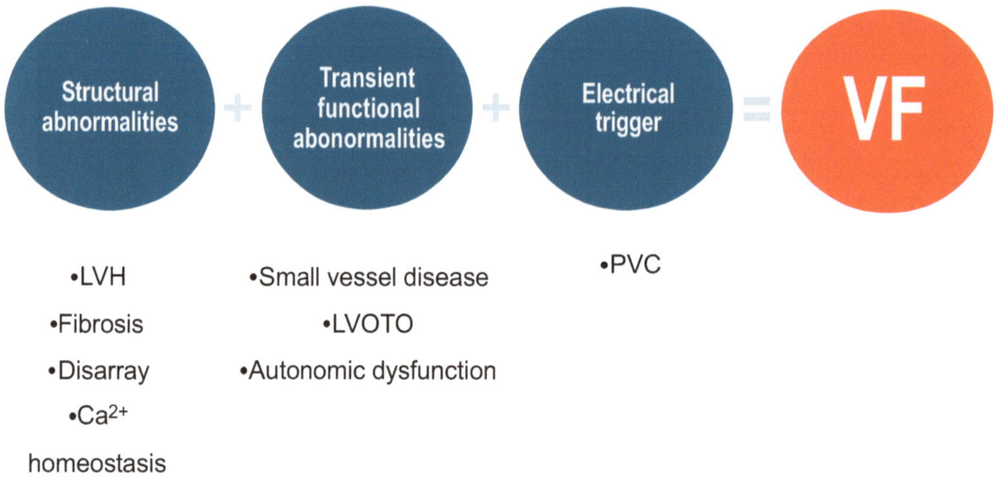

Fig. (4). Sudden cardiac death (SCD) in hypertrophic cardiomyopathy (HCM). Sarcomeric protein gene mutations cause structural and functional abnormalities promoting ventricular arrhythmias. Potent modulators which transiently act on this substrate reduce the threshold for ventricular arrhythmias. The majority of ventricular arrhythmias in HCM are precipitated by premature ventricular complexes. LVH, left ventricular hypertrophy; LVOTO, left ventricular outflow tract obstruction; PVC, premature ventricular contraction; VF, ventricular fibrillation.

Reflex Syncope: Reflex syncope has an uncertain and absent triggers on presentation. Its diagnosis solely relies on history taking and the absence of other structural heart diseases that can produce syncope and on reproducing similar symptoms with tilt-table testing and carotid sinus massage. Furthermore, the diagnostic workup of patients with reflex syncope should follow the 2009 ESC guidelines for the diagnosis and management of syncope [70].

Carotid Sinus Syncope It is defined as syncope with carotid sinus massage yielding either a fall in systolic blood pressure of .50 mmHg or asystole of .3 secs, or both, and the reproduction of spontaneous syncope. Massage is recommended in both upright and supine positions to be as diagnostic as possible. However, cases for adjusting the diagnostic criteria, particularly for the duration of asystole to .6 secs to be as symptomatic as possible has been raised [71].

Tilt-Induced Vasovagal Syncope: Typically, the vasovagal reflex induced during tilt table testing is both hypotensive and bradycardic. However, the lack of reproducibility of tilt testing limits its utility as a means of assessing therapy. Moreover, the mechanism of tilt-induced syncope is frequently different from that of spontaneous syncope.

Unexplained Syncope and Fall: Sometimes even after a thorough and complete work-up performed in a patient with HCM following the 2009 ESC guidelines for diagnosis and management of syncope, the cause of syncope may remain unexplained [70].

HYPERTROPHIC CARDIOMYOPATHY IN SPECIFIC SPECIAL GROUPS

Pregnancy: It implies increased loading pressures, and in the last trimester, the cardiovascular demand irreversibly increases the risk. HCM is a complex disease, and the risk of SCD during pregnancy needs to be addressed based on individual factors. In some situations, the lady may have to give up her wish of becoming a biological mother someday. In such cases, planned pregnancy and counseling should be offered to expectant mothers during the pregnancy and delivery by a multidisciplinary team. In rare instances in which an ICD implant is needed during pregnancy, specialized care, efforts and protection need to be provided against radiation or using echocardiography to assess the position of leads.

Driving: Though HCM patients driving [buses, trucks, taxis, trains and also piloting airplanes] in most countries have no driving restrictions nor any found to be published in European registries and guidelines, patients with ICD devices, either way, need special considerations. We (the authors) advise that survivors of cardiac arrest do not drive for the first six to eight months after the event. The risk after an arrhythmic event is high during the first few months, which makes six to eight months' restriction quite reasonable. However, this advice needs to be in harmony with the national laws of the individual country in question.

END-STAGE HEART FAILURE AND OTHER FORMS OF HYPERTROPHIC CARDIOMYOPATHY

It is imperative to recognize the beginning of this stage (Fig. **5**) and take prompt action, including optimal pharmacologic treatments and device therapy as this is the burnout phase of HCM (Fig. **6**). Ejection fraction (EF) <50% in HCM is the turning point and a marker for an ICD therapy as an EF <50% also predicts the risk of life-threatening ventricular arrhythmias [72, 73]. On the other hand, it is also vital to distinguish the different forms of HCM though classified as the minority and rare group namely; RASO-pathies (Costello syndrome and Noonan syndrome), lysosomal-associated membrane protein 2 (LAMP2) mutation, certain glycogen storage diseases [Pompe disease], glycogen storage disease type II and acid maltase deficiency (PRKAG2) mutations constitute an essential minority of HCM conditions.

These conditions highlight the importance of a holistic medical approach to the newly diagnosed patient with HCM; for example, coexisting Wolff-Parkinso--White patterns should raise the question of a PRKAG2 or LAMP2 mutation.

Skeletal muscle weakness should prompt consideration of mitochondrial variation or Pompe disease. Elevated liver enzymes and intellectual deficiencies suggest the diagnosis of LAMP2 mutation. Characteristic facial features will direct the clinician to evaluate for Costello or Noonan syndrome. Once the diagnosis is confirmed by enzymatic or genetic analysis, clinical surveillance and intervention may dramatically diverge from that typically used for sarcomeric forms of HCM.

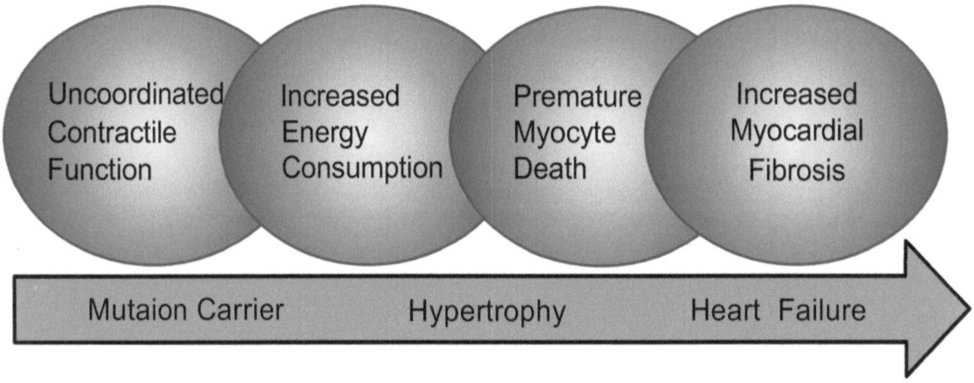

Fig. (5). The pathway from sarcomere gene mutation to heart failure.

IMAGING

The crucial goals of imaging are to evaluate ischemia, delineate cardiac anatomy, assess the implications of the anatomic findings on cardiac function, and monitor therapeutic efficacies [74] (Fig. 7). The anatomic considerations at initial diagnosis include assessment of location and severity of intraventricular obstruction, quantification, and qualification of hypertrophy, evaluation of the mitral apparatus, and the assessment of tissue characteristics that may signify the ongoing underlying fibrotic changes. Echocardiography has and remains the gold standard of imaging evaluation in HCM. It's portable and provides the best characterization of the physiologic abnormalities related to valvular abnormalities, intraventricular obstruction, systolic, and diastolic functions (**Box 1**).

Box 1| What an echo report in HCM should include. EF, ejection fraction; DMI, Doppler myocardial imaging; HCM, hypertrophic cardiomyopathy; SAM, the systolic anterior motion of the mitral valve; LA, left atria; STE, speckle tracking echocardiography; PM, papillary muscles.

However, cardiovascular magnetic resonance (CMR) imaging can characterize tissue changes which gives a chance for a more detailed description of the morphologic abnormalities seen in HCM, providing a further understanding of the disease pathology thereby, supporting risk stratification algorithms (**Box 2**). 2D echocardiography is the initial step in evaluating hypertrophy but its, however, dependent on the available acoustic windows, and it is also limited by constraints of lateral resolution. In instances like this, CMR should be considered as an alternative initial imaging investigation as it is more sensitive to detecting apical and segmental wall abnormalities than echocardiography.

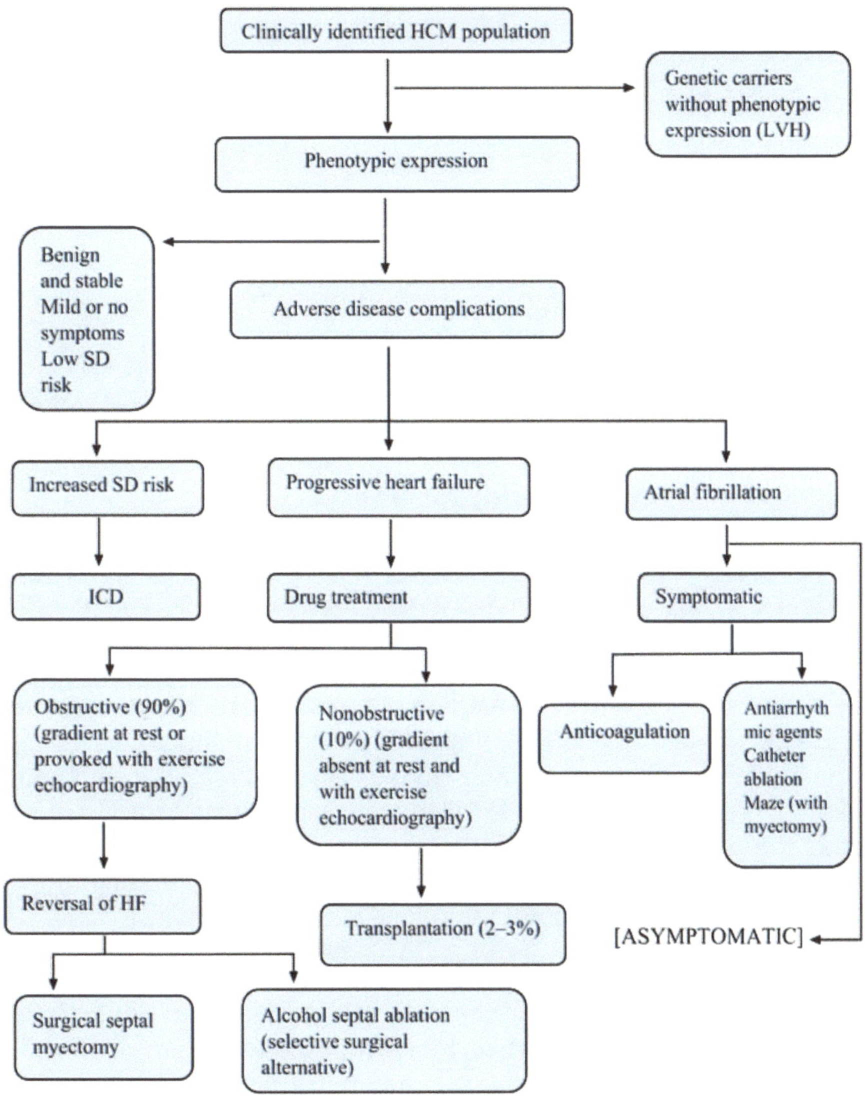

Fig. (6). Management Algorithm for the Clinical Spectrum of HCM. SD denotes sudden death.

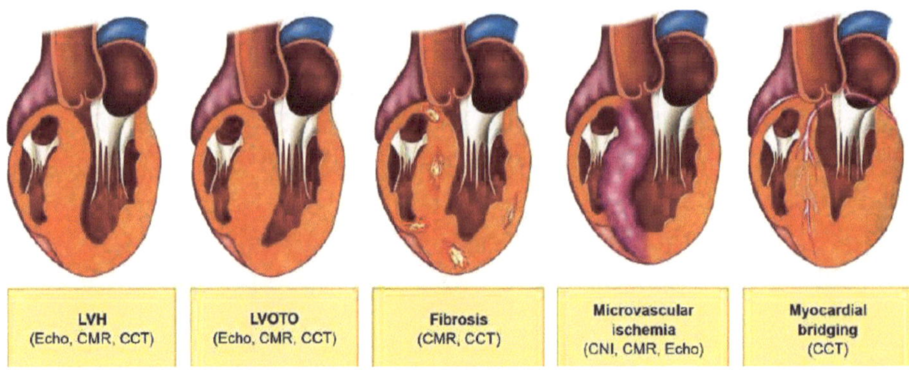

Fig. (7). Imaging phenotypes. LVH- left ventricular hypertrophy, LVOTO- left ventricular outflow tract obstruction, fibrosis, microvascular ischemia, and myocardial bridging).

Box 2| What a CMR report in HCM should include. HCM, hypertrophic cardiomyopathy; CMR, cardiac magnetic resonance; LVOT, left ventricular outflow tract; RV, right ventricle; LGE, late gadolinium enhancement.

DIAGNOSTIC IMPLICATIONS OF HYPERTROPHIC GENETIC TESTING

Identification of HCM Susceptibility Genes: It is over two decades since the first chromosome locus for familial HCM and the subsequent mutations involving the MYH7-encoded beta-myosin heavy chain were elucidated as the pathogenic basis for HCM [75, 76]. Moving forward over the years, hundreds of variations scattered among at least 27 putative HCM susceptibility genes encoding various sarcomeric, mitochondrial and calcium-handling, proteins have been identified. The most common genetically mediated form of HCM is myofilament [sarcomeric]-HCM with hundreds of disease-associated mutations in 9 genes encoding proteins [myofilaments] critical to the cardiac sarcomere which includes beta-myosin heavy chain (MYH7) [76], myosin binding protein C (MYBPC3) [77], cardiac troponin I (TNNI3) [78], regulatory (MYL2) and essential myosin light chains (MYL3) [79], cardiac troponin C (TNNC1) [80], cardiac troponin T (TNNT2), alpha-tropomyosin (TPM1) [81], and actin (ACTC) [82].

Approaches and New Insights to Genomics of HCM and Cardiac Hypertrophy: In the field of '-omics,' novel pathways underlying the pathophysiology of HCM and cardiac hypertrophy have been identified using several new techniques to study large-scale transcriptional changes [83]. A transcriptomic approach can be performed using a snapshot view expression, which can identify genes that seem to be co-regulated or differentially regulated, thereby forming a transcriptional network of genes and pathways which was further studied by Hwang *et al.* [84]. Another exciting and looming aspect in the field is that of micro-ribonucleic acids (miRNAs) and their role in hypertrophic heart disease.

HCM Genetic Testing in Clinical Practice: HCM has recently gone past its two decades wait in research laboratories into an era of clinically diagnostical available gene testing for physicians evaluating and treating patients with this disease. Significant HCM susceptible HCM genes are now commercially available for genetic testing (Table **1**).

Echocardiography-Guided Genetic Testing: As observed by Solomon *et al.* [85], patients with mutations in the beta-myosin heavy chain (MYH7-HCM) generally had reverse curve contour HCM. Echocardiography-guided genetic testing helps identify, differentiate, and classify the various septal morphologies of HCM where the septal contour is classified as a reverse curve, apical, sigmoidal, and neutral contour HCM (Fig. **8**).

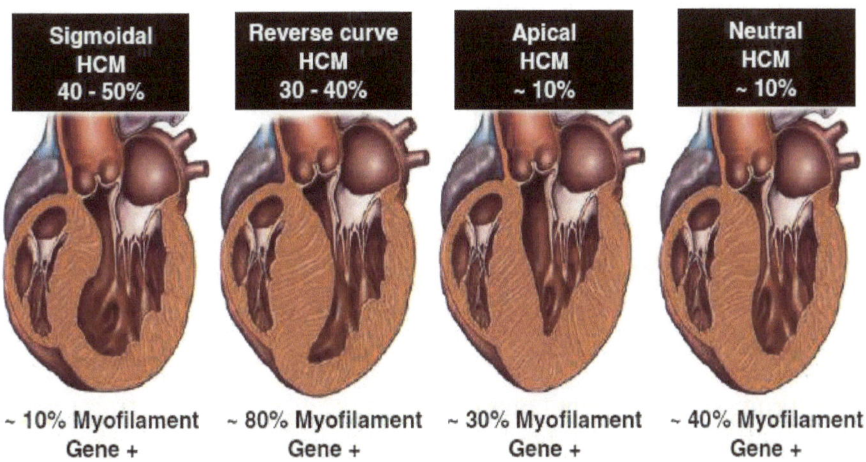

Fig. (8). Common Septal Morphologies in Hypertrophic Cardiomyopathy (HCM).

Novel Imaging Techniques in HCM Disease Gene Expression for Early Detection: Tissue Doppler echocardiography [86] and CMR [87] are the imaging modalities showing high potentials in the early detection of genetic substrates. With the rapid growth in basic theoretical and clinical knowledge on genetic and other pathogenetic pathways in HCM, early identification of genetic substrate in pre-clinical and pre-hypertrophic expression is vital for a better fundamental understanding of HCM progression.

Therapeutic Implications (Pharmacogenomics) of HCM Genetic Testing: There is currently no single therapy designed to target specific HCM-causing gene mutations or particular HCM genotypes. Further, no treatments have been shown to reverse the hypertrophic process in humans.

DOUBTS AND QUESTIONS ARISING IN RISK STRATIFICATION AND THERAPEUTIC MANAGEMENT IN HCM PATIENTS

At what Age Is Risk Greatest?

Much confusion has arisen in the literature from the uncritical habit of many authors of merely assuming that SCD risk is uniform over the whole childhood, and thus calculating annual death rates without any consideration of the age composition of the cohort. The published Swedish–British cohort [88] study helps to clarify the general perception that risk of SCD in HCM is at its highest just after puberty and in young adults, which has led to suggestions that family screening for HCM should be commenced after 12 years [89]. The study clearly shows that SCD is extremely low below 8 years of age, and rapidly increases from 8 years then rises to a maximum in 10- to 10.9-year-old where it reaches an annual mortality of 9.7% and is averaging 7.2% between 9 to 13.9 years, notably dropping to an average yearly death of 1.7% after the age of 16 years. Although this ongoing grave error is less likely inevitable in the field, age consideration is critical in SCD risk stratification and assessment [90].

Which Child and Adolescent Should Be Screened to Rule Out HCM?

The group with the highest risk of having overt HCM is, of course, children with one parent with HCM and thereby at 50-70% risk of being a mutation carrier. it is therefore essential and advantageous to have a window for therapeutic interventions before a child arrives in the high-risk age range. Bearing this in mind, we the authors strongly again suggest that the initial screening of a child with a parent who is an HCM patient should be carried out no later than five to six years of age. However, after initial screening, subsequent follow-up regimen should be set up by the physician, particularly during the pubertal growth spurt of the child.

Beta-adrenoceptor Antagonist Therapy

Unfortunately, there is a complete absence in the literature and published guidelines of long-term prospective randomized drug treatment trials in the treatment of HCM patients, which have used mortality as an end-point, both in adult and in pediatric patients. Below, we the authors give an equivalent and a contemporary view at the same time, try to answer the lingering doubts and question as to the pharmacotherapeutic management of patients with HCM based on our experience and expert opinions in the field.

Which Beta Blocker to be Chosen? Propranolol and metoprolol are our first line choice in patients with risk for SCD as propranolol especially has in addition to its beta-adrenoceptor blocking effects a membrane stabilizing action and tends to increase the threshold for Ventricular Fibrillation (VF) [91, 92] compared to hydrophilic beta-blockers (atenolol).

How Can One Titrate Beta-Blocker Dose Effectively in an Individual Patient? The best way to ascertain if a beta-blocker dose receptor therapy is adequate is with the use of a 24 Holter monitoring. In children with severe HCM, efforts should be directed towards preventing the heart rate from exceeding 120bpm during significant periods. However, in adolescents with severe HCM, to achieve a full therapeutic effect, maximal heart rate of 90bpm is non-negotiable. As for adults, the therapeutic goals are the same as that for adolescents, but the R-R interval should remain below 5-6%.

Calcium-Channel Blocker Therapy

Although still used by some physicians, we (the authors), however, do not recommend its use due to its fetal adverse effects, especially in pediatric HCM patients who fulfill high-risk criteria. In recent research carried out by O¨ stman-Smith I. *et al.* [93], verapamil use leads to an increase in heart failure mortality in patients who have a marked and generalized LV hypertrophy.

Disopyramide Therapy and Dose Range

The use of disopyramide is highly beneficial in outflow obstruction, especially in children and diastolic function in HCM patient. It is also an antiarrhythmic drug too, which reduces risk of paroxysmal atrial fibrillation although not the most preferable class of medication to treat non-sustained ventricular tachycardias by a cardiologist, we the authors recommend its use especially in the management of LVOT obstruction in HCM patients which also significantly decreases sudden cardiac mortality [94]. The disopyramide clearance rate is fast in children than in adults, dosing in both adult and pediatric patients should be targeted towards achieving therapeutic levels and monitoring of QT prolongation. We (the authors) recommend a daily dose of 2-4mg/kg twice daily and no more than 15 to 20% plasma levels.

Amiodarone Therapy

Although mostly used by practicing physicians, it is only useful in short-term treatment to control paroxysmal atrial fibrillation and for ventricular arrhythmias but its, however, not suitable for long-term therapy in pediatric HCM patients. Furthermore, it does not protect against sudden arrhythmia death. Moreover, it does not protect against sudden arrhythmia death.

NOVEL APPROACHES IN MEDICAL THERAPY

Although the therapies mentioned above which sure do have a place in the treatment of symptomatic LVOT obstruction [2, 20], there are however emerging alternative treatment options for HCM patients in the field namely;

Calcium Channel Blockers in The Preclinical State: There is a claim otherwise suggestive by researchers in the domain that there is a "preclinical" period in HCM. Where a family member may be found to have a sarcomeric mutation but a structurally healthy heart which provides an ample time to modify the disease progression. Diltiazem was, however, used to explore and modify the progress of the disease to clarify these claims [95].

Antifibrotic Agents: Modulating fibrosis pathogenesis was active with the use of spironolactone in animal models, but efficacy in human models is still yet to be elucidated. However, the randomized controlled trial INHERIT did not appear to show any difference in the burden of fibrosis as assessed by LGE [along with many other clinical outcome measures] with the use of losartan [96, 97].

Molecular Therapy: Since the initial recognition that HCM was a disease of the sarcomere that causes hypercontractility, there has been some focus on trying to improve the abnormalities at a molecular level [98]. MYK-461 is a small molecule inhibitor of sarcomere power which attenuate the development of some of the hallmark features of HCM such as hypercontractility, LV hypertrophy, and fibrosis when used early in the disease in murine models [99]. The same molecule was also shown to reduce LVOT obstruction when used in cats with obstructive HCM [100].

Metabolic Modulators: This modulation pathway was proposed by Abozguia K *et al.* to improve the contraction-relaxation cycle in HCM patients. Perhexiline is a metabolic modulator promoting the use of carbohydrates as a substrate for myocardial energy by inhibiting carnitine-palmitoyl-transferase, which enhances the contraction [101].

SEPTAL REDUCTION THERAPY

HCM patients with presenting with highly symptomatic LVOT obstruction despite maximal medical therapy, septal reduction therapy is the necessary next course of treatment. Obstruction is relieved by the initial introduction of negatively inotropic medications [2, 20] which is associated with an instant improvement in symptoms and outcome [102 - 105] as the constraint of LVOT obstruction in HCM patient doubles the risk of morbidity and mortality rate [106, 107]. Surgical myectomy has been considered the standard gold therapy in a septal reduction for decades [108]. The relief of LVOT obstruction was achieved years ago by removing 5-10g of myocardium from the basal interventricular septum [109] however, the marrow procedure has been extended down to the mid-septum providing a much more improved relief of obstruction [110]. On the other hand, ASA therapy was introduced as an alternative to surgical myectomy [111] which involves the injection of 1-3ml of desiccated alcohol [112] into an appropriate septal branch resulting in myocardial necrosis, scarring and subsequent septal shrinking [102, 104, 111 - 113]. The alcohol-induced scar of the septum widens the LVOT, reduces systolic anterior motion of the MV and thereby relieves the obstruction.

QUALITY OF LIFE AND THE PSYCHOLOGICAL WELL BEING OF PATIENTS WITH HYPERTROPHIC CARDIOMYOPATHY

HCM is a chronic condition with a substantial social and emotional ramification as many patients complain of diminished social interactions, curtailed and remarkably decreased physical activity levels due to the potentially life-threatening problem faced with HCM including sexual activity and body image concerns related to the appearance of ICD devices. HCM is familial in a substantial proportion of cases, giving rise to fear of transmission and issues surrounding genetic counseling. Many patients are diagnosed following a sudden death in the family so they may be suffering the pain of grief while attempting to come to terms with their own health risk. Although, unlike in the adult population, children with ICDs tend to be much more depressed as they also express concerns about receiving shocks and fear that the device would fail [114].

MISCONCEPTIONS

HCM is a rare disease relevant only to subspecialty care. This is however absolutely not true as the prevalence and actual burden of the disease is significantly underestimated [31] which could either be as a result of poor surveillance and risk stratification and inadequate research of the disease itself. Therefore, clinicians should be aware of HCM to diagnose, manage, and treat such patients properly.

1. HCM is a disease of cardiac muscle only. This is, however, absolutely incorrect as HCM is a genetic disease attributed to various sarcomere gene mutations and

also typically described as a non-physiologic LV muscle thickening without an apparent clinical cause. Apart from the commonly known feature of HCM, *i.e.*, dynamic obstruction LVOT, the abnormal mitral valve apparatus is underappreciated. However, understanding the contribution of the mitral valve apparatus abnormalities to the pathophysiology of the dynamic LVOT obstruction is essential too.

2. Hypertensive patients with HCM should be treated with traditional first-line antihypertensive agents. Treatment of patients with coexisting HCM and hypertension is indeed quite challenging [20], the first-line medications used for the treatment of hypertension exacerbate outflow obstruction in patients with obstructive HCM (especially those with possible obstruction) is potentially harmful, even in some non-obstructed patients with small left ventricular cavity [115]. However, a well-structured framework for treating HCM with hypertension should be individualized and well thought off before therapy is initiated [116].

PREVALENT ISSUES

Although, with the current progress and developments made over the years, the lack of improved risk stratification, algorithms and the uncertainties facing the use of defibrillator device therapies in both adult and pediatric population combine remains a lingering issue in the primary, secondary and tertiary health care providers. Also, with the growing indications for ICD placement, the needs of children will significantly have to be addressed too. However, many of the limitations faced today are due to technical considerations in using a device that is not intended for use in small patients or patients with structurally abnormal hearts. Apart from the technical difficulties, the devices are bulkily contributing to the increase psychosocial issues faced by children in some cases, causing a decreased range of motion primarily due to the shape of the generator can. Another growing concern is the battery life of these devices as a child who receives an ICD implant at a young age would have to undergo multiple generator change surgeries for the rest of his/her life which can be a daunting prospect and quite worrisome. That been said, in patients undergoing operations, there is a significant obstacle faced with defibrillator lead extractions due to the scar tissue formation formed around the lead body and in particular, the defibrillation coils too.

Finally, as more children receive devices and grow into young adulthood with the near lack or weak algorithms used so far in the field, there would be a significant need for a specialized pediatric algorithm to discriminate supraventricular tachycardia from malignant ventricular arrhythmias to prevent inappropriate shocks.

CONCLUSION AND FUTURE PERSPECTIVES

Once regarded as a rare and challenging heart condition with a grim prognosis and limited management options, its, however, now relatively common, treatable and recognized worldwide with a favorable life expectancy which is as a result of advances in innovative clinical science and an improved management paradigm. HCM awareness is driven by the particular attention being given to family screening and the number of patients being diagnosed. Although the majority are classified as low risk, rigorous and proper risk stratification is pivotal to identifying high-risk patients. Be it as it may, there remains some regional variability in standard of care available due to the multiple facets, diagnostic approach, and therapeutic management faced with HCM as a single entity. It can, however, be addressed by creating international standards and centers of excellence to concentrate on the complex care that is often required. Notwithstanding, there is significant progress in the field of HCM from laboratory and clinical research to applied theoretical and clinical scientific results gotten, which are translated into present-day clinical practice. It is therefore and however crucial for a 21st century clinician to be aware of the current state-of-the-art translational genetics, new techniques and developments achieved so far, and their applications as this would provide him/her, the opportunity to treat HCM patients adequately before some of the advanced complications occur.

Appendix. Outcome of randomized controlled trials of dual-chamber versus ventricular pacing HF-heart failure; HR, hazard ratio; SSS- sick sinus syndrome.

Outcome	Dual-chamber Benefit Over Ventricular Pacing	Notes	References
All-cause deaths	No benefit	HR 0.80.[12] Benefits higher in SSS	[117, 118 - 122]
Stroke, embolism	Benefit (in meta-analysis only, not in the single trial)	HR 0.81.[12] and 0.78.[13] Benefits higher in SSS	[117, 118 - 120]
Atrial fibrillation	Benefit		[117, 118 - 120]
HF, hospitalization for HF	No benefit		[117, 118 - 122]
Exercise capacity	Benefit		[122]
Pacemaker syndrome	Benefit	The overall standardized mean improvement of 35%. Not significantly compared to VVIR	[118 - 120]
Functional status	No benefit	Documented in up to 25% of VVI patients.	[118, 119 - 122]

Cont.....

Quality of life	Variable	Consistent direction of effect on the quality of life, but the size cannot be estimated in confidence	[118 - 120, 122]
Complications	More complications with dual-chamber	Higher rate of lead dislodgment (4.25 *vs.* 1.4%) and inadequate pacing (1.3 *vs.* 0.3%).	[117, 119 - 120, 122]

LIST OF ABBREVIATIONS

ACC/AHA/NASPE	American College of Cardiology/American Heart Association/National Association for Sport and Physical Education guidelines 2002
CRT	Cardiac Resynchronization Therapy
CMR	Cardiovascular Magnetic Resonance
EF	Ejection Fraction
HCM	Hypertrophic Cardiomyopathy
HCOM	Hypertrophic Obstructive Cardiomyopathy
ICD	Implantable Cardioverter Defibrillator
LVOT	Left Ventricular Obstructive Tract
LV	Left Ventricular
SCD	Sudden Cardiac Death
VT	Ventricular Tachycardia
VF	Ventricular Fibrillation

CONSENT FOR PUBLICATION

Not applicable.

CONFLICT OF INTEREST

The authors confirm that this chapter contents have no conflict of interest.

ACKNOWLEDGEMENTS

Declared none.

REFERENCES

[1] Teare D. Asymmetrical hypertrophy of the heart in young adults. Br Heart J 1958; 20(1): 1-8. [http://dx.doi.org/10.1136/hrt.20.1.1] [PMID: 13499764]

[2] Elliott PM, Anastasakis A, Borger MA, *et al.* 2014 ESC Guidelines on diagnosis and management of hypertrophic cardiomyopathy: the Task Force for the Diagnosis and Management of Hypertrophic Cardiomyopathy of the European Society of Cardiology (ESC). Eur Heart J 2014; 35(39): 2733-79. [http://dx.doi.org/10.1093/eurheartj/ehu284] [PMID: 25173338]

[3] Writing Committee Members. Gersh BJ, Maron BJ, Bonow RO et al. 2011 ACCF/AHA Guideline for the Diagnosis and Treatment of hypertrophic cardiomyopathy: a report of the American College of Cardiology Foundation/American Heart Association Task Force on Practice Guidelines. Circulation 2011; 124: e783-831.

[4] Schoendube FA, Klues HG, Reith S, Flachskampf FA, Hanrath P, Messmer BJ. Long-term clinical and echocardiographic follow-up after surgical correction of hypertrophic obstructive cardiomyopathy with extended myectomy and reconstruction of the subvalvular mitral apparatus. Circulation 1995; 92(9) (Suppl.): II122-7.
[http://dx.doi.org/10.1161/01.CIR.92.9.122] [PMID: 7586394]

[5] Braunwald E, Brockenbrough EC, Morrow AG. Hypertrophic subaortic stenosis-a broadened concept. Circulation 1962; 26: 161-5.
[http://dx.doi.org/10.1161/01.CIR.26.2.161] [PMID: 13872648]

[6] Pollick C, Morgan CD, Gilbert BW, Rakowski H, Wigle ED. Muscular subaortic stenosis: the temporal relationship between systolic anterior motion of the anterior mitral leaflet and the pressure gradient. Circulation 1982; 66(5): 1087-94.
[http://dx.doi.org/10.1161/01.CIR.66.5.1087] [PMID: 7127693]

[7] Braunwald E, Lambrew CT, Rockoff SD, Ross J Jr, Morrow AG. Idiopathic hypertrophic subaortic stenosis. I. A description of the disease based on an analysis of 64 patients. Circulation 1964; 30 (Suppl. 4): 4-, 3-119.
[http://dx.doi.org/10.1161/01.CIR.29.5S4.IV-3] [PMID: 14227306]

[8] Maron BJ, Rowin EJ, Casey SA, Maron MS. How hypertrophic cardiomyopathy became a contemporary treatable genetic disease with low mortality: shaped by 50 years of clinical research and practice. JAMA Cardiol 2016; 1(1): 98-105.
[http://dx.doi.org/10.1001/jamacardio.2015.0354] [PMID: 27437663]

[9] Elliott PM, Anastasakis A, Borger MA, *et al.* 2014 ESC Guidelines on diagnosis and management of hypertrophic cardiomyopathy: the Task Force for the Diagnosis and Management of Hypertrophic Cardiomyopathy of the European Society of Cardiology (ESC). Eur Heart J 2014; 35(39): 2733-79.
[http://dx.doi.org/10.1093/eurheartj/ehu284] [PMID: 25173338]

[10] Maron BJ, Ommen SR, Semsarian C, Spirito P, Olivotto I, Maron MS. Hypertrophic cardiomyopathy: present and future, with translation into contemporary cardiovascular medicine. J Am Coll Cardiol 2014; 64(1): 83-99.
[http://dx.doi.org/10.1016/j.jacc.2014.05.003] [PMID: 24998133]

[11] Maron BJ, Towbin JA, Thiene G, *et al.* Council on Clinical Cardiology, Heart Failure and Transplantation Committee; Quality of Care and Outcomes Research and Functional Genomics and Translational Biology Interdisciplinary Working Groups; Council on Epidemiology and Prevention. Contemporary definitions and classification of the cardiomyopathies. Circulation 2006; 113: 1807-16.
[http://dx.doi.org/10.1161/CIRCULATIONAHA.106.174287] [PMID: 16567565]

[12] Maron BJ. Hypertrophic cardiomyopathy: a systematic review. JAMA 2002; 287(10): 1308-20.
[http://dx.doi.org/10.1001/jama.287.10.1308] [PMID: 11886323]

[13] Maron BJ, Doerer JJ, Haas TS, Tierney DM, Mueller FO. Sudden deaths in young competitive athletes: analysis of 1866 deaths in the United States, 1980-2006. Circulation 2009; 119(8): 1085-92.
[http://dx.doi.org/10.1161/CIRCULATIONAHA.108.804617] [PMID: 19221222]

[14] Sugishita Y, Matsuda M, Iida K, Koshinaga J, Ueno M. Sudden cardiac death at exertion. Jpn Circ J 1983; 47(5): 562-72.
[http://dx.doi.org/10.1253/jcj.47.562] [PMID: 6854913]

[15] Kato TS, Noda A, Izawa H, *et al.* Discrimination of nonobstructive hypertrophic cardiomyopathy from hypertensive left ventricular hypertrophy on the basis of strain rate imaging by tissue Doppler ultrasonography. Circulation 2004; 110(25): 3808-14.
[http://dx.doi.org/10.1161/01.CIR.0000150334.69355.00] [PMID: 15583080]

[16] Maron BJ. Distinguishing hypertrophic cardiomyopathy from athlete's heart physiological remodelling: clinical significance, diagnostic strategies and implications for preparticipation screening. Br J Sports Med 2009; 43(9): 649-56.
[http://dx.doi.org/10.1136/bjsm.2008.054726] [PMID: 19734498]

[17] Arad M, Maron BJ, Gorham JM, *et al.* Glycogen storage diseases presenting as hypertrophic cardiomyopathy. N Engl J Med 2005; 352(4): 362-72.
[http://dx.doi.org/10.1056/NEJMoa033349] [PMID: 15673802]

[18] Nakamura T, Sugihara H, Kinoshita N, Yoneyama S, Azuma A, Nakagawa M. Can serum carnitine levels distinguish hypertrophic cardiomyopathy from hypertensive hearts? Hypertension 2000; 36(2): 215-9.
[http://dx.doi.org/10.1161/01.HYP.36.2.215] [PMID: 10948080]

[19] Maron MS, Olivotto I, Zenovich AG, *et al.* Hypertrophic cardiomyopathy is predominantly a disease of left ventricular outflow tract obstruction. Circulation 2006; 114(21): 2232-9.
[http://dx.doi.org/10.1161/CIRCULATIONAHA.106.644682] [PMID: 17088454]

[20] Gersh BJ, Maron BJ, Bonow RO, *et al.* 2011 ACCF/AHA guideline for the diagnosis and treatment of hypertrophic cardiomyopathy: a report of the American College of Cardiology Foundation/American Heart Association Task Force on Practice Guidelines. Circulation 2011; 124(24): e783-831.
[http://dx.doi.org/10.1161/CIR.0b013e318223e2bd] [PMID: 22068434]

[21] O'Mahony C, Jichi F, Pavlou M, *et al.* A novel clinical risk prediction model for sudden cardiac death in hypertrophic cardiomyopathy (HCM risk-SCD). Eur Heart J 2014; 35(30): 2010-20.
[http://dx.doi.org/10.1093/eurheartj/eht439] [PMID: 24126876]

[22] Maron BJ, Shen WK, Link MS, *et al.* Efficacy of implantable cardioverter-defibrillators for the prevention of sudden death in patients with hypertrophic cardiomyopathy. N Engl J Med 2000; 342(6): 365-73.
[http://dx.doi.org/10.1056/NEJM200002103420601] [PMID: 10666426]

[23] O'Mahony C, Tome-Esteban M, Lambiase PD, *et al.* A validation study of the 2003 American College of Cardiology/European Society of Cardiology and 2011 American College of Cardiology Foundation/American Heart Association risk stratification and treatment algorithms for sudden cardiac death in patients with hypertrophic cardiomyopathy. Heart 2013; 99(8): 534-41.
[http://dx.doi.org/10.1136/heartjnl-2012-303271] [PMID: 23339826]

[24] Schinkel AF, Vriesendorp PA, Sijbrands EJ, Jordaens LJ, ten Cate FJ, Michels M. Outcome and complications after implantable cardioverter defibrillator therapy in hypertrophic cardiomyopathy: systematic review and meta-analysis. Circ Heart Fail 2012; 5(5): 552-9.
[http://dx.doi.org/10.1161/CIRCHEARTFAILURE.112.969626] [PMID: 22821634]

[25] Syska P, Przybylski A, Chojnowska L, *et al.* Implantable cardioverter-defibrillator in patients with hypertrophic cardiomyopathy: efficacy and complications of the therapy in long-term follow-up. J Cardiovasc Electrophysiol 2010; 21(8): 883-9.
[http://dx.doi.org/10.1111/j.1540-8167.2009.01716.x] [PMID: 20132378]

[26] Vriesendorp PA, Schinkel AF, Van Cleemput J, *et al.* Implantable cardioverter-defibrillators in hypertrophic cardiomyopathy: patient outcomes, rate of appropriate and inappropriate interventions, and complications. Am Heart J 2013; 166(3): 496-502.
[http://dx.doi.org/10.1016/j.ahj.2013.06.009] [PMID: 24016499]

[27] Maron BJ, Spirito P, Shen WK, *et al.* Implantable cardioverter-defibrillators and prevention of sudden cardiac death in hypertrophic cardiomyopathy. JAMA 2007; 298(4): 405-12.
[http://dx.doi.org/10.1001/jama.298.4.405] [PMID: 17652294]

[28] Maron MS, Kalsmith BM, Udelson JE, Li W, DeNofrio D. Survival after cardiac transplantation in patients with hypertrophic cardiomyopathy. Circ Heart Fail 2010; 3(5): 574-9.
[http://dx.doi.org/10.1161/CIRCHEARTFAILURE.109.922872] [PMID: 20736440]

[29] Biagini E, Spirito P, Leone O, *et al.* Heart transplantation in hypertrophic cardiomyopathy. Am J Cardiol 2008; 101(3): 387-92.
[http://dx.doi.org/10.1016/j.amjcard.2007.09.085] [PMID: 18237606]

[30] Maron BJ, Gardin JM, Flack JM, Gidding SS, Kurosaki TT, Bild DE. Prevalence of hypertrophic cardiomyopathy in a general population of young adults. Echocardiographic analysis of 4111 subjects in the CARDIA Study. Coronary Artery Risk Development in (Young) Adults. Circulation 1995; 92(4): 785-9.
[http://dx.doi.org/10.1161/01.CIR.92.4.785] [PMID: 7641357]

[31] Semsarian C, Ingles J, Maron MS, Maron BJ. New perspectives on the prevalence of hypertrophic cardiomyopathy. J Am Coll Cardiol 2015; 65(12): 1249-54.
[http://dx.doi.org/10.1016/j.jacc.2015.01.019] [PMID: 25814232]

[32] Maron BJ, Olivotto I, Spirito P, *et al.* Epidemiology of hypertrophic cardiomyopathy-related death: revisited in a large non-referral-based patient population. Circulation 2000; 102(8): 858-64.
[http://dx.doi.org/10.1161/01.CIR.102.8.858] [PMID: 10952953]

[33] Maron BJ, Rowin EJ, Maron MS. Global burden of hypertrophic cardiomyopathy. JACC Heart Fail 2018; 6(5): 376-8.
[http://dx.doi.org/10.1016/j.jchf.2018.03.004] [PMID: 29724362]

[34] Daniel C, Iroegbu , Zhou , *et al.* Mitral Valve Insufficiency, a Constituent of Left Atrial Myxoma: Pathobiology, Physiopathology, and Pathophysiology of Left Atrial Myxoma. Are Long-Term Results Still Feasible 2018.

[35] Iroegbu DC, Zhou Z. Huge pedunculated left atrial myxoma with mitral valve replacement due to annular dilatation and concomitant coronary artery disease: A literature review. Ital J Vasc Endovasc Surg 2017; 24: 70-5.
[http://dx.doi.org/10.23736/S1824-4777.17.01289-X]

[36] Fifer MA, Vlahakes GJ. Management of symptoms in hypertrophic cardiomyopathy. Circulation 117(3): 429-439.
[http://dx.doi.org/10.1161/CIRCULATIONAHA.107.694158]

[37] Lopes LR, Rahman MS, Elliott PM. A systematic review and meta-analysis of genotype-phenotype associations in patients with hypertrophic cardiomyopathy caused by sarcomeric protein mutations. Heart 2013; 99(24): 1800-11.
[http://dx.doi.org/10.1136/heartjnl-2013-303939] [PMID: 23674365]

[38] Morita H, Nagai R, Seidman JG, *et al.* The impact of genetic testing on hypertrophic cardiomyopathy and heart failure. J Cardiovasc Transl Res 2010; 3: 297-303.
[http://dx.doi.org/10.1007/s12265-010-9188-4] [PMID: 20559778]

[39] Sébillon P, Bouchier C, Bidot LD, *et al.* Expanding the phenotype of LMNA mutations in dilated cardiomyopathy and functional consequences of these mutations. J Med Genet 2003; 40(8): 560-7.
[http://dx.doi.org/10.1136/jmg.40.8.560] [PMID: 12920062]

[40] Maron BJ, Piccininno M, Casey SA, Bernabò P, Spirito P. Relation of extreme left ventricular hypertrophy to age in hypertrophic cardiomyopathy. Am J Cardiol 2003; 91(5): 626-8.
[http://dx.doi.org/10.1016/S0002-9149(02)03326-X] [PMID: 12615280]

[41] Spirito P, Bellone P, Harris KM, Bernabo P, Bruzzi P, Maron BJ. Magnitude of left ventricular hypertrophy and risk of sudden death in hypertrophic cardiomyopathy. N Engl J Med 2000; 342(24): 1778-85.
[http://dx.doi.org/10.1056/NEJM200006153422403] [PMID: 10853000]

[42] Elliott PM, Gimeno Blanes JR, Mahon NG, Poloniecki JD, McKenna WJ. Relation between severity of left-ventricular hypertrophy and prognosis in patients with hypertrophic cardiomyopathy. Lancet 2001; 357(9254): 420-4.
[http://dx.doi.org/10.1016/S0140-6736(00)04005-8] [PMID: 11273061]

[43] Christiaans I, van Engelen K, van Langen IM, *et al.* Risk stratification for sudden cardiac death in hypertrophic cardiomyopathy: systematic review of clinical risk markers. Europace 2010; 12(3): 313-21.
[http://dx.doi.org/10.1093/europace/eup431] [PMID: 20118111]

[44] Maron MS, Olivotto I, Betocchi S, *et al.* Effect of left ventricular outflow tract obstruction on clinical outcome in hypertrophic cardiomyopathy. N Engl J Med 2003; 348(4): 295-303.
[http://dx.doi.org/10.1056/NEJMoa021332] [PMID: 12540642]

[45] Berruezo A, Vatasescu R, Mont L, *et al.* Biventricular pacing in hypertrophic obstructive cardiomyopathy: a pilot study. Heart Rhythm 2011; 8(2): 221-7.
[http://dx.doi.org/10.1016/j.hrthm.2010.10.010] [PMID: 20951231]

[46] Lenarczyk R, Woźniak A, Kowalski O, *et al.* Effect of cardiac resynchronization on gradient reduction in patients with obstructive hypertrophic cardiomyopathy: preliminary study. Pacing Clin Electrophysiol 2011; 34(11): 1544-52.
[http://dx.doi.org/10.1111/j.1540-8159.2011.03193.x] [PMID: 21834852]

[47] van Dockum WG, Beek AM, ten Cate FJ, *et al.* Early onset and progression of left ventricular remodeling after alcohol septal ablation in hypertrophic obstructive cardiomyopathy. Circulation 2005; 111(19): 2503-8.
[http://dx.doi.org/10.1161/01.CIR.0000165084.28065.01] [PMID: 15867172]

[48] Brignole M, Auricchio A, Baron-Esquivias G, *et al.* 2013 ESC guidelines on cardiac pacing and cardiac resynchronization therapy: the task force on cardiac pacing and resynchronization therapy of the European Society of Cardiology (ESC). Developed in collaboration with the European Heart Rhythm Association (EHRA). Europace 2013; 15(8): 1070-118.
[http://dx.doi.org/10.1093/europace/eut206] [PMID: 23801827]

[49] Gregoratos G, Abrams J, Epstein AE, *et al.* ACC/AHA/NASPE 2002 guideline update for implantation of cardiac pacemakers and antiarrhythmia devices: summary article. A report of the American College of Cardiology/American Heart Association Task Force on Practice Guidelines (ACC/AHA/NASPE Committee to Update the 1998 Pacemaker Guidelines). J Cardiovasc Electrophysiol 2002; 13(11): 1183-99.
[http://dx.doi.org/10.1046/j.1540-8167.2002.01183.x] [PMID: 12475117]

[50] Gregoratos G, Abrams J, Epstein AE, *et al.* ACC/AHA/NASPE 2002 guideline update for implantation of cardiac pacemakers and antiarrhythmia devices summary article: a report of the American College of Cardiology/American Heart Association Task Force on Practice Guidelines (ACC/AHA/NASPE Committee to Update the 1998 Pacemaker Guidelines). J Am Coll Cardiol 2002; 40(9): 1703-19. [Most recently updated guidelines for implantation of pacemakers and defibrillators in adults and children]
[http://dx.doi.org/10.1016/S0735-1097(02)02528-7] [PMID: 12427427]

[51] Chatrath R, Porter CB, Ackerman MJ. Role of transvenous implantable cardioverter-defibrillators in preventing sudden cardiac death in children, adolescents, and young adults. Mayo Clin Proc 2002; 77(3): 226-31.
[http://dx.doi.org/10.4065/77.3.226] [PMID: 11888025]

[52] Gradaus R, Wollmann C, Köbe J, *et al.* Potential benefit from implantable cardioverter-defibrillator therapy in children and young adolescents. Heart 2004; 90(3): 328-9.
[http://dx.doi.org/10.1136/hrt.2003.014266] [PMID: 14966061]

[53] Lee JC, Shannon K, Boyle NG, Klitzner TS, Bersohn MM. Evaluation of safety and efficacy of pacemaker and defibrillator implantation by axillary incision in pediatric patients. Pacing Clin Electrophysiol 2004; 27(3): 304-7.
[http://dx.doi.org/10.1111/j.1540-8159.2004.00432.x] [PMID: 15009854]

[54] Trappe HJ. The 'modern' implantable cardioverter-defibrillator: comparing it to those of the late 1980s. Am J Cardiol 1996; 78(5A): 3-8.

[http://dx.doi.org/10.1016/S0002-9149(96)00495-X] [PMID: 8820829]

[55] Calkins H, Ramza BM, Brinker J, *et al.* Prospective randomized comparison of the safety and effectiveness of placement of endocardial pacemaker and defibrillator leads using the extrathoracic subclavian vein guided by contrast venography versus the cephalic approach. Pacing Clin Electrophysiol 2001; 24(4 Pt 1): 456-64.
[http://dx.doi.org/10.1046/j.1460-9592.2001.00456.x] [PMID: 11341082]

[56] Gradaus R, Hammel D, Kotthoff S, Böcker D. Nonthoracotomy implantable cardioverter defibrillator placement in children: use of subcutaneous array leads and abdominally placed implantable cardioverter defibrillators in children. J Cardiovasc Electrophysiol 2001; 12(3): 356-60.
[http://dx.doi.org/10.1046/j.1540-8167.2001.00356.x] [PMID: 11291811]

[57] Magnusson P, Gadler F, Liv P, Mörner S. Causes of death and mortality in hypertrophic cardiomyopathy patients with implantable defibrillators in Sweden. J Cardiovasc Med (Hagerstown) 2016; 17(7): 478-84.
[http://dx.doi.org/10.2459/JCM.0000000000000359] [PMID: 26808417]

[58] Fishman GI, Chugh SS, Dimarco JP, *et al.* Sudden cardiac death prediction and prevention: report from a National Heart, Lung, and Blood Institute and Heart Rhythm Society Workshop. Circulation 2010; 122(22): 2335-48.
[http://dx.doi.org/10.1161/CIRCULATIONAHA.110.976092] [PMID: 21147730]

[59] Decker JA, Rossano JW, Smith EO, *et al.* Risk factors and mode of death in isolated hypertrophic cardiomyopathy in children. J Am Coll Cardiol 2009; 54(3): 250-4.
[http://dx.doi.org/10.1016/j.jacc.2009.03.051] [PMID: 19589438]

[60] Ostman-Smith I, Wettrell G, Keeton B, Riesenfeld T, Holmgren D, Ergander U. Echocardiographic and electrocardiographic identification of those children with hypertrophic cardiomyopathy who should be considered at high-risk of dying suddenly. Cardiol Young 2005; 15(6): 632-42.
[http://dx.doi.org/10.1017/S1047951105001824] [PMID: 16297259]

[61] Cupples LA, Gagnon DR, Kannel WB. Long- and short-term risk of sudden coronary death. Circulation 1992; 85(1) (Suppl.): I11-8.
[PMID: 1370216]

[62] Chiuve SE, Korngold EC, Januzzi JL Jr, Gantzer ML, Albert CM. Plasma and dietary magnesium and risk of sudden cardiac death in women. Am J Clin Nutr 2011; 93(2): 253-60.
[http://dx.doi.org/10.3945/ajcn.110.002253] [PMID: 21106914]

[63] Tomaschitz A, Pilz S, Ritz E, *et al.* Associations of plasma renin with 10-year cardiovascular mortality, sudden cardiac death, and death due to heart failure. Eur Heart J 2011; 32(21): 2642-9.
[http://dx.doi.org/10.1093/eurheartj/ehr150] [PMID: 21606079]

[64] Deo R, Katz R, Shlipak MG, *et al.* Vitamin D, parathyroid hormone, and sudden cardiac death: results from the Cardiovascular Health Study. Hypertension 2011; 58(6): 1021-8.
[http://dx.doi.org/10.1161/HYPERTENSIONAHA.111.179135] [PMID: 22068871]

[65] Patton KK, Sotoodehnia N, DeFilippi C, Siscovick DS, Gottdiener JS, Kronmal RA. N-terminal pro-B-type natriuretic peptide is associated with sudden cardiac death risk: the Cardiovascular Health Study. Heart Rhythm 2011; 8(2): 228-33.
[http://dx.doi.org/10.1016/j.hrthm.2010.10.038] [PMID: 21044699]

[66] Deo R, Vittinghoff E, Lin F, Tseng ZH, Hulley SB, Shlipak MG. Risk factor and prediction modeling for sudden cardiac death in women with coronary artery disease. Arch Intern Med 2011; 171(19): 1703-9.
[http://dx.doi.org/10.1001/archinternmed.2011.328] [PMID: 21788534]

[67] Cerrone M, Priori SG. Genetics of sudden death: focus on inherited channelopathies. Eur Heart J 2011; 32(17): 2109-18.
[http://dx.doi.org/10.1093/eurheartj/ehr082] [PMID: 21478491]

[68] Whang W, Kubzansky LD, Kawachi I, *et al.* Depression and risk of sudden cardiac death and coronary heart disease in women: results from the Nurses' Health Study. J Am Coll Cardiol 2009; 53(11): 950-8.
[http://dx.doi.org/10.1016/j.jacc.2008.10.060] [PMID: 19281925]

[69] Arntz HR, Willich SN, Schreiber C, Brüggemann T, Stern R, Schultheiss HP. Diurnal, weekly and seasonal variation of sudden death. Population-based analysis of 24,061 consecutive cases. Eur Heart J 2000; 21(4): 315-20.
[http://dx.doi.org/10.1053/euhj.1999.1739] [PMID: 10653679]

[70] Moya A, García-Civera R, Croci F, *et al.* Diagnosis, management, and outcomes of patients with syncope and bundle branch block. Eur Heart J 2011; 32(12): 1535-41.
[http://dx.doi.org/10.1093/eurheartj/ehr071] [PMID: 21444367]

[71] Sawhney NS, Waggoner AD, Garhwal S, Chawla MK, Osborn J, Faddis MN. Randomized prospective trial of atrioventricular delay programming for cardiac resynchronization therapy. Heart Rhythm 2004; 1(5): 562-7.
[http://dx.doi.org/10.1016/j.hrthm.2004.07.006] [PMID: 15851220]

[72] Ponikowski P, Voors AA, Anker SD, *et al.* 2016 ESC Guidelines for the diagnosis and treatment of acute and chronic heart failure: the Task Force for the diagnosis and treatment of acute and chronic heart failure of the European Society of Cardiology (ESC). Developed with the special contribution of the Heart Failure Association (HFA) of the ESC. Eur J Heart Fail 2016; 39(3): 291-301.

[73] Magnusson P, Gadler F, Liv P, Mörner S. Risk markers and appropriate implantable defibrillator therapy in hypertrophic cardiomyopathy. Pacing Clin Electrophysiol 2016; 39(3): 291-301.
[http://dx.doi.org/10.1111/pace.12801] [PMID: 26681505]

[74] Cardim N, Galderisi M, Edvardsen T, *et al.* Role of multimodality cardiac imaging in the management of patients with hypertrophic cardiomyopathy: an expert consensus of the European Association of Cardiovascular Imaging Endorsed by the Saudi Heart Association. Eur Heart J Cardiovasc Imaging 2015; 16(3): 280.
[http://dx.doi.org/10.1093/ehjci/jeu291] [PMID: 25650407]

[75] Jarcho JA, McKenna W, Pare JA, *et al.* Mapping a gene for familial hypertrophic cardiomyopathy to chromosome 14q1. N Engl J Med 1989; 321(20): 1372-8.
[http://dx.doi.org/10.1056/NEJM198911163212005] [PMID: 2811944]

[76] Geisterfer-Lowrance AA, Kass S, Tanigawa G, *et al.* A molecular basis for familial hypertrophic cardiomyopathy: a beta cardiac myosin heavy chain gene missense mutation. Cell 1990; 62(5): 999-1006.
[http://dx.doi.org/10.1016/0092-8674(90)90274-I] [PMID: 1975517]

[77] Watkins H, Conner D, Thierfelder L, *et al.* Mutations in the cardiac myosin binding protein-C gene on chromosome 11 cause familial hypertrophic cardiomyopathy. Nat Genet 1995; 11(4): 434-7.
[http://dx.doi.org/10.1038/ng1295-434] [PMID: 7493025]

[78] Kimura A, Harada H, Park JE, *et al.* Mutations in the cardiac troponin I gene associated with hypertrophic cardiomyopathy. Nat Genet 1997; 16(4): 379-82.
[http://dx.doi.org/10.1038/ng0897-379] [PMID: 9241277]

[79] Poetter K, Jiang H, Hassanzadeh S, *et al.* Mutations in either the essential or regulatory light chains of myosin are associated with a rare myopathy in human heart and skeletal muscle. Nat Genet 1996; 13(1): 63-9.
[http://dx.doi.org/10.1038/ng0596-63] [PMID: 8673105]

[80] Landstrom AP, Parvatiyar MS, Pinto JR, *et al.* Molecular and functional characterization of novel hypertrophic cardiomyopathy susceptibility mutations in TNNC1-encoded troponin C. J Mol Cell Cardiol 2008; 45(2): 281-8.
[http://dx.doi.org/10.1016/j.yjmcc.2008.05.003] [PMID: 18572189]

[81] Thierfelder L, Watkins H, MacRae C, *et al.* Alpha-tropomyosin and cardiac troponin T mutations cause familial hypertrophic cardiomyopathy: a disease of the sarcomere. Cell 1994; 77(5): 701-12. [http://dx.doi.org/10.1016/0092-8674(94)90054-X] [PMID: 8205619]

[82] Olson TM, Karst ML, Whitby FG, Driscoll DJ. Myosin light chain mutation causes autosomal recessive cardiomyopathy with mid-cavitary hypertrophy and restrictive physiology. Circulation 2002; 105(20): 2337-40. [http://dx.doi.org/10.1161/01.CIR.0000018444.47798.94] [PMID: 12021217]

[83] Holland MJ. Transcript abundance in yeast varies over six orders of magnitude. J Biol Chem 2002; 277(17): 14363-6. [http://dx.doi.org/10.1074/jbc.C200101200] [PMID: 11882647]

[84] Hwang JJ, Allen PD, Tseng GC, *et al.* Microarray gene expression profiles in dilated and hypertrophic cardiomyopathic end-stage heart failure. Physiol Genomics 2002; 10(1): 31-44. [http://dx.doi.org/10.1152/physiolgenomics.00122.2001] [PMID: 12118103]

[85] Solomon SD, Wolff S, Watkins H, *et al.* Left ventricular hypertrophy and morphology in familial hypertrophic cardiomyopathy associated with mutations of the beta-myosin heavy chain gene. J Am Coll Cardiol 1993; 22(2): 498-505. [http://dx.doi.org/10.1016/0735-1097(93)90055-6] [PMID: 8335820]

[86] Nagueh SF, Kopelen HA, Lim DS, *et al.* Tissue Doppler imaging consistently detects myocardial contraction and relaxation abnormalities, irrespective of cardiac hypertrophy, in a transgenic rabbit model of human hypertrophic cardiomyopathy. Circulation 2000; 102(12): 1346-50. [http://dx.doi.org/10.1161/01.CIR.102.12.1346] [PMID: 10993850]

[87] Germans T, Wilde AA, Dijkmans PA, *et al.* Structural abnormalities of the inferoseptal left ventricular wall detected by cardiac magnetic resonance imaging in carriers of hypertrophic cardiomyopathy mutations. J Am Coll Cardiol 2006; 48(12): 2518-23. [http://dx.doi.org/10.1016/j.jacc.2006.08.036] [PMID: 17174192]

[88] O¨ stman-Smith I., Wettrell G., Keeton B. *et al.* Age-and gender specific mortality rates in childhood hypertrophic cardiomyopathy. Eur Heart J 2008; 29: 1160–1167.

[89] Maron BJ, Seidman JG, Seidman CE. Proposal for contemporary screening strategies in families with hypertrophic cardiomyopathy. J Am Coll Cardiol 2004; 44(11): 2125-32. [http://dx.doi.org/10.1016/j.jacc.2004.08.052] [PMID: 15582308]

[90] Wren C, O'Sullivan JJ, Wright C. Sudden death in children and adolescents. Heart 2000; 83(4): 410-3. [http://dx.doi.org/10.1136/heart.83.4.410] [PMID: 10722539]

[91] Hjalmarson A. Cardioprotection with beta-adrenoceptor blockers. Does lipophilicity matter? Basic Res Cardiol 2000; 95 (Suppl. 1): I41-5. [http://dx.doi.org/10.1007/s003950070008] [PMID: 11192352]

[92] Chorro FJ, Trapero I, Such-Miquel L, *et al.* Pharmacological modifications of the stretch-induced effects on ventricular fibrillation in perfused rabbit hearts. Am J Physiol Heart Circ Physiol 2009; 297(5): H1860-9. [Epub ahead of print, Sept 11]. [http://dx.doi.org/10.1152/ajpheart.00144.2009] [PMID: 19749168]

[93] O¨ stman-Smith I., Keeton B., Wettrell G. Effect of medical therapy in childhood hypertrophic cardiomyopathy with risk factors for heart-failure related death. Cardiol Young 2008; 18 (Suppl. 1): 10.

[94] Sherrid MV, Barac I, McKenna WJ, *et al.* Multicenter study of the efficacy and safety of disopyramide in obstructive hypertrophic cardiomyopathy. J Am Coll Cardiol 2005; 45(8): 1251-8. [http://dx.doi.org/10.1016/j.jacc.2005.01.012] [PMID: 15837258]

[95] Ho CY, Cirino AL, Lakdawala NK, *et al.* Evolution of hypertrophic cardiomyopathy in sarcomere mutation carriers. Heart (British Cardiac Society) 2016. [http://dx.doi.org/10.1136/heartjnl-2016-310015]

[96] Marian AJ. Experimental therapies in hypertrophic cardiomyopathy. J Cardiovasc Transl Res 2009; 2(4): 483-92.
[http://dx.doi.org/10.1007/s12265-009-9132-7] [PMID: 20560006]

[97] Axelsson A, Iversen K, Vejlstrup N, *et al.* Efficacy and safety of the angiotensin II receptor blocker losartan for hypertrophic cardiomyopathy: the INHERIT randomised, double-blind, placebo-controlled trial. Lancet Diabetes Endocrinol 2015; 3(2): 123-31.
[http://dx.doi.org/10.1016/S2213-8587(14)70241-4] [PMID: 25533774]

[98] Adhikari AS, Kooiker KB, Sarkar SS, *et al.* Early-onset hypertrophic cardiomyopathy mutations significantly increase the velocity, force, and actin-activated atpase activity of human β-cardiac myosin. Cell Rep 2016; 17(11): 2857-64.
[http://dx.doi.org/10.1016/j.celrep.2016.11.040] [PMID: 27974200]

[99] Green EM, Wakimoto H, Anderson RL, *et al.* A small-molecule inhibitor of sarcomere contractility suppresses hypertrophic cardiomyopathy in mice. Science 2016; 351(6273): 617-21.
[http://dx.doi.org/10.1126/science.aad3456] [PMID: 26912705]

[100] Stern JA, Markova S, Ueda Y, *et al.* A small molecule inhibitor of sarcomere contractility acutely relieves left ventricular outflow tract obstruction in feline hypertrophic cardiomyopathy. PLoS One 2016; 11(12)e0168407.
[http://dx.doi.org/10.1371/journal.pone.0168407] [PMID: 27973580]

[101] Abozguia K, Elliott P, McKenna W, *et al.* Metabolic modulator perhexiline corrects energy deficiency and improves exercise capacity in symptomatic hypertrophic cardiomyopathy. Circulation 2010; 122(16): 1562-9.
[http://dx.doi.org/10.1161/CIRCULATIONAHA.109.934059] [PMID: 20921440]

[102] Jensen MK, Prinz C, Horstkotte D, *et al.* Alcohol septal ablation in patients with hypertrophic obstructive cardiomyopathy: low incidence of sudden cardiac death and reduced risk profile. Heart 2013; 99(14): 1012-7.
[http://dx.doi.org/10.1136/heartjnl-2012-303339] [PMID: 23644300]

[103] Sherrid MV, Shetty A, Winson G, *et al.* Treatment of obstructive hypertrophic cardiomyopathy symptoms and gradient resistant to first-line therapy with β-blockade or verapamil. Circ Heart Fail 2013; 6(4): 694-702.
[http://dx.doi.org/10.1161/CIRCHEARTFAILURE.112.000122] [PMID: 23704138]

[104] Sorajja P, Ommen SR, Holmes DR Jr, *et al.* Survival after alcohol septal ablation for obstructive hypertrophic cardiomyopathy. Circulation 2012; 126(20): 2374-80.
[http://dx.doi.org/10.1161/CIRCULATIONAHA.111.076257] [PMID: 23076968]

[105] Altarabsheh SE, Dearani JA, Burkhart HM, *et al.* Outcome of septal myectomy for obstructive hypertrophic cardiomyopathy in children and young adults. Ann Thorac Surg 2013; 95(2): 663-9.
[http://dx.doi.org/10.1016/j.athoracsur.2012.08.011] [PMID: 23040828]

[106] Maron BJ, Maron MS, Wigle ED, Braunwald E. The 50-year history, controversy, and clinical implications of left ventricular outflow tract obstruction in hypertrophic cardiomyopathy from idiopathic hypertrophic subaortic stenosis to hypertrophic cardiomyopathy: from idiopathic hypertrophic subaortic stenosis to hypertrophic cardiomyopathy. J Am Coll Cardiol 2009; 54(3): 191-200.
[http://dx.doi.org/10.1016/j.jacc.2008.11.069] [PMID: 19589431]

[107] Ommen SR, Nishimura RA. What causes outflow tract obstruction in hypertrophic cardiomyopathy? Heart 2009; 95(21): 1725-6.
[http://dx.doi.org/10.1136/hrt.2009.174292] [PMID: 19628468]

[108] Maron BJ, Maron MS. The 20 advances that have defined contemporary hypertrophic cardiomyopathy. Trends Cardiovasc Med 2015; 25(1): 54-64.
[http://dx.doi.org/10.1016/j.tcm.2014.09.004] [PMID: 25446045]

[109] Morrow AG, Reitz BA, Epstein SE, *et al.* Operative treatment in hypertrophic subaortic stenosis. Techniques, and the results of pre and postoperative assessments in 83 patients. Circulation 1975; 52(1): 88-102.
[http://dx.doi.org/10.1161/01.CIR.52.1.88] [PMID: 1169134]

[110] Dearani JA, Ommen SR, Gersh BJ, Schaff HV, Danielson GK. Surgery insight: Septal myectomy for obstructive hypertrophic cardiomyopathy-the Mayo Clinic experience. Nat Clin Pract Cardiovasc Med 2007; 4(9): 503-12.
[http://dx.doi.org/10.1038/ncpcardio0965] [PMID: 17712363]

[111] Sigwart U. Non-surgical myocardial reduction for hypertrophic obstructive cardiomyopathy. Lancet 1995; 346(8969): 211-4.
[http://dx.doi.org/10.1016/S0140-6736(95)91267-3] [PMID: 7616800]

[112] Veselka J, Tomašov P, Zemánek D. Long-term effects of varying alcohol dosing in percutaneous septal ablation for obstructive hypertrophic cardiomyopathy: a randomized study with a follow-up up to 11 years. Can J Cardiol 2011; 27(6): 763-7.
[http://dx.doi.org/10.1016/j.cjca.2011.09.001] [PMID: 22000583]

[113] Veselka J, Jensen MK, Liebregts M, *et al.* Low procedure-related mortality achieved with alcohol septal ablation in European patients. Int J Cardiol 2016; 209: 194-5.
[http://dx.doi.org/10.1016/j.ijcard.2016.02.077] [PMID: 26896622]

[114] DeMaso DR, Lauretti A, Spieth L, *et al.* Psychosocial factors and quality of life in children and adolescents with implantable cardioverter-defibrillators. Am J Cardiol 2004; 93(5): 582-7.
[http://dx.doi.org/10.1016/j.amjcard.2003.11.022] [PMID: 14996583]

[115] Topol EJ, Traill TA, Fortuin NJ. Hypertensive hypertrophic cardiomyopathy of the elderly. N Engl J Med 1985; 312(5): 277-83.
[http://dx.doi.org/10.1056/NEJM198501313120504] [PMID: 2857050]

[116] Argulian E, Messerli FH, Aziz EF, *et al.* Antihypertensive therapy in hypertrophic cardiomyopathy. Am J Cardiol 2013; 111(7): 1040-5.
[http://dx.doi.org/10.1016/j.amjcard.2012.12.026] [PMID: 23340036]

[117] Healey JS, Toff WD, Lamas GA, *et al.* Cardiovascular outcomes with atrial-based pacing compared with ventricular pacing: meta-analysis of randomized trials, using individual patient data. Circulation 2006; 114(1): 11-7.
[http://dx.doi.org/10.1161/CIRCULATIONAHA.105.610303] [PMID: 16801463]

[118] Connolly SJ, Kerr CR, Gent M, *et al.* Effects of physiologic pacing versus ventricular pacing on the risk of stroke and death due to cardiovascular causes. N Engl J Med 2000; 342(19): 1385-91.
[http://dx.doi.org/10.1056/NEJM200005113421902] [PMID: 10805823]

[119] Lamas GA, Lee KL, Sweeney MO, *et al.* Ventricular pacing or dual-chamber pacing for sinus-node dysfunction. N Engl J Med 2002; 346(24): 1854-62.
[http://dx.doi.org/10.1056/NEJMoa013040] [PMID: 12063369]

[120] Lamas GA, Orav EJ, Stambler BS, *et al.* Quality of life and clinical outcomes in elderly patients treated with ventricular pacing as compared with dual-chamber pacing. N Engl J Med 1998; 338(16): 1097-104.
[http://dx.doi.org/10.1056/NEJM199804163381602] [PMID: 9545357]

[121] Toff WD, Camm AJ, Skehan JD. Single-chamber versus dual-chamber pacing for high-grade atrioventricular block. N Engl J Med 2005; 353(2): 145-55.
[http://dx.doi.org/10.1056/NEJMoa042283] [PMID: 16014884]

[122] Castelnuovo E, Stein K, Pitt M, Garside R, Payne E. The effectiveness and cost-effectiveness of dual-chamber pacemakers compared with single-chamber pacemakers for bradycardia due to atrioventricular block or sick sinus syndrome: systematic review and economic evaluation. Health Technol Assess 2005; 9(43): iii-, xi-xiii, 1-246. [http://dx.doi.org/10.3310/hta9430] [PMID: 16266560]

CHAPTER 5

Restrictive Cardiomyopathy and Heart Failure in Children: Inheritance, Structural, and the Morpho-molecular Changes

Iroegbu Chukwuemeka Daniel[1], **Qing Guan**[1], **Xun Wu**[1], **Wasti Binaya**[2] and **Jinfu Yang**[1,*]

[1] *Department of Cardiovascular Surgery, The Second Xiangya Hospital, Central South University, Middle Renmin Road 139, 410011 Changsha, China*

[2] *Department of Respiratory Internal Medicine, The Second Xiangya Hospital, Central South University, Middle Renmin Road 139, 410011 Changsha, China*

Abstract: Restrictive cardiomyopathy is an uncommon heart muscle disorder characterized by reduced diastolic volume and an impaired ventricular filling in the presence of a normal systolic function and normal or near normal myocardial thickness (progressive symptoms of heart failure) with various gene mutations having been identified in cardiac genes (desmin, α-actin, troponin I and troponin T). It is a clinically challenging type of cardiomyopathy due to it is diverse etiopathogenesis, and a heterogeneous group of myocardial diseases which usually result from an increased myocardial stiffness leading to impaired ventricular filling with an often-poor prognosis in infants, and children. Despite advances in resynchronization and pharmacological therapy, many patients progress to end-stage heart failure as congestive heart failure continue to remain a severe burden even in the Western World with patients been either candidate for a heart transplant or a left ventricular assist device therapy. This chapter will focus primarily on clinical practice for primary care physicians and pediatric heart failure cardiologist. It will also go further to highlight the clinical and functional characteristics of restrictive cardiomyopathy linked mutations within the troponin complex, as well as address both clinical and reported functional studies for known troponin mutations associated with restrictive cardiomyopathy.

Keywords: Adolescents, Cardiomyopathies, Children, Diagnosis, Diastolic dysfunction, Genetic diseases, Heart failure, Infants, Outcome, Prognosis, Pulmonary hypertension, Restrictive cardiomyopathy, Syncope, Surgery, Sudden cardiac death, Structural and functional changes, Transplantation, Treatment, Ventricular assist device.

* **Corresponding author Jinfu Yang:** Department of Cardiovascular Surgery, The Second Xiangya Hospital, Central South University, Middle Renmin Road 139, 410011 Changsha, China; E-mails: yjf19682005@csu.edu.cn, Dr.iroegbu_daniel@yahoo.com and Dr.iroegbu_daniel@csu.edu.cn

Jinfu Yang & Iroegbu Chukwuemeka Daniel (Eds.)

INTRODUCTION

Restrictive cardiomyopathy (RCM) is a myocardial disease characterized by reduced diastolic volume and an impaired ventricular filling in the presence of a normal systolic function and normal or near normal myocardial thickness [1]. RCM is also characterized by symptoms of progressive right- and left-sided heart failure. Although it is characteristics can manifest at any period in life (Neonates/infancy to adulthood), it is general overall prognosis, however, is poor in childhood especially in neonates and infants as most patients often require cardiac transplantation [2, 3]. Several acquired and inherited disorders may cause RCM, many cases remain idiopathic [4, 5]. Familial restrictive cardiomyopathy (FRCM) has been reported, but whether a distinct genetic entity exists remains uncertain [6]. The cardiac contractility of the human heart is governed by cardiac troponin (cTn; plays a vital role in the contraction and regulation of striated muscle) and tropomyosin (Tm), regulated available levels of intracellular free calcium ([Ca^{2+}] i), and thin filament regulatory proteins. These thin filaments are composed of cTn consisting of three subunit is which are located at regular intervals:

I. cardiac troponin C (cTnC)

II. Troponin I (cTnI; the inhibitory subunit, whose primary function is to prevent actin and myosin interaction in the absence of Ca^{2+}), and

III. Troponin T (cTnT; binds to Tm and also responsible for the transmission of Ca^{2+} binding signal from cTn to Tm).

Within the cTn complex, cTnC acts as a Ca^{2+} sensor which confers Ca^{2+} sensitivity to muscle contraction [7]. During systole, the rise in [Ca^{2+}] I allow binding of Ca^{2+} to the regulatory site of cTnC, which leads to the movement of Tm over the actin filament. It enables myosin to interact with actin, subsequently leading to the generation of muscle tension [8]. Alternatively, in diastole, the [Ca^{2+}] I levels decline, and Ca^{2+} dissociates from cTnC, allowing Mg^{2+} to bind to the C-terminal sites. It allows the muscle to relax and enables ventricular filling to occur. However, only cTnI and cTnT have been linked to RCM as no mutations in cTnC are yet to be identified. Furthermore, mutations in sarcomeric proteins disrupt the complex thin filament regulatory protein interactions which lead to enhanced contraction due to Ca^{2+} increased sensitivity, arrhythmogenesis, cardiomyopathies and even sudden cardiac death (SCD) [9].

RCM is a clinically challenging type of cardiomyopathy (due to it is diverse etiopathogenesis), and a heterogeneous group of myocardial diseases which usually result from an increased myocardial stiffness leading to impaired ventricular filling with an often-poor prognosis in infants, and children. It could be classified/divided into primary and secondary RCM, in which genetic inheritance could exist in both types. Primary RCM is usually inherited, and several mutations have been identified. Most of which are autosomal dominant (AD) [10]. According to the location of the lesion, secondary RCM is divided into myocardial diseases and endocardial diseases. Myocardial diseases are subclassified as Storage disorders such as hemochromatosis, and glycogen storage disorder (accumulated deposit is within the cells), and infiltrative disorders such as amyloidosis (abnormal accumulation of proteins "amyloid proteins" in the interstitial space). Endocardial diseases include hematologic diseases (Sickle cell anemia), chemotherapy-induced (anthracyclines), carcinoid, medication-induced (serotonin, ergotamine), and drug-induced restrictive cardiomyopathy. Other rare causes include post-viral myocarditis and muscular dystrophies [11], diabetic cardiomyopathy (mainly describing restrictive phenotype with concentric left ventricular (LV) remodeling and diastolic LV dysfunction). FRCM (primary RCM) will be discussed in the chapter.

This chapter will focus primarily on clinical practice for primary care physicians and pediatric heart failure (HF) cardiologist. It will also go further to highlight the clinical and functional characteristics of RCM linked mutations within the troponin complex, as well as address both clinical and reported functional studies for known troponin mutations associated with RCM.

EPIDEMIOLOGY AND PREVALENCE

The prevalence of FRCM is unknown. Within the broad category of cardiomyopathy, RCM a rare form of heart muscle disease and also, the least common in children, accounting for 2-5% of the diagnosed cardiomyopathies (occurs in less than one per million children). The average age at diagnosis is 3 to 6 years. In Europe and the United States, RCM accounts for less than 5% of all cardiomyopathies. However, RCM somewhat often affects girls more than boys. There is approximately 35% family history of cardiomyopathic cases worldwide. In most cases, the cause of the disease is idiopathic, although a genetic cause is suspected in most cases of pediatric RCM [12].

PATHOPHYSIOLOGY

For the heart to beat normally, the cardiac muscles must contract and relax in a coordinated way. Oxygen-rich blood from the lungs first travels through the atria (upper chambers), and then to the ventricles (lower chambers) of the heart. Though RCM was once often considered as an extreme form of HCM [13], the pathogenesis of primary RCM is mainly due to the accumulation of desmin and type III collagen and the increased sensitivity of muscle filament to calcium [14 -

16]. Familial cases are commonly manifested in an autosomal dominant inheritance pattern with incomplete penetrance. There are, however, over twenty reported genes known to be associated with RCM, but familial RCM caused by a single gene defect is the least common. Genes related to primary RCM include troponin (cTnI and cTnT), myosin light chain 3 (MYL2, MYL3), desmin (DES), myosin binding protein C (MyBP-C), and myopalladin (MYPN) [17]. The TNNI3 (one of the major causes of this condition) gene provides instructions for making cTnI, which is found solely in the heart. Therefore, mutations in the gene result in the production of a defective cTn complex. The cTn protein complex function is disrupted by the altered protein, which, in turn, prevents the heart muscle from completely relaxing. As a result, blood getting into the ventricles is not sufficient enough, leading to a buildup in the atria and lungs. Mutations in other genes associated with FRCM each account for a small percentage of cases of this condition.

FAMILIAR RESTRICTIVE CARDIOMYOPATHY

In individuals with FRCM, the heart muscle is stiff and cannot fully relax after each contraction. Hence, the inability to relax and fill with blood results in a "back up" of blood into the atria, lungs, and body reducing the amount of blood in the ventricles causing the symptoms and signs of HF. First signs and symptoms in children are extreme tiredness, fainting, and failure to gain weight and failure to thrive. Children who are severely affected often have increased blood pressure, an abnormal buildup of fluid in the abdominal cavity (ascites), unusual swelling or puffiness (edema), an enlarged liver, and lung congestion.

In some cases, however, the child may not have any apparent signs or symptoms, but they may die suddenly due to HF. Affected children only survive a few years after they are diagnosed without treatment. Also, children with RCM often present with symptoms of "asthma" or "repeated lung infections" and constrictive pericarditis (masking RCM) which could prove difficult for physicians to diagnose at first especially in 2-6 years old children. Furthermore, SCD is more prevalent in pediatric RCM with a two-year mean survival rate for pediatric cases reaching approximately 50% after diagnosis [18 - 21]. SCD is also prevalent in pediatric RCM cases that display ECG evidence of ischemia [18] (discussed in detail further in the chapter).

TROPONIN AND CARDIAC MUSCLE REGULATION

The functional roles of each cTn subunit is are distinct and involve complex short- and long-range protein interactions. The binding of Ca^{2+} to the regulatory site of cTnC evokes the minimal exposure of a hydrophobic cleft within the N-domain of cTnC. It enables the regulatory region of cTnI (residues 148–163) to associate with cTnC [22, 23]. Structural analysis shows that cTnI interacts with cTnC in an antiparallel manner [24, 25]. However, the association of cTnI with cTnC in the presence of Ca^{2+} facilitates the release of cTnI's inhibitory region (residues 128–147) from actin. When cTnI dissociates from actin, Tm changes it is conformation and allows for the full interaction of myosin heads with actin. Cardiac TnI has a unique feature absent in the fast and slow skeletal muscle isoforms such that it possesses a 30- amino acid N-terminal extension which contains two Protein Kinase A (PKA) phosphorylation sites (Ser 22 and 23) [26, 27]. Activation of PKA by β-adrenergic stimulation enhances the rate of cross-bridge cycling and increases the rate of Ca^{2+} uptake by the sarcoplasmic reticulum [28 - 30]. Both of these phenomena contribute to the lusitropic effect associated with phosphorylation by PKA [31 - 33]. Occasionally, troponin mutations may interfere with the processes involved with thin filament phosphorylation and diminish the subsequent Ca^{2+} desensitizing effects. The thin filament undergoes activation due to relevant associations coordinated by cTnT. The N-terminal region of cTnT anchors cTn to Tm and this interaction modulates ATPase activation when Ca^{2+} concentrations achieve threshold levels [34]. Cardiac TnT has two main interactions with Tm. The first is located in the N-terminus of cTnT and is Ca^{2+} dependent [35], and the second is located in the C terminal portion of cTnT which also interacts with cTnC and cTnI [36]. In addition to anchoring cTn to the thin filament, cTnT has a critical role in the activation of actomyosin ATPase activity [37]. When cTnT is combined with cTnI-cTnC, the actomyosin ATPase is activated in a Ca^{2+}-dependent manner. Critical to this process is the region of overlap that exists between TnT1 (residues 1–158) at the head-to-tail junction of two adjacent Tm molecules [38, 39]. These interactions confer cooperativity to muscle activation when Ca^{2+} reaches threshold levels [40]. Inhibition of contraction is dependent on cTnI; however, in the absence of TnI, both TnT and TnT1 can inhibit the actin-activated myosin subfragment-1 (S1) ATPase [41].

ISOFORM SWITCH, DISEASE ONSET, AND LETHALITY

During the development of the fetal heart, the presence, and expression of different isoforms of cTnT and cTnI vary. These changes expressed, underlines the various aggressive and early onset course of pediatric cardiomyopathies. The slow skeletal isoform of TnI is thereby a product of a distinct gene which is expressed and incorporated in the fetal heart. The effects of mutations in the cardiac isoform of TnI appear later, as regulated by the activation of cTnI gene expression. Mutations in the cardiac TnI gene that change cTn function would consequently alter the Ca^{2+} homeostasis of the cell and manifesting their deleterious effects shortly after birth. Cardiac TnT also undergoes an isoform switch. The fetal heart expresses a different isoform by alternative splicing of the

TNNT2 gene. The fetal isoform of cTnT (cTnT1) contains both exons 4 and 5, while the adult isoform (cTnT3) contains only exon 4 [42 - 44].

HEART FAILURE

Regardless of etiology, RCM patients have poor overall prognostic features with increased mortality due to progressive heart failure characterized by the impaired ventricular filling of either or both ventricles [5, 45 - 47]. Continuous-flow LV assist device (LVAD) therapeutic option should be considered at first in children with an HF (advanced or not) in order to improve survival and quality of life whether they are awaiting transplantation or as destination therapy [48, 49]. Although limited data exist in pediatric patients.

LVAD PUMP TYPES

The LVAD is systemically structured with cannulas (driveline) placed at the pump itself, the apex of the heart, and the aorta with an outflow conduit. The pump is tunneled with a cannula out of the body through an exit site to the batteries and a belt controller [49]. The use of HM II pump system is suitable for children compared to the HM XVE pump system because of the absence of a reservoir chamber and it is 1-way valves which making the device smaller [50 - 52]. Although, the ventricular continuous-flow output negatively impacts organ microcirculation [53, 54], endothelial function [55 - 57], inflammatory biomarkers [55], and nitric oxide production [58].

Indications, Risk Factors, and Exclusion Criteria for LVAD Therapy

Optimal and efficient LVAD implantation and outcomes depend on early recognition of HF symptoms by non-HF cardiologists, primary care physicians, and referral of patients to an HF specialist. Advanced HF is clinically defined as severe circulatory compromise requiring special care, mechanical cardiac support, continuous inotropic therapy, or heart transplant [59]. In pediatric patients with RCM, a heart transplant is always indicated to improve survival outcomes as compared to adult patients despite optimal medical therapy. Hence, patients listed for heart transplant irrespective of age are potential candidates for an LVAD implantation. The main clinical focus and the decision to proceed with LVAD implantation should conform to the projected trajectory of life. Various clinical scoring systems have been developed to predict HF prognosis (The Heart Failure Survival Score, and the Seattle Heart Failure Model score) although, no single parameter is a perfect predictor. At first, psychosocial state (intellectual disability, previous nonadherence, and chemical dependencies) of the child should be an integral part of the pre-implant evaluation which should be achieved with the help of a psychiatrist and a social worker. Although obesity increases the risk of driveline infection [60], it is only relative in children. However, the nutritional issues of the child should also be addressed before implantation to optimize outcomes [61]. Other relative specific exclusion criteria include adolescents and younger patients with severe pulmonary hypertension which could reverse after unloading the left ventricle with an LVAD [62, 63], or patients who have been treated for cancer and may require time before transplant [64, 65]. Of note, age does increase the risk for complications in children during and after LVAD implantation irrespective of the stratification scoring system/parameters used.

Further parameters indicating caution in LVAD implantation include recent septicemia, intracerebral bleeding, and coagulopathy. An active infection is contraindicated for an LVAD implantation. Aggressive treatment with an infectious disease specialist is advised as to it is often challenging to sterilize a seeded device with antibiotics [66]. Also, aortic regurgitation has been considered a contraindication to LVAD placement in the past. However, the aortic valve can be closed if necessary, by placing a coaptation stitch at the central portion of the cusps to ensure aortic valve competence [67, 68]. Atrial septal defects and patent foramen ovale not detected postoperatively can lead to right-to-left shunting after LVAD implantation and the development of paradoxical emboli. Therefore, proper investigations should be carried out preoperatively or intraoperatively, and repair should be performed during LVAD implantation [69].

LVAD as A Bridge to Decision

An LVAD can be used as a bridge to the decision in children unsuitable initially for a heart transplant. LVAD implantations help improve specific physiologic parameters (pulmonary hypertension) and/or gain enough malignancy-free time to be considered for transplantation [70].

LVAD as A Bridge to Recovery

The use of LVAD therapy leads to cellular and echocardiographic improvements [71] though, minimal clinical recovery occurs. However, the Harefield group reports sustained recovery [72, 73]; it is use as a bridge to recovery remains controversial and even an area of ongoing clinical investigation [74].

Complications Related to LVAD Therapy

Despite the therapeutic benefit is and improved outcomes with the use of LVADs, adverse post-therapeutic complications occur in patients during it is transient use phase (awaiting transplantation) or as destination therapy in others:

I. Right-sided HF [75, 76]
II. Pump thrombosis [77, 78]
III. Gastrointestinal tract bleeding [79].

OVERVIEW ON MYOCARDIAL INFARCTION AND CONSTRUCTIVE PERICARDITIS IN RELATION TO RESTRICTIVE CARDIOMYOPATHY

Raised cTn concentration in clinical practice are usually attributed to acute myocardial infarction and a crucial and invaluable step forward in the identification of high-risk patients with acute coronary syndromes. However, this typically generates diagnostic dilemmas for clinicians especially in children presenting with such increase cTn levels which often blind sights the attending physician to the fact that, cTn are also raised in heart failures caused by cardiomyopathies [80 - 82]. On the other hand, the differentiation of RCM and constrictive pericarditis has been a perennial problem in clinical cardiology (Table **1**). It is further bolstered by the fact that, though constrictive pericarditis requires surgical treatment and is usually curable, while RCM can be treated adequately only with medical therapy which often responds unsatisfactorily is however only favorable in adult patients. This is only compounded by the fact that; (i) an implanted LVAD and a compulsory surgical therapy (heart transplant) is key to improvement and survival in pediatric patients and (ii) an exploratory operation is the only feasible way to distinguish the two although only in a few cases.

Varieties of Constrictive Pericarditis (Table 2)

I. Typical forms

(a) chronic (calcific, rigid shell)

(b) subacute (non-calcific, elastic)

II. Localized

III. Effusive-constrictive

IV. Occult

Clinical Parameters Which Help differentiate Constrictive Pericarditis from Restrictive Cardiomyopathy (Table 3)

I. History—active pericarditis

II. Examination— paradoxical pulse, Friedreich's sign

III. Electrocardiography (ECG)—the absence of intraventricular conduction defect

IV. Chest radiograph—pericardial calcification

V. Computer tomography/Magnetic resonance imaging—thickened pericardium

VI. Echocardiogram—septal notch

VII. Doppler—ventricular interdependence

VIII. Cardiac catheterization—close equilibration of diastolic pressures

IX. Biopsy—the absence of amyloid or other infiltrative diseases

Table 1. Comparison of specific features in subacute (elastic) and chronic (rigid shell) constrictive pericarditis AF- Atrial fibrillation.

Subacute	Chronic
Paradoxical pulse usually present, other signs of interdependence often prominent	Paradoxical pulse typically minimal or absent, other signs of reliance less prominent
Usually an XY waveform ("M" or "W" waveform)	Y is predominant, X sometimes minimal
Dip–plateau pattern less conspicuous, because the early diastolic nadir may not approach zero	Dip–plateau usually noticeable, because early diastolic nadir often reaches zero
Calcification usually absent	Calcification often present
Pericardial effusion sometimes present, generalized or loculated. Constriction is by the visceral pericardium	Absent pericardial effusion. The two layers of the pericardium are fused, and jointly constrict the heart
Normal P waves	Wide, notched and low amplitude P waves
Flutter rare or AF	Flutter common or AF

Table 2. Variant forms and features of constrictive pericarditis.

Effusive-constrictive pericarditis	Pericardial effusion is present, sometimes loculated, with constriction by the visceral pericardium
Occult constrictive pericarditis	Hemodynamics is normal at rest but assume the features of constriction after an acute volume load
Localized form	Limited constriction either to the right or left ventricle. Ventricular interdependence reduced or absent
Transient form	During the resolution of acute pericarditis with effusion, constriction develops but then resolves spontaneously over a few weeks

DIAGNOSIS OF RESTRICTIVE CARDIOMYOPATHY

The diagnosis of RCM is often challenging to establish and identify early in it is clinical course most notably in children due to either lack of symptoms or clarity of symptoms, and presenting differentials as seen in constrictive pericarditis. Therefore, once suspected, certain tests can help confirm it is diagnoses such as the use of an ECG (show abnormally large electrical forces due to enlargement of the atria) or electrocardiogram/ultrasound (identify the enlarged atria, normal sized ventricles, and normal heart function). In a more advanced state of the disease, blood pressure in the lungs (pulmonary artery pressure) can be estimated during echocardiographic studies. Cardiac catheterization is another valuable diagnostic tool and a step forward in confirming the diagnosis which helps measure the pressures within the heart chambers (relaxation period) and blood pressure in the lungs (help establish echo estimates) in the absence of any other structural heart disease. Although, this, however, should only be done in a much older child who is in a more stable hemodynamic state. Finally, once the diagnosis is certain, parents, siblings, and close relatives of the patient should be screened with an echocardiogram and examined for already presenting symptoms such as a new heart sound (gallop), chest pain with exercise, syncope, and decreased exercise tolerance.

TREATMENT OF RESTRICTIVE CARDIOMYOPATHY AND ASSOCIATED HEART FAILURE

Some children with RCM present with signs and symptoms of HF due to the abnormal relaxation properties of the heart muscle. Medications should include:

I. Diuretics oral or intravenously, *e.g.*, spironolactone, furosemide, metolazone, and bumetanide. Common side effects of diuretics include potassium loss and dehydration. Caution should be applied when diuretics are used. it is should only be given in doses to treat extra-abdominal and lung fluid without inducing excessive fluid loss as it would symptomatically cause low blood pressure.

II. Beta-blockers oral, *e.g.*, metoprolol, atenolol, propranolol, and carvedilol (slow the heartbeat and increase the relaxation time of the heart giving the heart time to fill better with blood before each pulse and decreasing symptoms created by the stiff pumping chambers). Common side effects of beta-blockers include low blood pressure, low heart rate, dizziness, depression, impaired school performance, and fatigue.

III. Anticoagulation medications, *e.g.*, Less stronger anticoagulants (dipyridamole and aspirin) or much stronger anticoagulants (Heparin, warfarin, and enoxaparin). They require careful monitoring with regular blood testing and are only included in medical therapy when there is a reasonable suspicion of the risk of blood clots, which can eventually lead to stroke. The choice of anticoagulants used also depends on the risk score of blood clots formation. Common side effects include excessive bruising or bleeding from otherwise minor skin injuries and interaction with other medications. Dietary intake of the child should also be monitored as dietary changes affect anticoagulation blood levels such as in warfarin.

Table 3. Features useful in differentiating constrictive pericarditis from restrictive cardiomyopathy.

Feature	Constrictive Pericarditis	Restrictive Cardiomyopathy
Past medical history	Previous pericarditis, cardiac surgery, trauma, radiotherapy, connective tissue disease	These items are rare
Jugular venous waveform	X and Y dips brief and "flicking," not conspicuous positive waves	X and Y dips less brief may have conspicuous A wave or V wave
Extra sounds in diastole	Early S3, and No S4	Later S3, and S4 in some cases
Mitral or tricuspid regurgitation	Usually absent	Often present
ECG	P waves reflect intra-atrial conduction delay. AV or IV conduction defects rare	P waves reflect left or right atrial hypertrophy or overload. AV or IV conduction defects not unusual
Chest radiograph	18–25%	Rare
Septal ventricular movement in diastole	Seen in most cases	Seen only occasionally
Ventricular septal movement towards the left ventricle with respiration	notable movement	Little movement
Atrial enlargement	Mild or moderate	Obvious
Mitral and tricuspid respiratory velocity flow variation	> 23%	<13%
Diastolic pressures equilibrium in all cardiac chambers	Within 5 mm Hg in all cases	Within 5 mm Hg in few cases
Dip–plateau waveform	End-diastolic pressure more than one-third of systolic pressure in many cases	End-diastolic pressure often less than one-third of systolic pressure
Right ventricular systolic peak pressures	<60 mm Hg/< 40 mm Hg	<40/>60mm Hg
Discordant ventricular respiratory systolic peak pressures	out-of-phase	in-phase
Paradoxical pulse	Mild to a moderate degree	Nearly absent

(Table 3) cont.....

Feature	Constrictive Pericarditis	Restrictive Cardiomyopathy
MR/CT imaging	In some cases, it shows thick a pericardium	Shows thick pericardium only rarely
EMB	Normal	In some cases, it indicates amyloid disease

EMB- Endomyocardial biopsy, CT- Computer Tomography, ECG-Electrocardiography, AV-Atrioventricular, IT-Intraventricular.

HEART TRANSPLANTATION

Heart transplantation is the only effective surgery and known intervention for the disease as there are currently, no practical, proven therapies for children with RCM particularly children who already have symptoms at the time of diagnosis or in whom increased lung blood pressure and HF exists. A heart transplant address both abnormal heart function as well as associated HF and increased lung blood pressure, giving the child a chance to return to a normal lifestyle. Although a heart transplant can cure symptoms of HF and significantly improve the child survival, it is a significant operation with considerable risks and long-term complications such as coronary artery disease, infection, side effects of medications, and organ rejection.

PROGNOSIS

The long-term prognosis for children with RCM varies depending on the symptoms at the time of diagnosis, associated HF, and the presence of increased blood pressure in the lung vessels. Once diagnosed, approximately 10 to 20% develop thrombotic or embolic events. The average 2-year survival rate for children with RCM without a heart transplant is 30–70%. Survival, however, increases significantly for children who are transplanted. Irreversible pulmonary hypertension has been the only significant risk factor associated with poor prognosis. Hence, it is of great importance that a heart transplant is given due consideration early to improve the survival rate of patients, as the waiting time for a donor's heart can be unpredictable.

LIVING WITH RESTRICTIVE CARDIOMYOPATHY

RCM affects many areas of a child's life, and it is essential that specific recommendations are developed and employed by the team caring for the child.

Psychological Issues

Adjusting to a chronic illness even for an adult is stressful, let alone a child. However, a child's reaction to having RCM mostly depends on the age of the child and the stage of his/her development. Discussions about the disease should be directed towards the specific concerns of the child. Pediatric psychiatrists play crucial roles at this point, helping children cope during their entire childhood life.

Family

Once a diagnosis is made, it is impact is felt throughout the child's entire family members. Psychologist, psychiatrist and other caregivers involved should try there possible best to let the family know they are not alone both in feeling and sharing the weight of responsibility when it comes to taking care of the child. it is the job of the whole medical team involved in the treatment and care of the child, including the psychologist and psychiatrist. The medical team should also, help the parents and caregivers keep track of clinic/hospital appointments, and maintain a normal family life too.

Physical Activity

The child should not be involved in competitive sports. Competitive sport is defined as an organized team activity for which training is required. However, a child with no associated symptoms of HF can be selectively allowed (individualized by the treating cardiologist) to participate only in recreational athletic activities (low-dynamic or low-static sports) which should be in a non-competitive situation.

Friends and School

All efforts should be made to allow the child to spend time with friends and also participate in recreational activities whenever possible for as much as he/she can. Also, the social, intellectual, and psychological benefit is of attending school cannot be overestimated. If medications and clinic/hospital appointments would interfere with school activities, it should, however, be adjusted and knowledge of both the patient and the physician responsible for the child's care. The school authority, teachers and the physical training tutor in school should all be aware of the child's health condition in order to help the child stay in school and keep up with his/her peers academically.

Diet

The child should keep a healthy diet. A low salt diet is recommended to avoid excessive fluid retention. In most cases, children with HF have delayed or poor growth; therefore, a diet that increases calories should be supported. Vegetables and cereals high in both potassium and magnesium should be added to the child's diet as some medications the child take leads to poor levels of potassium and magnesium. it is vital that the cardiologist works with a dietician to achieve satisfactory results.

CONCLUSION AND FUTURE DIRECTIONS

Though a rare type of pediatric cardiomyopathy, progress is being made in our ability to diagnose RCM in both molecular and clinical arenas. Therefore, it is knowledge and treatment can, however, not be overestimated for pediatricians. it is features and outcome are yet complicated when associated with HF in children. However, LVADs have revolutionized advanced HF treatment with newer devices allowing long-term treatment and transitioning patients not initially deemed to be transplant candidates transplant eligible.

Although complications and multiple challenges still linger in the field, future directions should be directed towards developing strategies to make LVAD devices much smaller and more durable for pediatric practice to diminish thrombosis, and minimize the complication rates which would further improve prognosis after surgery. Further future research directions should be aimed at:

I. Understanding RCM better as a disease process and it is characteristic features in relation to the disease outcome, which will only help improve management strategies

II. The identification of a more precise diagnostic genetic screening/testing methods, and novel genetic, molecular mutations which will result in a more accurate diagnosis and help guide the medical therapy.

III. Increase clinical trials which will lead to new drug development and more effective therapies.

LIST OF ABBREVIATIONS

cTn Cardiac Troponin

cTnC Cardiac Troponin C

ECG Electrocardiography

FRCM Familiar Restrictive Cardiomyopathy

HF Heart Failure

LV Intracellular Free Calcium [(Ca^{2+}) i] Left Ventricular

LVAD Left Ventricular Assist Device

RCM Restrictive Cardiomyopathy

SCD Sudden Cardiac Death

Tm Tropomyosin

cTnI Troponin I

cTnT Troponin T

CONSENT FOR PUBLICATION

Not applicable.

CONFLICT OF INTEREST

The authors confirm that this chapter contents have no conflict of interest.

ACKNOWLEDGEMENTS

Declared none.

REFERENCE

[1] Richardson P, McKenna W, Bristow M, *et al.* Report of the 1995 World Health Organization/International Society and Federation of Cardiology Task Force on the Definition and Classification of cardiomyopathies. Circulation 1996; 93(5): 841-2. [http://dx.doi.org/10.1161/01.CIR.93.5.841] [PMID: 8598070]

[2] Rivenes SM, Kearney DL, Smith EO, Towbin JA, Denfield SW. Sudden death and cardiovascular collapse in children with restrictive cardiomyopathy. Circulation 2000; 102(8): 876-82. [http://dx.doi.org/10.1161/01.CIR.102.8.876] [PMID: 10952956]

[3] Siegel RJ, Shah PK, Fishbein MC. Idiopathic restrictive cardiomyopathy. Circulation 1984; 70(2): 165-9. [http://dx.doi.org/10.1161/01.CIR.70.2.165] [PMID: 6733871]

[4] Keren A, Popp RL. Assignment of patients into the classification of cardiomyopathies. Circulation 1992; 86(5): 1622-33. [http://dx.doi.org/10.1161/01.CIR.86.5.1622] [PMID: 1423973]

[5] Kushwaha SS, Fallon JT, Fuster V. Restrictive cardiomyopathy. N Engl J Med 1997; 336(4): 267-76. [http://dx.doi.org/10.1056/NEJM199701233360407] [PMID: 8995091]

[6] Fitzpatrick AP, Shapiro LM, Rickards AF, Poole-Wilson PA. Familial restrictive cardiomyopathy with atrioventricular block and skeletal myopathy. Br Heart J 1990; 63(2): 114-8. [http://dx.doi.org/10.1136/hrt.63.2.114] [PMID: 2317404]

[7] Gordon AM, Homsher E, Regnier M. Regulation of contraction in striated muscle. Physiol Rev 2000; 80(2): 853-924. [http://dx.doi.org/10.1152/physrev.2000.80.2.853] [PMID: 10747208]

[8] Gordon AM, Regnier M, Homsher E. Skeletal and cardiac muscle contractile activation: tropomyosin "rocks and rolls". News Physiol Sci 2001; 16(2): 49-55. [http://dx.doi.org/10.1152/physiologyonline.2001.16.2.49] [PMID: 11390948]

[9] Knollmann BC, Kirchhof P, Sirenko SG, *et al.* Familial hypertrophic cardiomyopathy-linked mutant troponin T causes stress-induced ventricular tachycardia and Ca^{2+}-dependent action potential remodeling. Circ Res 2003; 92(4): 428-36. [http://dx.doi.org/10.1161/01.RES.0000059562.91384.1A] [PMID: 12600890]

[10] Edwards CQ, Griffen LM, Goldgar D, Drummond C, Skolnick MH, Kushner JP. Prevalence of

hemochromatosis among 11,065 presumably healthy blood donors. N Engl J Med 1988; 318(21): 1355-62.
[http://dx.doi.org/10.1056/NEJM198805263182103] [PMID: 3367936]

[11] JurcuŢ RO, Bastian AE, Militaru S, *et al.* Discovery of a new mutation in the desmin gene in a young patient with cardiomyopathy and muscular weakness. Rom J Morphol Embryol 2017; 58(1): 225-30. [PMID: 28523323]

[12] Crotty TB, Li CY, Edwards WD, Suman VJ. Amyloidosis and endomyocardial biopsy: Correlation of extent and pattern of deposition with amyloid immunophenotype in 100 cases. Cardiovasc Pathol 1995; 4(1): 39-42.
[http://dx.doi.org/10.1016/1054-8807(94)00023-K] [PMID: 25850778]

[13] Hinton RB, Michelfelder EC, Marino BS, Bove KE, Ware SM. A fetus with hypertrophic cardiomyopathy, restrictive, and single-ventricle physiology, and a beta-myosin heavy chain mutation. J Pediatr 2010; 157(1): 164-6.
[http://dx.doi.org/10.1016/j.jpeds.2010.02.044] [PMID: 20394946]

[14] Zhang J, Kumar A, Stalker HJ, *et al.* Clinical and molecular studies of a large family with desmin-associated restrictive cardiomyopathy Clin Genet. 2001; 59: 248-56.
[http://dx.doi.org/10.1034/j.1399-0004.2001.590406.x]

[15] Davis J, Wen H, Edwards T, Metzger JM. Allele and species dependent contractile defects by restrictive and hypertrophic cardiomyopathy-linked troponin I mutants. J Mol Cell Cardiol 2008; 44(5): 891-904.
[http://dx.doi.org/10.1016/j.yjmcc.2008.02.274] [PMID: 18423659]

[16] Yumoto F, Lu QW, Morimoto S, *et al.* Drastic Ca^{2+} sensitization of myofilament associated with a small structural change in troponin I in inherited restrictive cardiomyopathy. Biochem Biophys Res Commun 2005; 338(3): 1519-26.
[http://dx.doi.org/10.1016/j.bbrc.2005.10.116] [PMID: 16288990]

[17] Gu Q, Mendsaikhan U, Khuchua Z, *et al.* Dissection of Z-disc myopalladin gene network involved in the development of restrictive cardiomyopathy using system genetics approach. World J Cardiol 2017; 9(4): 320-31.
[http://dx.doi.org/10.4330/wjc.v9.i4.320] [PMID: 28515850]

[18] Rivenes SM, Kearney DL, Smith EO, Towbin JA, Denfield SW. Sudden death and cardiovascular collapse in children with restrictive cardiomyopathy. Circulation 2000; 102(8): 876-82.
[http://dx.doi.org/10.1161/01.CIR.102.8.876] [PMID: 10952956]

[19] Chen S-C, Balfour IC, Jureidini S. Clinical spectrum of restrictive cardiomyopathy in children. J Heart Lung Transplant 2001; 20(1): 90-2.
[http://dx.doi.org/10.1016/S1053-2498(00)00162-5] [PMID: 11166616]

[20] Kimberling MT, Balzer DT, Hirsch R, Mendeloff E, Huddleston CB, Canter CE. Cardiac transplantation for pediatric restrictive cardiomyopathy: presentation, evaluation, and short-term outcome. J Heart Lung Transplant 2002; 21(4): 455-9.
[http://dx.doi.org/10.1016/S1053-2498(01)00400-4] [PMID: 11927222]

[21] Peddy SB, Vricella LA, Crosson JE, *et al.* Infantile restrictive cardiomyopathy resulting from a mutation in the cardiac troponin T gene. Pediatrics 2006; 117(5): 1830-3.
[http://dx.doi.org/10.1542/peds.2005-2301] [PMID: 16651346]

[22] Li MX, Spyracopoulos L, Sykes BD. Binding of cardiac troponin-I147-163 induces a structural opening in human cardiac troponin-C. Biochemistry 1999; 38(26): 8289-98.
[http://dx.doi.org/10.1021/bi9901679] [PMID: 10387074]

[23] Takeda S, Yamashita A, Maeda K, Maéda Y. Structure of the core domain of human cardiac troponin in the Ca(2+)-saturated form. Nature 2003; 424(6944): 35-41.
[http://dx.doi.org/10.1038/nature01780] [PMID: 12840750]

[24] Farah CS, Miyamoto CA, Ramos CHI, *et al.* Structural and regulatory functions of the NH_2- and COOH-terminal regions of skeletal muscle troponin I. J Biol Chem 1994; 269(7): 5230-40. [PMID: 8106506]

[25] Murakami K, Yumoto F, Ohki S-Y, Yasunaga T, Tanokura M, Wakabayashi T. Structural basis for Ca^{2+}-regulated muscle relaxation at interaction sites of troponin with actin and tropomyosin. J Mol Biol 2005; 352(1): 178-201. [http://dx.doi.org/10.1016/j.jmb.2005.06.067] [PMID: 16061251]

[26] Moir AJG, Solaro RJ, Perry SV. The site of phosphorylation of troponin I in the perfused rabbit heart. The effect of adrenaline. Biochem J 1980; 185(2): 505-13. [http://dx.doi.org/10.1042/bj1850505] [PMID: 7396829]

[27] Noland TA Jr, Guo X, Raynor RL, *et al.* Cardiac troponin I mutants. Phosphorylation by protein kinases C and A and regulation of Ca(2+)-stimulated MgATPase of reconstituted actomyosin S-1. J Biol Chem 1995; 270(43): 25445-54. [http://dx.doi.org/10.1074/jbc.270.43.25445] [PMID: 7592712]

[28] Kentish JC, McCloskey DT, Layland J, *et al.* Phosphorylation of troponin I by protein kinase A accelerates relaxation and crossbridge cycle kinetics in mouse ventricular muscle. Circ Res 2001; 88(10): 1059-65. [http://dx.doi.org/10.1161/hh1001.091640] [PMID: 11375276]

[29] Ray KP, England PJ. Phosphorylation of the inhibitory subunit of troponin and it is effect on the calcium dependence of cardiac myofibril adenosine triphosphatase. FEBS Lett 1976; 70(1): 11-6. [http://dx.doi.org/10.1016/0014-5793(76)80716-8] [PMID: 136365]

[30] Solaro RJ, Moir AJG, Perry SV. Phosphorylation of troponin I and the inotropic effect of adrenaline in the perfused rabbit heart. Nature 1976; 262(5569): 615-7. [http://dx.doi.org/10.1038/262615a0] [PMID: 958429]

[31] Zhang R, Zhao J, Mandveno A, Potter JD. Cardiac troponin I phosphorylation increases the rate of cardiac muscle relaxation. Circ Res 1995; 76(6): 1028-35. [http://dx.doi.org/10.1161/01.RES.76.6.1028] [PMID: 7758157]

[32] Michele DE, Szatkowski ML, Albayya FP, Metzger JM. Parvalbumin gene delivery improves diastolic function in the aged myocardium *in vivo*. Mol Ther 2004; 10(2): 399-403. [http://dx.doi.org/10.1016/j.ymthe.2004.05.011] [PMID: 15294186]

[33] Zhang R, Zhao J, Potter JD. Phosphorylation of both serine residues in cardiac troponin I is required to decrease the Ca^{2+} affinity of cardiac troponin C. J Biol Chem 1995; 270(51): 30773-80. [http://dx.doi.org/10.1074/jbc.270.51.30773] [PMID: 8530519]

[34] Malnic B, Farah CS, Reinach FC. Regulatory properties of the NH_2- and COOH-terminal domains of troponin T. ATPase activation and binding to troponin I and troponin C. J Biol Chem 1998; 273(17): 10594-601. [http://dx.doi.org/10.1074/jbc.273.17.10594] [PMID: 9553120]

[35] Pearlstone JR, Smillie LB. Effects of troponin-I plus-C on the binding of troponin-T and it is fragments to α-tropomyosin. Ca^{2+} sensitivity and cooperativity. J Biol Chem 1983; 258(4): 2534-42. [PMID: 6822572]

[36] White SP, Cohen C, Phillips GN Jr. Structure of co-crystals of tropomyosin and troponin. Nature 1987; 325(6107): 826-8. [http://dx.doi.org/10.1038/325826a0] [PMID: 3102969]

[37] Zot AS, Potter JD. Structural aspects of troponin-tropomyosin regulation of skeletal muscle contraction. Annu Rev Biophys Biophys Chem 1987; 16: 535-59. [http://dx.doi.org/10.1146/annurev.bb.16.060187.002535] [PMID: 2954560]

[38] Maytum R, Geeves MA, Lehrer SS. A modulatory role for the troponin T tail domain in thin filament regulation. J Biol Chem 2002; 277(33): 29774-80.

[http://dx.doi.org/10.1074/jbc.M201761200] [PMID: 12045197]

[39] Tobacman LS. Structure-function studies of the amino-terminal region of bovine cardiac troponin T. J Biol Chem 1988; 263(6): 2668-72.
[PMID: 2963817]

[40] Hinkle A, Goranson A, Butters CA, Tobacman LS. Roles for the troponin tail domain in thin filament assembly and regulation. A deletional study of cardiac troponin T. J Biol Chem 1999; 274(11): 7157-64.
[http://dx.doi.org/10.1074/jbc.274.11.7157] [PMID: 10066775]

[41] Tobacman LS, Nihli M, Butters C, *et al.* The troponin tail domain promotes a conformational state of the thin filament that suppresses myosin activity. J Biol Chem 2002; 277(31): 27636-42.
[http://dx.doi.org/10.1074/jbc.M201768200] [PMID: 12011043]

[42] Perry SV. Troponin T: genetics, properties and function. J Muscle Res Cell Motil 1998; 19(6): 575-602.
[http://dx.doi.org/10.1023/A:1005397501968] [PMID: 9742444]

[43] Tobacman LS, Lee R. Isolation and functional comparison of bovine cardiac troponin T isoforms. J Biol Chem 1987; 262(9): 4059-64.
[PMID: 2951382]

[44] Gomes AV, Guzman G, Zhao J, Potter JD. Cardiac troponin T isoforms affect the Ca^{2+} sensitivity and inhibition of force development. Insights into the role of troponin T isoforms in the heart. J Biol Chem 2002; 277(38): 35341-9.
[http://dx.doi.org/10.1074/jbc.M204118200] [PMID: 12093807]

[45] Ammash NM, Seward JB, Bailey KR, Edwards WD, Tajik AJ. Clinical profile and outcome of idiopathic restrictive cardiomyopathy. Circulation 2000; 101(21): 2490-6.
[http://dx.doi.org/10.1161/01.CIR.101.21.2490] [PMID: 10831523]

[46] Mogensen J, Arbustini E. Restrictive cardiomyopathy. Curr Opin Cardiol 2009; 24(3): 214-20.
[http://dx.doi.org/10.1097/HCO.0b013e32832a1d2e] [PMID: 19593902]

[47] Kristen AV, Perz JB, Schonland SO, *et al.* Non-invasive predictors of survival in cardiac amyloidosis. Eur J Heart Fail 2007; 9(6-7): 617-24.
[http://dx.doi.org/10.1016/j.ejheart.2007.01.012] [PMID: 17350331]

[48] Miller LW, Pagani FD, Russell SD, *et al.* HeartMate II Clinical Investigators. Use of a continuous-flow device in patients awaiting heart transplantation. N Engl J Med 2007; 357(9): 885-96.
[http://dx.doi.org/10.1056/NEJMoa067758] [PMID: 17761592]

[49] Slaughter MS, Rogers JG, Milano CA, *et al.* HeartMate II Investigators. Advanced heart failure treated with continuous-flow left ventricular assist device. N Engl J Med 2009; 361(23): 2241-51.
[http://dx.doi.org/10.1056/NEJMoa0909938] [PMID: 19920051]

[50] Pagani FD, Miller LW, Russell SD, *et al.* HeartMate II Investigators. Extended mechanical circulatory support with a continuous-flow rotary left ventricular assist device. J Am Coll Cardiol 2009; 54(4): 312-21.
[http://dx.doi.org/10.1016/j.jacc.2009.03.055] [PMID: 19608028]

[51] Frazier OH, Rose EA, Oz MC, *et al.* HeartMate LVAS Investigators. Left Ventricular Assist System. Multicenter clinical evaluation of the HeartMate vented electric left ventricular assist system in patients awaiting heart transplantation. J Thorac Cardiovasc Surg 2001; 122(6): 1186-95.
[http://dx.doi.org/10.1067/mtc.2001.118274] [PMID: 11726895]

[52] Dembitisky WP, Tector AJ, Park S, *et al.* Left ventricular assist device performance with long-term circulatory support: lessons from the REMATCH trial. Ann Thorac Surg 2004; 78(6): 2123-9.
[http://dx.doi.org/10.1016/j.athoracsur.2004.02.030] [PMID: 15561049]

[53] Baba A, Dobsak P, Mochizuki S, *et al.* Evaluation of pulsatile and nonpulsatile flow in microvessels of the bulbar conjunctiva in the goat with an undulation pump artificial heart. Artif Organs 2003; 27(10):

875-81.
[http://dx.doi.org/10.1046/j.1525-1594.2003.00027.x] [PMID: 14616529]

[54] Sezai A, Shiono M, Orime Y, *et al.* Major organ function under mechanical support: comparative studies of pulsatile and nonpulsatile circulation. Artif Organs 1999; 23(3): 280-5. [http://dx.doi.org/10.1046/j.1525-1594.1999.06318.x] [PMID: 10198721]

[55] Hall JL, Fermin DR, Birks EJ, *et al.* Clinical, molecular, and genomic changes in response to a left ventricular assist device. J Am Coll Cardiol 2011; 57(6): 641-52. [http://dx.doi.org/10.1016/j.jacc.2010.11.010] [PMID: 21292124]

[56] Maltais S, Jaik NP, Feurer ID, *et al.* Mechanical circulatory support and heart transplantation: donor and recipient factors influencing graft survival. Ann Thorac Surg 2013; 96(4): 1252-8. [http://dx.doi.org/10.1016/j.athoracsur.2013.05.043] [PMID: 23915592]

[57] Thacher T, Gambillara V, da Silva RF, Silacci P, Stergiopulos N. Reduced cyclic stretch, endothelial dysfunction, and oxidative stress: an ex vivo model. Cardiovasc Pathol 2010; 19(4): e91-8. [http://dx.doi.org/10.1016/j.carpath.2009.06.007] [PMID: 19733484]

[58] Cheng A, Williamitis CA, Slaughter MS. Comparison of continuous-flow and pulsatile-flow left ventricular assist devices: is there an advantage to pulsatility? Ann Cardiothorac Surg 2014; 3(6): 573-81.
[PMID: 25512897]

[59] Jessup M, Abraham WT, Casey DE, *et al.* 2009 focused update: ACCF/AHA Guidelines for the Diagnosis and Management of Heart Failure in Adults: a report of the American College of Cardiology Foundation/American Heart Association Task Force on Practice Guidelines: developed in collaboration with the International Society for Heart and Lung Transplantation. Circulation 2009; 119(14): 1977-2016.
[http://dx.doi.org/10.1161/CIRCULATIONAHA.109.192064] [PMID: 19324967]

[60] Zahr F, Genovese E, Mathier M, *et al.* Obese patients and mechanical circulatory support: weight loss, adverse events, and outcomes. Ann Thorac Surg 2011; 92(4): 1420-6. [http://dx.doi.org/10.1016/j.athoracsur.2011.05.085] [PMID: 21958791]

[61] Holdy K, Dembitisky W, Eaton LL, *et al.* Nutrition assessment and management of left ventricular assist device patients. J Heart Lung Transplant 2005; 24(10): 1690-6. [http://dx.doi.org/10.1016/j.healun.2004.11.047] [PMID: 16210148]

[62] Slaughter MS. Implantation of the HeartWare left ventricular assist device. Semin Thorac Cardiovasc Surg 2011; 23(3): 245-7.
[http://dx.doi.org/10.1053/j.semtcvs.2011.07.008] [PMID: 22172363]

[63] Krabatsch T, Hennig E, Stepanenko A, *et al.* Evaluation of the HeartWare HVAD centrifugal pump for right ventricular assistance in an *in vitro* model. ASAIO J 2011; 57(3): 183-7. [http://dx.doi.org/10.1097/MAT.0b013e318211ba2b] [PMID: 21336105]

[64] Otterstad JE, Ford I. The effect of carvedilol in patients with impaired left ventricular systolic function following an acute myocardial infarction. How do the treatment effects on total mortality and recurrent myocardial infarction in CAPRICORN compare with previous beta-blocker trials? Eur J Heart Fail 2002; 4(4): 501-6.
[http://dx.doi.org/10.1016/S1388-9842(02)00099-5] [PMID: 12167391]

[65] Ootaki C, Yamashita M, Ootaki Y, *et al.* Reduced pulsatility induces periarteritis in kidney: role of the local renin-angiotensin system. J Thorac Cardiovasc Surg 2008; 136(1): 150-8. [http://dx.doi.org/10.1016/j.jtcvs.2007.12.023] [PMID: 18603068]

[66] Miller LW, Guglin M. Patient selection for ventricular assist devices: a moving target. J Am Coll Cardiol 2013; 61(12): 1209-21.
[http://dx.doi.org/10.1016/j.jacc.2012.08.1029] [PMID: 23290542]

[67] Park SJ, Liao KK, Segurola R, Madhu KP, Miller LW. Management of aortic insufficiency in patients

with left ventricular assist devices: a simple coaptation stitch method (Park's stitch). J Thorac Cardiovasc Surg 2004; 127(1): 264-6.
[http://dx.doi.org/10.1016/S0022-5223(03)01301-1] [PMID: 14752440]

[68] De Praetere H, Jacobs S, Rega F, Droogne W, Meyns B. Can a central stitch over the Arantius' nodules provide a solution for preoperative severe native AI in LVAD patients. Int J Artif Organs 2013; 36(3): 220-4.
[http://dx.doi.org/10.5301/ijao.5000200] [PMID: 23404643]

[69] Peura JL, Colvin-Adams M, Francis GS, *et al.* Recommendations for the use of mechanical circulatory support: device strategies and patient selection: a scientific statement from the American Heart Association. Circulation 2012; 126(22): 2648-67.
[http://dx.doi.org/10.1161/CIR.0b013e3182769a54] [PMID: 23109468]

[70] Daneshmand MA, Rajagopal K, Lima B, *et al.* Left ventricular assist device destination therapy versus extended criteria cardiac transplant. Ann Thorac Surg 2010; 89(4): 1205-9.
[http://dx.doi.org/10.1016/j.athoracsur.2009.12.058] [PMID: 20338335]

[71] Maybaum S, Mancini D, Xydas S, *et al.* LVAD Working Group. Cardiac improvement during mechanical circulatory support: a prospective multicenter study of the LVAD Working Group. Circulation 2007; 115(19): 2497-505.
[http://dx.doi.org/10.1161/CIRCULATIONAHA.106.633180] [PMID: 17485581]

[72] Birks EJ, Tansley PD, Hardy J, *et al.* Left ventricular assist device and drug therapy for the reversal of heart failure. N Engl J Med 2006; 355(18): 1873-84.
[http://dx.doi.org/10.1056/NEJMoa053063] [PMID: 17079761]

[73] Birks EJ, George RS, Hedger M, *et al.* Reversal of severe heart failure with a continuous-flow left ventricular assist device and pharmacological therapy: a prospective study. Circulation 2011; 123(4): 381-90.
[http://dx.doi.org/10.1161/CIRCULATIONAHA.109.933960] [PMID: 21242487]

[74] Klovaite J, Gustafsson F, Mortensen SA, Sander K, Nielsen LB. Severely impaired von Willebrand factor-dependent platelet aggregation in patients with a continuous-flow left ventricular assist device (HeartMate II). J Am Coll Cardiol 2009; 53(23): 2162-7.
[http://dx.doi.org/10.1016/j.jacc.2009.02.048] [PMID: 19497443]

[75] Topilsky Y, Oh JK, Shah DK, *et al.* Echocardiographic predictors of adverse outcomes after continuous left ventricular assist device implantation. JACC Cardiovasc Imaging 2011; 4(3): 211-22.
[http://dx.doi.org/10.1016/j.jcmg.2010.10.012] [PMID: 21414567]

[76] Drakos SG, Janicki L, Horne BD, *et al.* Risk factors predictive of right ventricular failure after left ventricular assist device implantation. Am J Cardiol 2010; 105(7): 1030-5.
[http://dx.doi.org/10.1016/j.amjcard.2009.11.026] [PMID: 20346326]

[77] Kirklin JK, Naftel DC, Kormos RL, *et al.* Interagency Registry for Mechanically Assisted Circulatory Support (INTERMACS) analysis of pump thrombosis in the HeartMate II left ventricular assist device. J Heart Lung Transplant 2014; 33(1): 12-22.
[http://dx.doi.org/10.1016/j.healun.2013.11.001] [PMID: 24418730]

[78] Starling RC, Moazami N, Silvestry SC, *et al.* Unexpected abrupt increase in left ventricular assist device thrombosis. N Engl J Med 2014; 370(1): 33-40.
[http://dx.doi.org/10.1056/NEJMoa1313385] [PMID: 24283197]

[79] Crow S, Milano C, Joyce L, *et al.* Comparative analysis of von Willebrand factor profiles in pulsatile and continuous left ventricular assist device recipients. ASAIO J 2010; 56(5): 441-5.
[http://dx.doi.org/10.1097/MAT.0b013e3181e5de0a] [PMID: 20613494]

[80] Sato Y, Yamada T, Taniguchi R, *et al.* Persistently increased serum concentrations of cardiac troponin t in patients with idiopathic dilated cardiomyopathy are predictive of adverse outcomes. Circulation 2001; 103(3): 369-74.
[http://dx.doi.org/10.1161/01.CIR.103.3.369] [PMID: 11157687]

[81] Setsuta K, Seino Y, Ogawa T, Arao M, Miyatake Y, Takano T. Use of cytosolic and myofibril markers in the detection of ongoing myocardial damage in patients with chronic heart failure. Am J Med 2002; 113(9): 717-22.
[http://dx.doi.org/10.1016/S0002-9343(02)01394-3] [PMID: 12517360]

[82] Sato Y, Taniguchi R, Nagai K, *et al.* Measurements of cardiac troponin T in patients with hypertrophic cardiomyopathy. Heart 2003; 89(6): 659-60.
[http://dx.doi.org/10.1136/heart.89.6.659] [PMID: 12748227]

CHAPTER 6

Arrhythmogenic Right Ventricular Cardiomyopathy

Iroegbu Chukwuemeka Daniel[1], Ming Wu[1], Zhang Hao[2], Liu Jingsong[2] and **Jinfu Yang[1,*]**

[1] *Department of Cardiovascular Surgery, The Second Xiangya Hospital, Central South University, Middle Renmin Road 139, 410011 Changsha, China*

[2] *Department of Thoracic and Cardiovascular Surgery, Affiliated Hospital of Xuzhou Medical University, Xuzhou, 99 Huaihai Road West Xuzhou, Jiangsu Province 221000, China*

Abstract: Arrhythmogenic right ventricular cardiomyopathy is a myocardial disease that primarily affects the right ventricle where the right ventricular free wall is partially or almost entirely replaced by fatty or fibrofatty tissue, providing a substrate for life-threatening ventricular arrhythmias in young, apparently healthy individuals and athletes. However, whether fatty or fibrofatty infiltration of the right ventricle has been considered to be a sufficient morphologic hallmark of arrhythmogenic right ventricular cardiomyopathy is still a source of controversy as it is crucial that arrhythmogenic right ventricular cardiomyopathy is kept distinct from both fatty infiltrations of the right ventricle and Adipositas cordis. The autosomal dominant inheritance pattern is typical of this myocardial disease, and the identification of causative mutations in cell adhesion proteins has shed new light on its pathogenesis with familiar studies highlighting the need to broaden the diagnostic criteria, which are highly specific but lacking in sensitivity. This chapter will provide a detailed insight into arrhythmogenic right ventricular cardiomyopathies pathology, pathophysiology, clinical presentations, diagnosis, and management. It will however also highlight the genetic basis of arrhythmogenic right ventricular cardiomyopathy, risk stratification, phenotypic manifestations, and arrhythmia mechanisms with an analytical review of the evolving role of cardiac magnetic resonance and late gadolinium enhancement with contrast-enhanced imaging in the diagnostic workup of arrhythmogenic right ventricular cardiomyopathy.

Keywords: Arrhythmia, Adipositas, Cardiomyopathy, Cather ablation, Desmosomes, Death, Defibrillator, Diagnosis, Electrocardiography, Electrophysiology, Genetics, Heart failure, Pathology, Pathophysiology, Prevention, Right ventricle, Sudden cardiac death, Tachyarrhythmias.

* **Corresponding author Jinfu Yang:** Department of Cardiovascular Surgery, The Second Xiangya Hospital, Central South University, Middle Renmin Road 139, 410011 Changsha, China; E-mails: yjf19682005@csu.edu.cn, Dr.iroegbu_daniel@yahoo.com andDr.iroegbu_daniel@csu.edu.cn

Jinfu Yang & Iroegbu Chukwuemeka Daniel (Eds.)

INTRODUCTION

Arrhythmogenic right ventricular cardiomyopathy (ARVC) is a myocardial disease that primarily affects the right ventricle (RV) where the RV free wall is partially or almost entirely replaced by fatty or fibrofatty tissue, providing a substrate for life-threatening ventricular arrhythmias [1 - 5]. The human heart usually contains a varying physiological amount of fat (also called cor adiposum and Adipositas cordis) found mainly in the subepicardial region. Huge credit has always been given to the original description of the disease which was published in an article in 1982 although, previous French reports and that of two Italian pathologists, had once been described a few years earlier [2, 3, 6 - 8]. The two Italian pathologists in 1959 made an in-depth study in a series of fourth cases affected by fatty heart, comparing them with sixty non-adipose hearts found out that, the epicardial fatty tissue was way more abundant on the RV surface, in the furrows, and along the margins [8]. Despite the fatty infiltration of the RV, the RV myocardial free wall of the human heart is usually surrounded by fatty tissue particularly at the level of the apical, and the anterolateral regions separating the myocardial fibers by strands of adipose tissue. However, the boundary between the outer subepicardial fat and the inner myocardium in the healthy human heart is usually distinct, although a slight fuzzy border may be observed. Notwithstanding, fatty infiltrations of the myocardium can be described and sectioned into three different modalities [8]: (I) fatty tissue localized only around the vessels and nerves; (II) fatty tissue separating the muscular fibers, which are then subject to intense regressive alterations and; (III) fatty tissue separating the myocardium into coarse bundles.

Marcus *et al.* [2] in 1982, reported the first clinical series pointing out the peculiar fatty histological composition of the RV free wall. In their original series, aneurysms were first described in the so-called triangle of dysplasia (*i.e.*, apex, inferoposterior wall, and the anterior RV outflow tract). Furthermore, a marked decrease in myocardial fibers with myocardium usually replaced by fat was evidenced, with a sclerotic whitish thickened endocardium together with an inconstant amount of intramyocardial fibrosis. Noteworthy apart from the three modalities described earlier, Thiene *et al.* [3] identified two distinct patterns of ARVC based upon the nature of myocardial replacement as mostly fatty tissue (lipomatous or fatty pattern) or fibrous and fatty tissue (fibro-lipomatous or fibrofatty pattern). However, the present-day pathologic diagnosis is now based on histologic and gross evidence of fibrofatty or fatty transmural myocardial replacement, defined as a wave-front phenomenon extending from the epicardium towards the endocardium, sparing the trabecular myocardium [4, 5]. In the fatty variant (or lipomatous), the adipose tissue reaches the endocardium (transmural infiltration), and the wall thickness may even increase (pseudo-hypertrophy)

[3 - 5]. The infundibular and anterolateral regions are usually affected, whereas the posteroinferior wall appears normal. This ARVC fatty pattern is typically confined to the RV, sparing both the left ventricle (LV) and the septum, with only rare cases of aneurysms. However, in the fibrofatty variant, the wall is translucent and thin. Here, saccular aneurysms are normally visible at the triangle of dysplasia [3 - 5]. The involvement of the LV occurs in 40% and the ventricular septum in 15% of cases, which is distinctively different from the fatty variant. The fibrofatty variant is more prone to electrical instability, sudden cardiac death (SCD), and may progress with time to heart failure. Be it as it may, ARVC marked fat replacement of the RV versus fatty infiltration is however not enough to diagnose ARVC and two important histologic features are essential to providing a precise diagnosis: (I) significant fibrosis (replacement-type) and/or (II) entrapped degenerative myocytes within areas of fatty/fibrous tissue.

Nonetheless, a fatty heart and the fatty pattern initially described should be kept distinct from the pure fatty infiltration of the RV [9]. Also, pathologic conditions associated with fatty infiltration such as inherited myopathies (Duchenne/Becker muscular dystrophy), and chronic alcohol consummation as massive fat infiltration of the RV without any evidence of myocyte degeneration and fibrosis does not indicate ARVC because the myocytes are instead pushed apart other than been replaced appearing structurally normal. However, the diagnosis of SCD in a patient with an extensive RV fatty infiltration Q would rather be better, as it clinically does not mean a cause-effect relationship thereby, leaving the door open for other hypotheses on the final cause of death.

This chapter will provide a detailed insight into ARVC pathology, pathophysiology, clinical presentations, diagnosis, and management. It will however also, highlight the genetic basis of ARVC, risk stratification, phenotypic manifestations, and arrhythmia mechanisms with an analytical review of the evolving role of cardiac magnetic resonance (CMR) and late gadolinium enhancement (LGE) with contrast-enhanced (CE) imaging in the diagnostic workup of ARVC.

DISEASES NAME AND SYNONYMS

I. Arrhythmogenic cardiomyopathy (ACM).
II. Arrhythmogenic right ventricular dysplasia (ARVD).
III. Arrhythmogenic left-dominant ventricular cardiomyopathy (ALDVC).
IV. Arrhythmogenic right ventricular cardiomyopathy/dysplasia (ARVC/D).
V. Arrhythmogenic right ventricular cardiomyopathy (ARVC) (used in the chapter)

BACKGROUND

Definition

ARVC is a unique myocardial disease that primarily affects the RV with progressive dystrophy and fibrofatty replacement of the RV myocardium, clinically characterized by non-ischemic ventricular arrhythmias originating from the RV, posing a higher risk for cardiac arrest. It is also one of the major causes of SDC in young individuals and athletes.

Historical Notes

ARVC was first described by Giovanni Maria Lancisi in his book "De Motu Cordis et Aneurysmatibus" in 1736, where he reported a family case with a stem disease recurrence in four generations [10]. In 1961, Dalla Volta *et al.* further reported a case of "auricularization" of the RV pressure curve thereby emphasizing the peculiar hemodynamic picture of this non-ischemic heart muscle disease with RV behaving like an atrium [11]. However, it was not until the early, and late 80's that the first clinicopathologic case series of patients were reported by Thiene, Drs Marcus, and Nava [1 - 3]. Marcus *et al.* in 1982 reported the disease in adults, laying emphases on the fibrofatty replacement of the RV free wall, accounting for epsilon wave and the persistent originating arrhythmias from the RV with left bundle branch block (LBBB) morphology [2]. Between 1987 and 1988, Nava *et al.* first proved the familiar occurrence with an autosomal dominant inheritance pattern [3, 4, 10 - 15]. In 1988, Thiene *et al.* studied case series of SCD in young patients (≤ 35 years), with ARVC pathology mostly occurring during effort. They all showed a similar characteristically inverted T-wave in the right precordial electrocardiographic (ECG) lead, and a benign ventricular arrhythmia of LBBB morphology [3, 16].

After that, diagnostic imaging was then implemented to visualize the RV, either invasively through angiography [17] or non-invasively through echocardiogram [18]. Furthermore, major and minor diagnostic criteria's where proposed based on arrhythmias seen on ECG readings, repolarization abnormalities, tissue characterization at biopsy, structural alterations at imaging, RV dysfunction, and family history of sudden death [12] as the search for improved in-depth knowledge on the diagnostic procedures of the disease increased. In 1985, the first recessive variant of the disease was discovered in Naxos island, Greece consisting of a cardiocutaneous form (palmoplantar keratosis and woolly hair) [19], hence the name Naxos disease. ARVC first gene locus (ARVD1) was found in 1994 by Rampazzo *et al.* at chromosome 14q23 [20], which was described in detail by Basso *et al.* in 1996 [4]. In 1995, ARVC was included among cardiomyopathies in the revised World Health Organization (WHO) classification [21]. Thereafter, other genes encoding cell junction proteins were found such as plakophilin-2 [22], desmoplakin [23], desmocollin-2 [24], and desmoglein-2 [25]. Other variants of the disease were explained by the transforming growth factor β3 genes [26], and mutation of the ryanodine 2 receptors [27] allowing preliminary genotype-phenotype correlations to be made [28, 29].

MORBID ANATOMY AND HISTOLOGY

The most distinctive morphological ARVC feature is the segmental or diffuse lack of myocardium in the RV free wall been replaced by fatty or fibrofatty tissue. After replacement, the myocardium is interspersed with fibrosis, and the persistent cardiomyocyte strands become visible in the epicardial and the media-mural fatty layers with only the subendocardial layers preserved. Although at this stage, the diagnosis of ARVC during autopsy are overlooked mainly due to the fact that, the presence of fat interspersed with cardiomyocytes can be seen generally in a healthy adult heart as myocardial fat increases with age and body size, and the limit between pathological and normal fatty infiltration (fatty heart) is unclear [30, 31]. Unlike the fibrotic, aneurysmal dilatation, RV wall thinning, and the inflammatory infiltrates distinctive for ARVC, the fatty heart is characterized by almost or partial replacement of the same RV wall by fatty tissue, with predominant involvement of the apex and the infundibulum [31]. However, patchy acute myocarditis with infiltrates (mostly lymphocytes) and myocyte death over time is inevitable in a fatty heart [32] and are always present in two third of every case.

EPIDEMIOLOGY

ARVC is a leading cause of SCD in young athletes accounting for 11-22% of all cases [33, 34]. Although, this significantly varies on geographical area, 17% in the States [35], and 22% in the northern Italy [36, 37]. However, the different mode of inheritance and the genes involved explain its ethnic variation [38]. The estimated prevalence of ARVC in the general population ranges from 1 in 2000 to 1 in 5000 individuals; men frequently more affected than women, with an approximate ratio of 3:1 [39, 40]. The disease rarely manifests before the age of twelve or after the age of sixty years, with the median age of the disease onset set about thirty years of age [33, 41].

PATHOLOGY AND PATHOPHYSIOLOGY

The pathologic hallmark lesion of ARVC should not be confounded with similar heart diseases such as Uhl anomaly, a congenital heart defect where the epicardium is attached directly to the endocardium in the absence of an intervening fat as a result of RV myocardial failure to develop during early life [42]. The myocardial atrophy in ARVC is a genetically determined process that occurs progressively with time (Fig. **1**), as it starts from the epicardium and extends towards the endocardium to become transmural, resulting into progressive wall thinning. As a result, its pathognomonic gross features consist of single or multiple aneurysms, predominantly located in the triangle of dysplasia. The LV is less commonly involved, and the septum is relatively spared. However, its pathologic features range from a grossly healthy heart where only a careful histopathologic investigation can reveal ARVC features in one or both ventricles, to hearts with massive biventricular disease involvement.

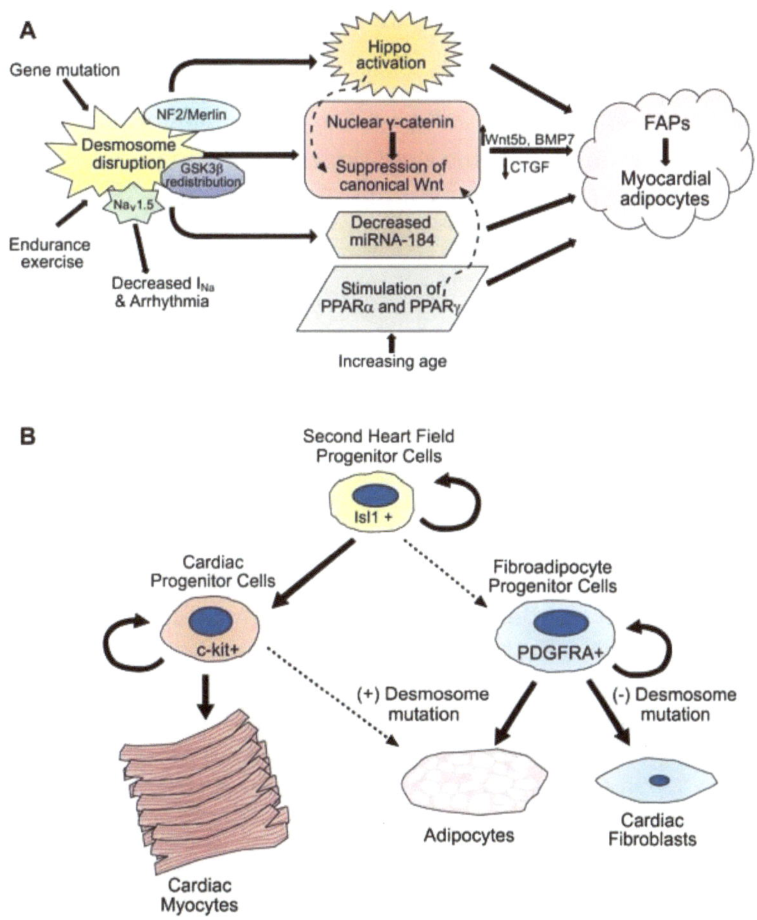

Fig. (1). Factors involved in the pathogenesis of arrhythmogenic cardiomyopathy (ARVC). A Progenitor cells area. B Simplified schematic of cardiac differentiation in ARVC. Sodium channel complex-(NaV1.5); NF2 (neurofibromin-2)/Merlin; Wnt (canonical Signaling); Wnt5b (noncanonical); BMP7 (bone morphogenetic protein-7); CTGF (connective tissue growth factor); PPARα (peroxisome proliferator–activated receptor-alpha); PPARγ (peroxisome proliferator–activated receptor gamma); FAPs (fibro-adipocyte progenitor cells).

CLINICAL PRESENTATION AND OTHER NON-FAMILIAR PRESENTING FORM OF ARVC IN DIFFERENT CIRCUMSTANCES/SITUATIONS

In the early description of ARVC classical form, RV is primarily mostly affected with possible later involvement of the LV. Recent clinico-genetic characterization of ARVC families have identified two new patterns; left dominant phenotype with early and predominant LV manifestation, and the biventricular phenotype with equal involvement of both ventricles. However, immunohistochemical studies show that ARVC is a global biventricular disease [43] although, overt functional manifestations of the disease usually start in the RV due to the RV poor ability to withstand (over) load in the presence of impaired function due to its thin wall. Physicians should also be alert to the possibility of ARVC in several non-familiar circumstances. However, the notion that ARVC is unlikely to manifest in later life is worth dispelling; as the condition may present at any age. Suspicion should be heightened by the presence of arrhythmia of RV origin, which can range from isolated ventricular extrasystoles to VT.

The Classical Form of ARVC

Typically, ARVC patients present with typical monomorphic ventricular tachycardia (VT) and rarely RV failure at first presentation. Initial presenting symptoms include dizziness, dyspnea, and syncope or near syncope. However, based on clinicopathologic and patient follow-up studies, four different phases can be described primarily affecting the RV namely;

I. Early or Concealed period, which is characterized lack of any apparent clinical change but subtle RV structural changes can be found. Although early, patients at this phase of the disease are still at risk of SCD, especially during heavy exercise.
II. Overt phase characterized by early symptoms but with palpitations and ventricular arrhythmias are ranging from isolated premature ventricular contractions to sustained VT and ventricular fibrillation (VF).
III. RV failure dominates the third phase, which manifests as reduced RV systolic function due to progressive loss of myocardium, RV dilatation but with a preserved LV function.
IV. The fourth phase also termed biventricular failure phase due to LV involvement. This phase may mimic dilated cardiomyopathy (DCM) and may require cardiac transplantation.

Non-Classic Form of ARVC

The non-classic form includes the cutaneous and the left dominant type of ARVC.

ARVC with Cutaneous Manifestations (Cardiocutaneous Disease): ARVC cardiocutaneous disease includes:

Naxos Disease: It is an inherited recessive stereotype association of ARVC with a cutaneous phenotype due to its characteristic palmoplantar keratoderma which develops in the first year of life when the infant starts making use of use their hands and feet, and the peculiar wooly hair which appears much later after birth [44]. Its cardiac manifestations are identical to ARVC in both histological and clinical studies [45] though, the cardiomyopathy clinically manifests in adolescence and shows 100% penetrance [46]. Clinical manifestations include typical syncope, dyspnea, VT but of LBBB configuration, ECG abnormalities, RV structural alterations, LV involvement, and SCD. Naxos disease is also a rapid progressive heart disease with adverse prognosis as compared to other classic and non-classic ARVC types, especially in young before the age of thirty [46].

Carvajal Syndrome: This syndrome also a recessive disease has been described in families from Ecuador, and India have similar cutaneous manifestations like that of Naxos disease with a predominantly LV involvement. A significant proportion of patient's symptoms clinically manifest in early childhood, and most of them died during adolescence [46, 47].

Arrhythmogenic Left-Dominant Ventricular Cardiomyopathy (ALDVC): ALDVC is distinguished from DCM by a propensity towards arrhythmia exceeding the degree of ventricular dysfunction [48]. Patients have fibrofatty changes, which predominantly involve the LV, syncope or presyncope, and shortness of breath [48, 49]. ALDVC is also characterized by ECG changes in the form of inferolateral T-wave inversion, and arrhythmias of LV origin sometimes explained by the patient as severe non-radiating chest pain.

Family Members of Patients with A Confirmed Diagnosis During Postmortem Examination or on Clinical Assessment

The incidence of SCD as the first clinical manifestation in some few cases coupled with the genetic etiology of ARVC underscores the importance of evaluating relatives for the disease. Though presentation in childhood is rare [50], systematic evaluation from early adolescence is recommended.

Family Members of Sudden Cardiac Death Victims in Whom ARVC Was Not Excluded During Postmortem Studies

In the absence of the indispensable opinion of a pathology expert when evaluating family members of an SCD victim, ARVC should be considered part of the differential diagnosis, as the disease may have been missed on postmortem without rigorous histologic and macroscopic examination of the RV.

Survivors of VF with No Previous Cardiac History

The exclusion of ARVD is mandatory in patients who have no evidence of ischemic heart disease. SCD and established diagnosis only after postmortem studies are observed in a few related cases, as cardiac arrest was the first manifestation of ARVD in less than 10% of live index cases [51, 52]. The underrepresentation of VT in some cases as a mode of presentation among patients reflects the poor rates of survival from many out-of-hospital cardiac arrests in ARVD patients.

Asymptomatic Patients, Especially Athletes, with Incidental Findings Compatible with ARVC during Cardiovascular Evaluation

ARVC is a well-documented and recognized cause of SCD during competitive sporting activities and endurance patients, though, not exclusive to these groups alone [3]. Screening conditions vary considerably among different countries, as ARVC is identified consistently in a substantial proportion of athletes, many of whom are asymptomatic [53], unfortunately, physiologic adaptations to obscure training diagnosis [54].

Relatives of Patients with Apparent DCM

Both advanced ARVC and familiar forms of the disease mimic DCM [51]. Therefore, the possibility of ARVC should be considered when assessing the relatives of patients with ARVC, particularly in the presence of a prominent family history of SCD.

EARLY HYPOTHESIS

I. The early first hypothesis by Basso *et al.* [4] suggested that the mechanism for myocardial atrophy and myocardial loss appeared to be the consequence of fibrofatty replacement (repair), and myocyte death (acquired injury) mediated by patchy myocarditis and
II. Trans-differentiation of the myocardium (This hypothesis assumes that myocardial cells can be changed from cardiac muscle to adipose tissue) [55].

CURRENT HYPOTHESIS

I. Abnormal cell-cell adhesion (desmosomal disease): Current understanding of ARVC indicates that it is a desmosomal disease. Desmosomes consist of three families of proteins (discussed further in the chapter) providing cells with the mechanical strength needed; hence, mediating cell-cell adhesion [56, 57].
II. Abnormal intracellular signaling and junction proteins: Suppression of the canonical Wnt/β-catenin signaling pathway [58] (also discussed further in the chapter).
III. Gap junction and ion channel remodeling [59] (also discussed further in the chapter).

MOLECULAR GENETICS

ARVC is primarily a disease of disturbed desmosomal function and a genetically determined heart disease because one or more first-degree relatives also display signs of the disease 50% of cases [60]. It is also been found to be encoded in different components of the cardiac desmosome, *i.e.*, desmocollin 2 (DSC2), desmoplakin (DSP), plakophilin 2 (PKP2), plakoglobin (JUP), and desmoglein 2 (DSG2). Noteworthy, mutations in other non-desmosomal genes have also been reported which includes; desmin (DES), titin (TTN), and transmembrane protein 43 (TMEM43), indicating genetic heterogeneity (Fig. **2**).

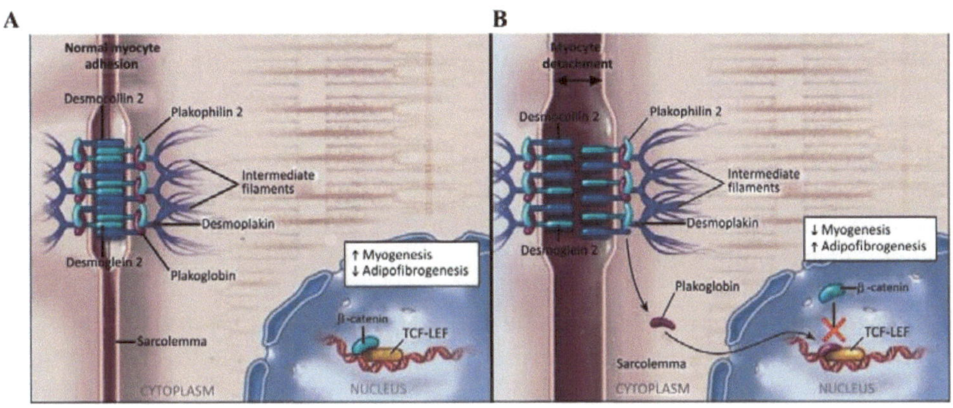

Fig. (2). Molecular genetics of arrhythmogenic cardiomyopathy. ARVC is caused by genetically defective desmosomes. The desmosome contains three major components: desmoplakin, transmembrane proteins, and linker proteins which mediate interactions between the desmosomal cadherin tails and desmoplakin, as shown in Panel A. Abnormal desmosomes confer a predisposition over time to disruption of the intercellular junction, as shown in Panel B (double-headed arrow), mostly under conditions of increased mechanical stress, such as sports activity.

Desmosomal ARVC

Autosomal Dominant Disease

Plakophilin-2: It is a protein encoded by the PKP2 gene [61] which is also expressed in cardiac muscle as well as skin, where it functions to link cadherins to intermediate cytoskeletal filaments. Plakophilin-2 is found in desmosome cardiac muscle structures located within intercalated discs [21]. Syrris *et al.* in 2004 [22] were the first to show that mutations in PKP2 constitute a significant cause of ARVC. Sensitive and Specific markers of PKP2 and plakoglobin mutation carriers in ARVC have been identified to include ventricular extrasystoles, right ventricular wall motion abnormalities, and T-wave inversions [62, 63].

Desmoplakin: Desmoplakin is an essential component of desmosome structure in epidermal cells and cardiac muscle and encoded by the DSP gene [64] which function to maintain the structural integrity at adjacent cell contacts. In cardiac myocardium, desmoplakin is centralized to intercalated discs, which enables cardiac cells to function in a mechanically syncytial coordinated structure. Mutations in this gene are the cause of ARVC and also DCM [65, 66].

Desmoglein-2: It is also highly expressed in epithelial cells and cardiomyocytes encoded by the DSG2 gene [67]. Desmoglein-2 is localized to desmosome structures structurally adhering adjacent cells together at regions of cell-cell contact. In cardiac muscle, these regions are specific regions known as intercalated discs. Mutations in desmoglein-2 are associated with ARVC [68] and also familial DCM [69].

Desmocollin-2: It is a cadherin-type protein linking adjacent cells together in desmosomes and encoded by the DSC2 gene [70]. Desmocollin-2 is the only desmocollin isoform widely expressed in cardiac muscle, where it localizes to intercalated discs. Mutations in DSC2 is linked to ARVC [22].

Plakoglobin: Plakoglobin was first described in a German family [71] where affected individuals carry an extra serine residue inserted at position 39 in the N-terminus of plakoglobin (S39_K40insS) [71]. However, none of the individuals affected by the S39_K40insS mutation showed apparent cutaneous abnormalities, in contrast to defects seen in patients with Naxos disease.

Autosomal Recessive Disease

Plakoglobin: It is also known as gamma-catenin or junction plakoglobin (JUP) encoded by the JUP gene is an adherence junction and a cytoplasmic component of desmosomes located within intercalated discs of cardiac muscles which function is to join adjacent cells and anchor sarcomeres in cardiac muscle. Mutations in JUP specifically cause an autosomal recessive form of the disease referred to as Naxos disease. Noninvasive cardiac screening identified frequent ventricular extrasystoles, abnormal RV wall motion, and T-wave inversion as a specific and sensitive marker of JUP mutations [62].

Desmoplakin: It is an autosomal recessive mutation as a result of a frameshift (7901delG) in DSP, which eventually results in Carvajal syndrome and DCM [46].

Non-desmosomal ARVC

Transforming Growth Factor Beta-3 (TGFβ3): It is a superfamily of cytokines mapped to chromosome 14 regulating different physiological processes, such as homeostasis, chemotaxis, embryonic development, wound healing, and cell cycle control [72]. TGFβs proliferate and stimulate mesenchymal cells to produce extracellular matrix components [73] and the mutation TGFβ3 gene genetically linked to ARVC [26].

Cardiac Ryanodine Receptor (RyR2): Mutations in RYR2 gene is associated with three inherited cardiac diseases: Familial polymorphic VT (FPVT) [74], catecholaminergic polymorphic VT (CPVT) [75], and ARVC type II (ARVC/D2) [76]. Though only been described in one Italian ARVC family [27], RyR2 receptor is responsible for calcium release from the sarcoplasmic reticulum.

Transmembrane Protein 43 (TMEM43): It is also called luma encoded by the TMEM43 gene [77], it plays a vital role in maintaining a nuclear envelope structure by organizing protein complexes at the inner nuclear membrane. With a sex-influenced pattern of inheritance, the TMEM43 gene contains the response element for PPAR gamma, an adipogenic transcription factor. A missense mutation in the TMEM43 gene and the dysregulation of the adipogenic pathway regulated by PPAR gamma as a result of TMEM43 gene mutation explains the fibrofatty replacement of myocardium in patients with ARVC [78, 79].

Others: Few isolated reports show causal mutations in other non-desmosomal genes, such as Lamin A/C (LMNA), titin (TTN), desmin (DES), αT-catenin (CTNNA3), and phospholamban (PLN), sometimes with a clinical phenotype similar but not identical to ARVC, as to be considered phenocopies or overlap syndromes [80].

DIAGNOSIS

Diagnostic Criteria

Although till date, no single gold diagnostic standard tool exists, the best strategy consists of achieving clinical diagnosis through multiple sources of clinical information, such as family history, histopathologic (Fig. **3**), ECG (Fig. **4**), arrhythmic, angiography, MRI, or radionuclide scintigraphy (Table **1**), morpho-functional, and genetic findings. A scoring system in 1994 was proposed by an International Task Force [ITF] for the diagnosis of ARVC where the diagnosis is fulfilled in the presence of two major criteria, one major plus two minor, or four minor criteria from different categories [12]. Be it as it may, the proposed criteria by the ITF lacked sensitivity for identification of early/minor phenotypes, especially in the setting of familial ARVC, and has also not been useful in differentiating ARVC, and DCM or idiopathic RV outflow tract tachycardia hence a reversed diagnostic guideline was made in 2010. The reversed diagnostic criteria improved the specificity by diagnosing probands and first-degree relatives [81] with the inclusion of molecular genetic information (disease-causing gene mutation) as a major criterion.

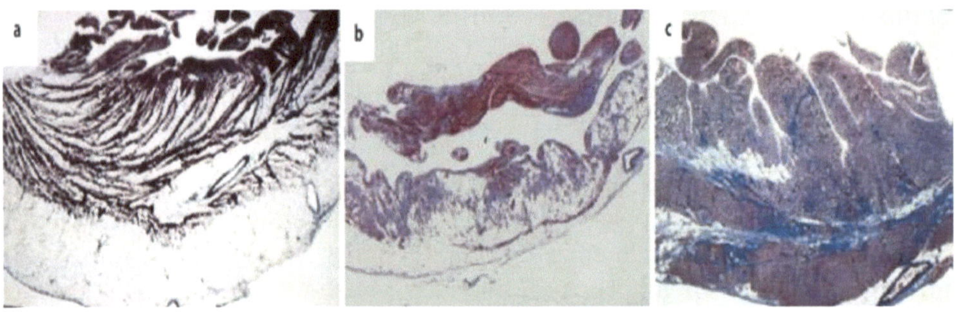

Fig. (3). Myocardial tissue characterization by histopathology. (a) Fatty infiltration of the right ventricular (RV) free wall in an obese patient; (b) transmural fibrofatty replacement of the RV free wall in a patient with arrhythmogenic right ventricular cardiomyopathy (ARVC); (c) mid-mural subepicardial fibrofatty (mostly fibrous) replacement of the left ventricular free wall in a patient with ARVC.

Clinical Manifestations

Clinical manifestations are essential in guiding diagnoses. However, the phenotypic expression of ARVC varies considerably, ranging from symptomatic patients experiencing various arrhythmic episodes or undergoing a heart transplant due to refractory heart failure to asymptomatic family members with no arrhythmias and concealed structural abnormalities [36, 82, 83]. Common clinical presentations include; syncopal episodes, palpitations and finally, cardiac arrest. SCD may occur though mostly in young people, competitive athletes, and unexpectedly in previously asymptomatic individuals [84].

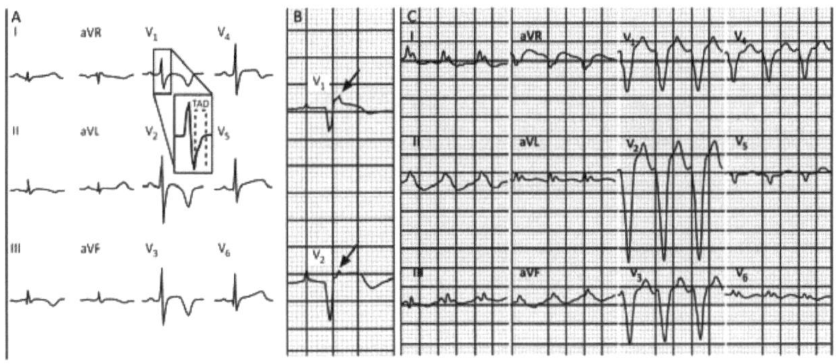

Fig. (4). Electrocardiographic (ECG) features of arrhythmogenic right ventricular cardiomyopathy (ARVC). Panel A shows abnormal repolarization that is characteristic of ARVC patients. Panel B shows a typical ECG example of an "epsilon waves" seen ARVC patients. Panel C shows ventricular tachycardia (160 beats per minute) with a left bundle-branch block pattern.

Histopathology and Endomyocardial Biopsy (EMB)

A definitive diagnosis of ARVC relies on EMB (*"in vivo"*), and the histologic demonstration of full-thickness substitution of the RV myocardium by fatty or fibrofatty tissue examination though, with several diagnostic limitations. In this regard, the histomorphometric criteria have been advanced to give a clear-cut diagnostic border between healthy hearts or DCM, and ARVC [85]. Also, the reversed ITF criteria introduced quantitative parameters for histopathologic evaluation of EMB samples, focusing on fibrous repair and the severity of myocyte loss rather than on fatty infiltration of the myocardium [81]. EMB represents a histologic validation of clinical findings, improves diagnostic accuracy by excluding another cardiomyopathy such as DCM, sarcoidosis, or myocarditis conditions, both idiopathic and specific. Although EMB cannot, however, be routinely recommended for the diagnosis of ARVC, if supported, procedures should be guided either by MRI or voltage mapping [85, 86].

Table 1. Diagnostic criteria for arrhythmogenic right ventricular cardiomyopathy (ARVC) (†-Detected by echocardiography, angiography, magnetic resonance imaging, or radionuclide scintigraphy). LBBB-left bundle branch block; VT- ventricular tachycardia; ECG- electrocardiography.

Criteria's	**Major**	**Minor**
Family history	Familial disease confirmed at surgery or autopsy.	*Family history of sudden premature death (<30-35 years of age) due to suspected ARVC. *Family history (diagnosis is clinically based on present criteria).

(Table 1) cont.....

Criteria's	Major	Minor
ECG depolarization/ conduction abnormalities	Epsilon waves or QRS complex prolongation in the right precordial leads (V1-V3).	Late potentials on signal-averaged ECG.
ECG repolarization abnormalities		Right precordial leads (V2 and V3) inverted T waves in people >12 years of age and in the absence of right bundle branch block.
Arrhythmias		*Sustained or Nonsustained LBBB-type VT documented on ECG or during exercise testing and Holter monitoring. *Frequent ventricular extrasystoles (>1000/24 h on Holter monitoring).
Global or regional dysfunction and structural alterations†	*Severe reduction and dilatation of right ventricular ejection fraction with no or mild left ventricular involvement. * Right ventricular localized aneurysms (dyskinetic or akinetic areas with diastolic bulging's). Severe segmental right ventricular dilatation.	* Global mild right ventricular dilatation or ejection fraction reduction with normal LV. *Mild right ventricular segmental dilatation. * Right ventricular regional hypokinesia.
Tissue characteristics of walls	Fibro-fatty replacement of myocardium on endomyocardial biopsy	

Depolarization and Repolarization Abnormalities

Twelve-lead ECG is an essential diagnostic test in ARVC because it records depolarization and repolarization abnormalities in probands with a definitive diagnosis of ARVC . Negative T waves in the anterior precordial leads (V1 through V4) is the most common finding [3, 4] although, it may extend to the precordial lateral leads (V5 and V6), suggesting a diffuse fibrofatty myocardial replacement with severe RV dilatation and LV involvement [87]. Depolarization abnormalities include incomplete right bundle branch block (RBBB), QRS fragmentation, prolongation of right precordial QRS duration with a delayed S-wave upstroke, and post-excitation epsilon waves [88, 89] although, a sizeable interobserver variability exist in the ECG diagnosis of epsilon waves [89].

Ventricular Arrhythmias

Arrhythmia severity varies during the entire course of the disease and from patient to patient. Its spectrum, however, ranges from isolated premature ventricular beats to sustained VT or VF leading to cardiac arrest [3, 4, 36, 82, 83]. In the revised

ITF diagnostic criteria, the morphology of VT, either non-sustained or sustained has a different diagnostic impact [81], and it is noteworthy that in left-sided variants of ARVC, ventricular arrhythmias show an RBBB morphology, which denotes their origin from the LV [49].

Imaging of RV Morphofunctional Abnormalities

Structural and functional abnormalities consist of segmental RV dilatation with or without bulging or aneurysms; global RV dilatation with or without LV involvement and ejection fraction reduction; and wall motion abnormalities such as dyskinesia. Demonstration of RV morphofunctional abnormalities by angiography, echocardiography, and MRI is a major criterion for diagnosing ARVC [1] although, they are associated with significant limitations in their diagnostic. Angiography helps in demonstrating dyskinetic or akinetic bulging's localized in the apical, infundibular, and sub-tricuspid regions [17]. Echocardiography, on the other hand, is widely non-invasively used technique representing first-line imaging approach in evaluating patients with suspected ARVC or in the serial examination of patients, and screening of family members to determine the disease progression during follow up. Furthermore, echocardiography is also a reliable diagnostic tool in the measurements of wall thickness, volume, and function, end diastolic cavity dimensions (mean ventricular body, inlet, outlet), and also in the differential diagnosis of ARVC to enhance diagnostic accuracy. Cardiac magnetic resonance imaging (CMR) is also another valuable and an attractive imaging method due to its unique ability to characterizing tissue, specifically by differentiating muscle from fat [90] (Figs. **5** & **6**).

DIFFERENTIAL DIAGNOSIS

The differential diagnosis of ARVC from other diseases affecting the RV is crucial as the management and prognosis are different. The differential diagnosis of ARVCD includes: (i) DCM (ii) myocarditis (ii) cardiac sarcoidosis (iv) right ventricular outflow tract (v) Uhl anomaly.

MANAGEMENT

Management of Symptomatic Patients

Pharmacological Therapy: Pharmaco-therapy is the first step in alleviating presenting symptoms, improving lifestyle, and possibly better long-term prognosis in ARVC patients. The below are necessary management strategy and plan which should be carried out by clinicians faced with diagnostic ARVC patients:

Beta-Blockers: We (the authors) recommend the use of Beta-blockers as they are useful in the treatment of heart failure, lowering the progression of RV wall stress, and preventing the effort load related VT. Since VT and cardiac arrest in ARVC patients mostly occur during or immediately after physical exercise [91, 92], the use of Beta-blockers as first-line therapy in ARVC patients with recurrent VTs is helpful and severs as an adjunct to implantable cardiac defibrillator (ICD) therapy. Also, it minimizes inappropriate ICD shock due to atrial fibrillation/flutter with high ventricular rate, sinus tachycardia, or supraventricular tachycardia [93].

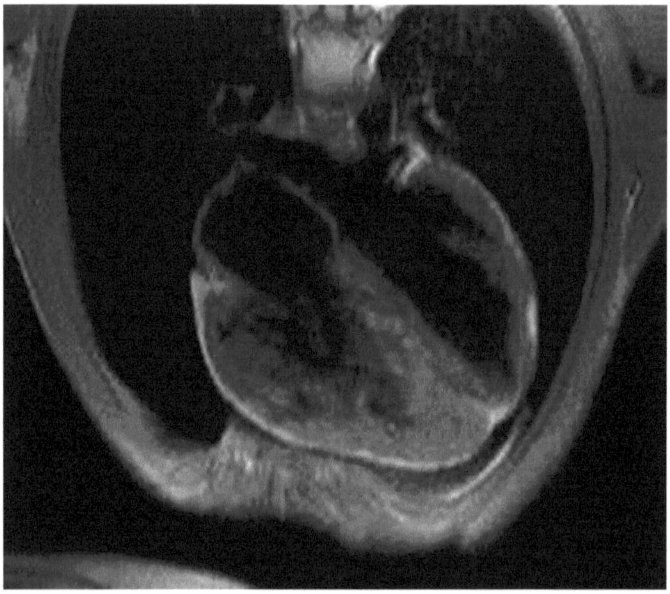

Fig. (5). Arrhythmogenic right ventricular cardiomyopathy fatty variant on cardiac magnetic resonance imaging. Spin-echo sequences, four-chamber view: Note the typical biventricular fatty replacement (bright white signal intensity) of the entire right ventricular wall and of the left ventricular lateral wall, coming from the epicardium toward the endocardium, most visible in the mid-apical lateral wall.

Heart Failure Therapy: We (the authors) recommend the use of angiotensin II receptor blockers, angiotensin-converting-enzyme inhibitors, and diuretics for ARVC patients with ether right- and/or left-sided heart failure [93] along with long-term antithrombotic therapy though only when indicated as patients with severe RV dilatation are at risk of thromboembolism (systemic/venous thromboembolism, and intra-cavitary thrombosis) [93, 94].

Antiarrhythmic Drug Therapy: The aim of antiarrhythmic drug therapy in patients with ARVC is to enhance the patient's quality of life by preventing symptomatic VT's and ICD shocks. We (the authors) recommend the use of amiodarone (loading dose of 400–600 mg daily for two to three weeks and then a maintenance dose of 200–400 mg daily), in combination with β-blockers, as It is (most) effective for preventing symptomatic VTs and has relatively low proarrhythmic risk even in patients with ventricular dysfunction. Although, sotalol administered at a dosage of 320–640 mg/day, is effective only achieving partial to complete arrhythmia suppression in approximately 60-68% of patients with ARVC [95].

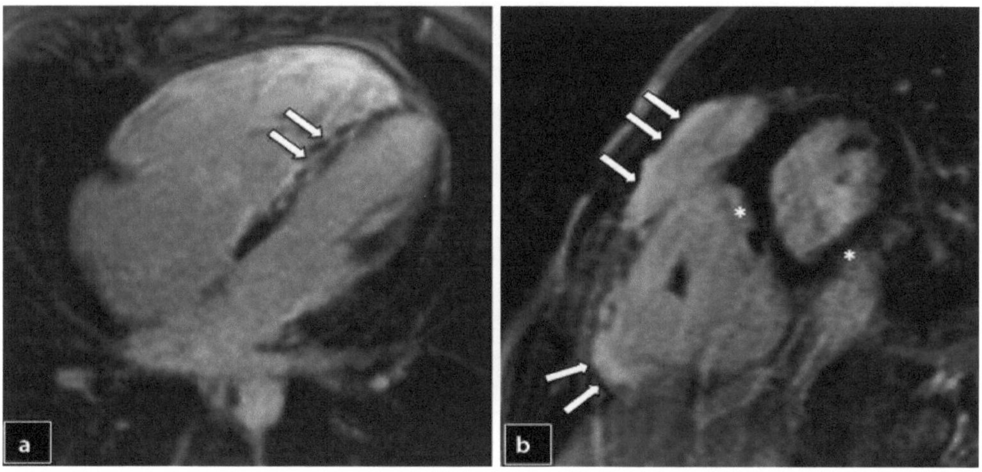

Fig. (6). Arrhythmogenic right ventricular cardiomyopathy fibrous variant on cardiac magnetic resonance imaging. T1 inversion recovery sequence, four-chamber view (a) and basal short-axis view (b): Widespread right ventricular late gadolinium enhancement (arrows) with septal and left ventricular involvement is notable (asterisk).

Catheter Ablation: Although, catheter ablation is a short-term therapy, it's highly effective in the treatment of reentry arrhythmias and VT due to the resultant scars created by the fibrofatty replacements of the RV myocardium, and reoccurring VTs are only as a result of the progressive nature of the disease [96] (Fig. **7**). However, the reoccurrence rate can further be decreased with the combination of epicardial and endocardial ablation approaches [97]. Although, we (the authors) do not, however, recommend the use of the epicardial-endocardial approach due to its potential adverse complications such as; bleeding, and coronary stenosis. Nevertheless, catheter ablation remains a very valuable therapeutic modality in decreasing patients' morbidity in conjunction with antiarrhythmic medication especially in ARVC patients with incessant VT despite maximal pharmacological therapy, including the use of amiodarone even after ICD implantation [93, 95].

ICD Therapy: Randomized trials to guide ICD therapy in ARVC patients are not available for ethical reasons, low disease prevalence, and small event rates. However, data collected from observational registries demonstrate ICD therapy efficacy to interrupt potentially fatal VTs [98 - 100], and the only treatment option shown to reduce high-risk markers for mortality in ARVC patients such as; syncope, severe RV dysfunction, and LV involvement [101] (Fig. **8**).

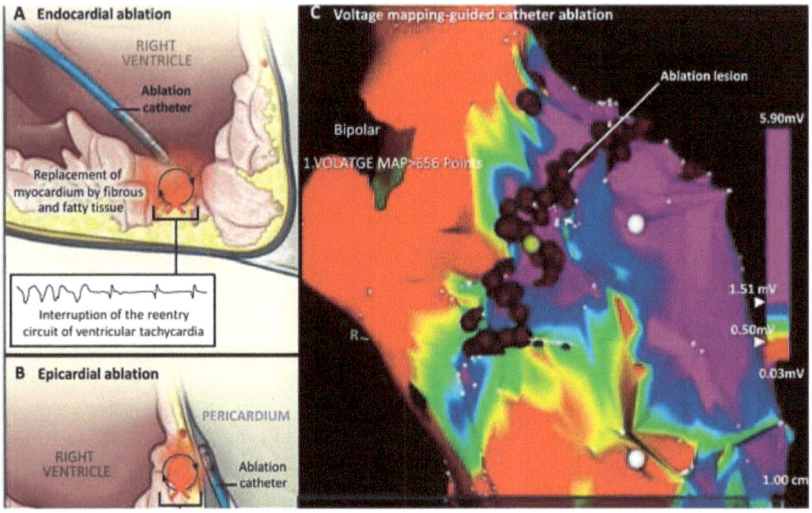

Fig. (7). Catheter Ablation of Ventricular Tachycardia in Patients with Arrhythmogenic right ventricular cardiomyopathy (ARVC) with the use of either an endocardial or an epicardial approach, depending on the site of the arrhythmia substrate. (Panel A), the catheter is advanced into the right ventricular cavity through the venous system; the black circular arrow shows a reentry circuit of ventricular tachycardia, and the red X indicates interruption by endocardial catheter ablation of the reentry circuit of ventricular tachycardia (inset). Epicardial ablation (Panel B) requires the introduction of the catheter into the pericardial space using pericardial puncture; the black circular arrow shows a reentry circuit, and the red X indicates interruption by epicardial catheter ablation of the reentry circuit of ventricular tachycardia (inset). Target sites for catheter ablation can be identified with the use of three-dimensional electro-anatomical voltage mapping (Panel C) to reconstruct regions of right ventricular scarring.

Lifestyle Changes: Lifestyle changes are defiantly mandatory for patients as competitive sporting activities promote the development and progression of ARVC phenotypes [93] thereby, increasing the risk of SCD by fivefold in adolescent and young adults [102]. Hence, patients with a definite diagnosis of ARVC should be encouraged and advised not to participate in endurance and competitive sports.

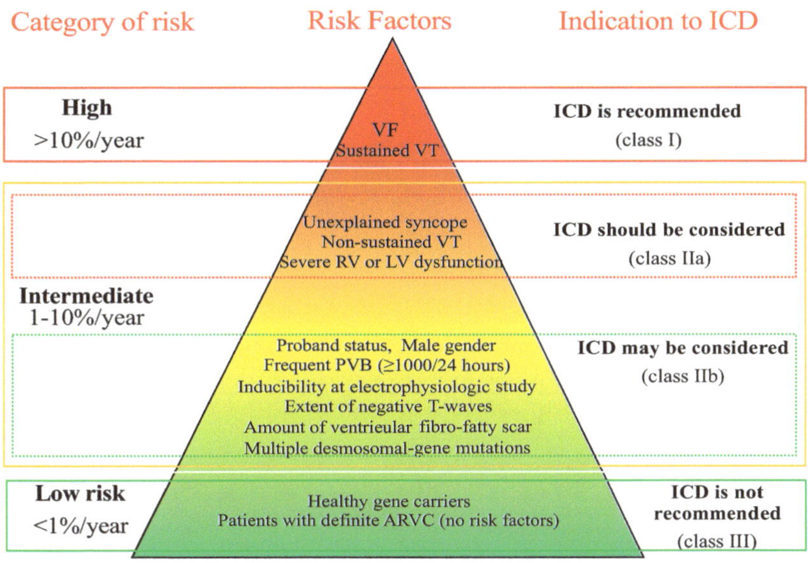

Fig. (8). Pyramid of risk and indications for implantable cardioverter defibrillator (ICD) therapy in arrhythmogenic cardiomyopathy (ARVC). The recommendations here are based on the 2015 International Task Force consensus document on the treatment of ARVC. LV (left ventricle); PVB (premature ventricular beats); RV (right ventricle); VF (ventricular fibrillation); and VT (ventricular tachycardia).

Management of Symptomatic Patients and Screening of Family Members

Although asymptomatic ARVC patients do not require specific antiarrhythmic and other specific cardiac treatment, they should, however, be carefully followed with noninvasive cardiac investigations which are key to early identification of ventricular arrhythmias and potential progression of the disease with worsening of regional or global myocardial dysfunction. It is also

Important that the follow-up visits include an adequate clerking of the patient concerning issues of arrhythmic symptoms or events, syncope or near syncope, and a quarterly cardiac examination (as the case may be) with a 24h Holter monitoring test, and a complete imaging analysis either by echocardiography and magnetic resonance imaging. Furthermore, patients should be advised not to participate in endurance and/or any other competitive sports at all if possible and family members of patients with a definite diagnosis of ARVC should visit their family physician (preferably a cardiologist) experienced with the disease at regular intervals every two to five years or with onset of symptoms [103].

SURGICAL INTERVENTIONS

The most common indication for a heart transplant in an ARVC patient is the progression of heart failure followed by intractable VTs [104]. It is however, recommended as the final therapeutic option available in patients with either recurrent episodes of VT/VF, which are refractory to a catheter (and surgical) ablation and ICD therapy or unresponsive severe congestive heart failure [93]. Although they currently have no clinical role, other surgical treatment includes; left cardiac sympathetic denervation, beating heart cryoablation [105], RV cardiomyoplasty [106], and RV disarticulation [107].

RISK STRATIFICATION

Identification of patients at risk of SCD is one of the critical issues in the management of ARVC (Table **2**) although, risk stratification largely depends on the evaluation of ARVC phenotypic expression in terms of the amount of fibrofatty replacement, and the severity of arrhythmia as it is evaluated by imaging and ECG tests, respectively. However, the most challenging clinical dilemma has not been treating malignant ventricular arrhythmic patients (secondary prevention) but instead, considering prophylactic treatment in patients who have already been diagnosed during a routine family screening or by chance (primary prevention) with no or only minor symptoms. Other risk profile includes; extensive RV disease with a decreased ejection fraction and LV involvement, competitive sports, syncope, malignant family background, and young age [3, 4].

Table 2. Proposed Scheme for Prognostic Stratification of Patients with Arrhythmogenic rightventricular cardiomyopathy (ARVC) According to the Clinical Presentation. The estimated annualrisk of more than 10% defines the high-risk group, a risk between 1% and 10% the intermediate riskgroup, and risk below 1% of the low-risk group. PVB denotes premature ventricular beats.

Major Arrhythmic Events *Cardiac arrest due to ventricular fibrillation *Sustained ventricular tachycardia	**High Risk >10%/years**
Major Risk Factors *Unexplained syncope *Nonsustained ventricular tachycardia *Severe right or left ventricular dysfunction	**Intermediate Risk 1–10%/years**
Minor Risk Factors *Proband status, male sex *Frequent PVBs (^{3}1000/24 hr) *Inducibility on electrophysiological study *Extent of negative T waves *Amount of right ventricular fibrofatty scarring *Multiple desmosomal gene mutations	**Intermediate Risk 1–10%/years**
No Events or Risk Factors *Healthy gene carriers *Patients with definite ARVC	**Low Risk <1%/years**

CMR TRADITIONAL AND EVOLVING ROLE IN THE DIAGNOSIS OF ARVC

CMR imaging provides vital information necessary for the diagnosis (definite/indefinite) and the prognosis of all ARVC patients in terms of morphofunctional and tissue characterization assessment due to the reversed 2010 Task Force Criteria with a specific quantitative cut-off values of RV dysfunction/dilatation combined with the qualitative evaluation of abnormalities on cine images (dyskinesia, dyssynchrony, RV regional akinesia) [81].

Morphofunctional Assessment

The morphofunctional assessment CMR sequences are the breath-hold, and the ECG-gated imaging which both offers excellent natural contrast between ventricular blood cavity, and the endocardial borders which are not only useful for an accurate volume evaluation, and specific abnormalities on cine images, but also valuable in the acquisition of the correct RV volumes too. The new combination of qualitative cine assessment plus dilatation/dysfunction decreases the possibility of any significant interobserver variability (over-diagnosis in this case) due to isolated RV minor cine-imaging abnormalities by correctly differentiating ARVC from clinical conditions characterized by isolated dilatation and dysfunction. However, apart from the huge step taken by the Taskforce in the diagnosis of ARVC and including the removal of hypokinesia from the diagnostic criterion, some limitations still exist;

I. The cut-offs included were obtained by comparing ARVC probands with regular healthy volunteers involved in the Multi-Ethnic Study of Atherosclerosis [81]. This study used suboptimal evaluation of subendocardial borders (the old gradient-echo sequences), compared with the more suitable breath-hold cine images used in the majority of ARVC studies.

I. The concealed form of ARVC, where the fibrofatty replacement is segmental, it is possible to detect localized dyskinetic or akinetic areas not determining a substantial RV dilatation/dysfunction.

II. Finally, the inter-reader variability in the RV function and volume mostly relates to the correct inclusion of RV endocardium and the evaluation of basal slice, and the partial volume effects for apical slice or artifacts.

Therefore, in this setting, detecting early LV involvement is crucial, not in terms of function but in terms of tissue characterization (discussed below), which is not yet included in the current Task Force Criteria.

Tissue Characterization

Taking into account the difficulties in distinguishing between pathologic and physiologic fatty infiltration, tissue characterization demonstrated on histological analyses of EMB remains the hallmark of ARVC [81, 86]. One of the huge steps forward, made in the diagnosis of ARVC has been the introduction of LGE with CE imaging which is based on the ability of LGE to identify areas of intramyocardial fibrosis [108]. The disruption and extension of the demarcated line (white as epicardial fat and gray as RV myocardium) by the hyperintense signals into the RV myocardium are interpreted as infiltration of epicardial fat into the RV wall. These are, however, frequently noted in ARVC patients whereas, in healthy individuals, epicardial fat overlies the RV, and is abundant toward the RV apex and also in the atrioventricular groove. These, however, lead to the application of CMR in the diagnostic work-up of ARVC for RV wall tissue characterization in detecting fatty tissues [109].

Furthermore, the use of CE-LGE imaging offers a great possibility to visualize fibrofatty scars. An intermediate signal similar to skeletal muscles can be seen in a normal myocardium as fat appears to be a hyperintense signal (bright) on spin-echo black-blood images. Consequently, It is essential to note already that, the presence of intramyocardial fatty infiltration is not specific, particularly with fatty heart, and in obese patients with metabolic diseases.

Be it as it may, the difficulty sometimes faced in diagnosing thin RV wall with the use of LGE are among the other reasons the Task Force made the decision not to include LGE as a work-up diagnostic parameter:

I. The histological basis of LGE
II. LGE in the LV myocardium
III. The cine-imaging abnormalities and LGE and
IV. The role of LGE in the differential diagnosis of ARVC.

CONCLUSION AND FUTURE DIRECTIONS

Fat infiltration per se is probably a different process, and the least reliable criterion which should not be considered synonymous with ARVC, and also for the diagnosis of ARVC patients too. Histopathologic features that refer to both myocytes and fibrous tissue deposition, and a multiparametric approach combining all clinical data, including twelve lead- and signal-averaged ECG, EMB, family history including genetics, CMR, and electroanatomic mappings help in the definitive diagnosis of ARVC. It is also essential that both general or forensic pathologist dealing with a case of SCD avoid overdiagnosis of ARVC.

However, such instances occur where the only morphologic finding consists of a high amount of intramyocardial or epicardial fat. Hence, a more convincing arrhythmogenic substrate, such as fibrosis, anomalous pathways, ion channel disease, and myocardial inflammatory infiltrates should always be searched for pathologically. Also, the differential diagnosis should include the so-called phenocopies when dealing with sporadic forms, bearing in mind that, there is currently no gold standard criterion sufficient enough to give a definite diagnosis of ARVC. Meanwhile, the need to adopt a strict diagnostic criterion is warranted not only in clinical settings but also in the general pathology, and in forensic medicine as the lack of specific diagnostic guidelines contribute to the under-recognition of the non-classic variants of ARVC, *i.e.,* isolated or dominant LV disease.

Future revision and Task Force set up for the diagnoses of ARVC patients should consider this disparity, various gaps, and limitations in the diagnostic criteria's which would represent the starting point for epidemiological, and clinical implication, familial screening and SCD prevention.

LIST OF ABBREVIATIONS

ARVC Arrhythmogenic right ventricular cardiomyopathy

CMR Cardiac magnetic resonance>

CE Contrast-enhanced

DCM Dilated cardiomyopathy

ECG Electrocardiography

ITF International Task Force

LV Left ventricle

LBBB Left bundle branch block

LGE Late gadolinium enhancement

RV Right ventricle

RBBB Right bundle branch block

SCD Sudden cardiac death

VT Ventricular tachycardia

VF Ventricular fibrillation

WHO World Health Organization

CONSENT FOR PUBLICATION

Not applicable.

CONFLICT OF INTEREST

The authors confirm that this chapter contents have no conflict of interest.

ACKNOWLEDGEMENTS

Declared none.

REFERENCE

[1] Nava A, Rossi L, Thiene G, Eds. Arrhythmogenic right ventricular cardiomyopathy/dysplasia. Amsterdam: Elsevier 1997.

[2] Marcus FI, Fontaine GH, Guiraudon G, *et al.* Right ventricular dysplasia: a report of 24 adult cases. Circulation 1982; 65(2): 384-98. [http://dx.doi.org/10.1161/01.CIR.65.2.384] [PMID: 7053899]

[3] Thiene G, Nava A, Corrado D, Rossi L, Pennelli N. Right ventricular cardiomyopathy and sudden death in young people. N Engl J Med 1988; 318(3): 129-33. [http://dx.doi.org/10.1056/NEJM198801213180301] [PMID: 3336399]

[4] Basso C, Thiene G, Corrado D, Angelini A, Nava A, Valente M. Arrhythmogenic right ventricular cardiomyopathy. Dysplasia, dystrophy, or myocarditis? Circulation 1996; 94(5): 983-91. [http://dx.doi.org/10.1161/01.CIR.94.5.983] [PMID: 8790036]

[5] Thiene G, Basso C. Arrhythmogenic right ventricular cardiomyopathy: An update. Cardiovasc Pathol 2001; 10(3): 109-17. [http://dx.doi.org/10.1016/S1054-8807(01)00067-9] [PMID: 11485854]

[6] Foale RA, Nihoyannopoulos P, Ribeiro P, *et al.* Right ventricular abnormalities in ventricular tachycardia of right ventricular origin: relation to electrophysiological abnormalities. Br Heart J 1986; 56(1): 45-54. [http://dx.doi.org/10.1136/hrt.56.1.45] [PMID: 3730207]

[7] Frank R, Fontaine G, Vedel J, *et al.* Electrocardiology of 4 cases of right ventricular dysplasia inducing arrhythmia. Arch Mal Coeur Vaiss 1978; 71(9): 963-72. [PMID: 102297]

[8] Bronzini E, Novi AM. Contributo anatomopatologico allo studio del cuore adiposo Studio su 100 casi. Arch Maragliano 1959; 15: 1045-70.

[9] d'Amati G, Leone O, di Gioia CR, *et al.* Arrhythmogenic right ventricular cardiomyopathy: Clinicopathologic correlation based on a revised definition of pathologic patterns. Hum Pathol 2001; 32(10): 1078-86. [http://dx.doi.org/10.1053/hupa.2001.28232] [PMID: 11679942]

[10] Lancisi GM. De Motu Cordis et Aneurysmatibus. Naples 1736.

[11] Dalla Volta S, Battaglia G, Zerbini E. "Auricularization' of right ventricular pressure curve. Am Heart J 1961; 61: 25-33. [http://dx.doi.org/10.1016/0002-8703(61)90513-0] [PMID: 13719440]

[12] McKenna WJ, Thiene G, Nava A, *et al.* Task Force of the Working Group Myocardial and Pericardial Disease of the European Society of Cardiology and of the Scientific Council on Cardiomyopathies of the International Society and Federation of Cardiology. Diagnosis of arrhythmogenic right ventricular dysplasia/cardiomyopathy. Br Heart J 1994; 71(3): 215-8. [http://dx.doi.org/10.1136/hrt.71.3.215] [PMID: 8142187]

[13] Wichter T, Borggrefe M, Haverkamp W, Chen X, Breithardt G. Efficacy of antiarrhythmic drugs in patients with arrhythmogenic right ventricular disease. Results in patients with inducible and

noninducible ventricular tachycardia. Circulation 1992; 86(1): 29-37. [http://dx.doi.org/10.1161/01.CIR.86.1.29] [PMID: 1617780]

[14] Rampazzo A, Danieli GA. Arrhythmogenic in right ventricular cardiomyopathy/dysplasia. Advances in genetics: Dominant forms. Arrhythmogenic Right Ventricular Cardiomyopathy/Dysplasia. Milano: Springer 2007; pp. 7-14. [http://dx.doi.org/10.1007/978-88-470-0490-0_2]

[15] Nava A, Thiene G, Canciani B, *et al.* Familial occurrence of right ventricular dysplasia: A study involving nine families. J Am Coll Cardiol 1988; 12(5): 1222-8. [http://dx.doi.org/10.1016/0735-1097(88)92603-4] [PMID: 3170963]

[16] Maron BJ. Right ventricular cardiomyopathy: Another cause of sudden death in the young. N Engl J Med 1988; 318(3): 178-80. [http://dx.doi.org/10.1056/NEJM198801213180309] [PMID: 3336404]

[17] Daliento L, Rizzoli G, Thiene G, *et al.* Diagnostic accuracy of right ventriculography in arrhythmogenic right ventricular cardiomyopathy. Am J Cardiol 1990; 66(7): 741-5. [http://dx.doi.org/10.1016/0002-9149(90)91141-R] [PMID: 2399893]

[18] Scognamiglio R, Fasoli G, Nava A, Miraglia G, Thiene G, Dalla-Volta S. Contribution of cross-sectional echocardiography to the diagnosis of right ventricular dysplasia at the asymptomatic stage. Eur Heart J 1989; 10(6): 538-42. [http://dx.doi.org/10.1093/oxfordjournals.eurheartj.a059524] [PMID: 2759115]

[19] Protonotarios N, Tsatsopoulou A, Patsourakos P, *et al.* Cardiac abnormalities in familial palmoplantar keratosis. Br Heart J 1986; 56(4): 321-6. [http://dx.doi.org/10.1136/hrt.56.4.321] [PMID: 2945574]

[20] Rampazzo A, Nava A, Danieli GA, *et al.* The gene for arrhythmogenic right ventricular cardiomyopathy maps to chromosome 14q23-q24. Hum Mol Genet 1994; 3(6): 959-62. [http://dx.doi.org/10.1093/hmg/3.6.959] [PMID: 7951245]

[21] Richardson P. McKenna, Bristow M, Maisch B, Mautner B, O'Connel J, Olsen E, Thiene G, Goodwin J, Gyarfas I, Martin I, Nordet P: Report of the 1995 WHO/ISFC Task Force on the definition and classification of cardiomyopathies. Circulation 1996; 93: 841-2. [PMID: 8598070]

[22] Gerull B, Heuser A, Wichter T, *et al.* Mutations in the desmosomal protein plakophilin-2 are common in arrhythmogenic right ventricular cardiomyopathy. Nat Genet 2004; 36(11): 1162-4. [http://dx.doi.org/10.1038/ng1461] [PMID: 15489853]

[23] Rampazzo A, Nava A, Malacrida S, *et al.* Mutation in human desmoplakin domain binding to plakoglobin causes a dominant form of arrhythmogenic right ventricular cardiomyopathy. Am J Hum Genet 2002; 71(5): 1200-6. [http://dx.doi.org/10.1086/344208] [PMID: 12373648]

[24] Syrris P, Ward D, Evans A, *et al.* Arrhythmogenic right ventricular dysplasia/cardiomyopathy associated with mutations in the desmosomal gene desmocollin-2. Am J Hum Genet 2006; 79(5): 978-84. [http://dx.doi.org/10.1086/509122] [PMID: 17033975]

[25] Pilichou K, Nava A, Basso C, *et al.* Mutations in desmoglein-2 gene are associated with arrhythmogenic right ventricular cardiomyopathy. Circulation 2006; 113(9): 1171-9. [http://dx.doi.org/10.1161/CIRCULATIONAHA.105.583674] [PMID: 16505173]

[26] Beffagna G, Occhi G, Nava A, *et al.* Regulatory mutations in transforming growth factor-beta3 gene cause arrhythmogenic right ventricular cardiomyopathy type 1. Cardiovasc Res 2005; 65(2): 366-73. [http://dx.doi.org/10.1016/j.cardiores.2004.10.005] [PMID: 15639475]

[27] Tiso N, Stephan DA, Nava A, *et al.* Identification of mutations in the cardiac ryanodine receptor gene in families affected with arrhythmogenic right ventricular cardiomyopathy type 2 (ARVD2). Hum Mol

Genet 2001; 10(3): 189-94.
[http://dx.doi.org/10.1093/hmg/10.3.189] [PMID: 11159936]

[28] Bauce B, Basso C, Rampazzo A, *et al.* Clinical profile of four families with arrhythmogenic right ventricular cardiomyopathy caused by dominant desmoplakin mutations. Eur Heart J 2005; 26(16): 1666-75.
[http://dx.doi.org/10.1093/eurheartj/ehi341] [PMID: 15941723]

[29] Sen-Chowdhry S, Syrris P, Ward D, Asimaki A, Sevdalis E, McKenna WJ. Clinical and genetic characterization of families with arrhythmogenic right ventricular dysplasia/cardiomyopathy provides novel insights into patterns of disease expression. Circulation 2007; 115(13): 1710-20.
[http://dx.doi.org/10.1161/CIRCULATIONAHA.106.660241] [PMID: 17372169]

[30] Fontaliran F, Fontaine G, Fillette F, Aouate P, Chomette G, Grosgogeat Y. Frontières nosologiques de la dysplasie arythmogène. Variations quantitatives du tissu adipeux ventriculaire droit normal. Arch Mal Coeur Vaiss 1991; 84(1): 33-8.
[PMID: 2012483]

[31] Burke AP, Farb A, Tashko G, Virmani R. Arrhythmogenic right ventricular cardiomyopathy and fatty replacement of the right ventricular myocardium: are they different diseases? Circulation 1998; 97(16): 1571-80.
[http://dx.doi.org/10.1161/01.CIR.97.16.1571] [PMID: 9593562]

[32] Thiene G, Corrado D, Nava A, *et al.* Right ventricular cardiomyopathy: Is there evidence of an inflammatory aetiology? Eur Heart J 1991; 12 (Suppl. D): 22-5.
[http://dx.doi.org/10.1093/eurheartj/12.suppl_D.22] [PMID: 1915454]

[33] Dalal D, Nasir K, Bomma C, *et al.* Arrhythmogenic right ventricular dysplasia: A United States experience. Circulation 2005; 112(25): 3823-32.
[http://dx.doi.org/10.1161/CIRCULATIONAHA.105.542266] [PMID: 16344387]

[34] Corrado D, Fontaine G, Marcus FI, *et al.* Study Group on Arrhythmogenic Right Ventricular Dysplasia/Cardiomyopathy of the Working Groups on Myocardial and Pericardial Disease and Arrhythmias of the European Society of Cardiology and of the Scientific Council on Cardiomyopathies of the World Heart Federation. Arrhythmogenic right ventricular dysplasia/cardiomyopathy: need for an international registry. Circulation 2000; 101(11): E101-6.
[http://dx.doi.org/10.1161/01.CIR.101.11.e101] [PMID: 10725299]

[35] Shen WK, Edwards WD, Hammill SC, Gersh BJ. Right ventricular dysplasia: a need for precise pathological definition for interpretation of sudden death (abstr). J Am Coll Cardiol 1994; 23 (Suppl.): 34A.

[36] Groeneweg JA, Bhonsale A, James CA, *et al.* Clinical presentation, longterm follow-up, and outcomes of 1001 arrhythmogenic right ventricular dysplasia/cardiomyopathy patients and family members. Circ Cardiovasc Genet 2015; 8(3): 437-46.
[http://dx.doi.org/10.1161/CIRCGENETICS.114.001003] [PMID: 25820315]

[37] Fressart V, Duthoit G, Donal E, *et al.* Desmosomal gene analysis in arrhythmogenic right ventricular dysplasia/cardiomyopathy: Spectrum of mutations and clinical impact in practice. Europace 2010; 12(6): 861-8.
[http://dx.doi.org/10.1093/europace/euq104] [PMID: 20400443]

[38] Romero J, Mejia-Lopez E, Manrique C, Lucariello R. Arrhythmogenic right ventricular cardiomyopathy (ARVC/D): A systematic literature review. Clin Med Insights Cardiol 2013; 7: 97-114.
[http://dx.doi.org/10.4137/CMC.S10940] [PMID: 23761986]

[39] Gemayel C, Pelliccia A, Thompson PD. Arrhythmogenic right ventricular cardiomyopathy. J Am Coll Cardiol 2001; 38(7): 1773-81.
[http://dx.doi.org/10.1016/S0735-1097(01)01654-0] [PMID: 11738273]

[40] Corrado D, Thiene G. Arrhythmogenic right ventricular cardiomyopathy/dysplasia: Clinical impact of

molecular genetic studies. Circulation 2006; 113(13): 1634-7.
[http://dx.doi.org/10.1161/CIRCULATIONAHA.105.616490] [PMID: 16585401]

[41] Al-Ghamdi B, Shafquat A, Mallawi Y. Arrhythmogenic right ventricular cardiomyopathy/dysplasia in Saudi Arabia: A single-center experience with long-term follow-up. Ann Saudi Med 2014; 34(5): 415-26.
[http://dx.doi.org/10.5144/0256-4947.2014.415] [PMID: 25827699]

[42] Uhl HS. A previously undescribed congenital malformation of the heart: Almost total absence of the myocardium of the right ventricle. Bull Johns Hopkins Hosp 1952; 91(3): 197-209.
[PMID: 12978573]

[43] Ross SE, Hemati N, Longo KA, *et al.* Inhibition of adipogenesis by Wnt signaling. Science 2000; 289(5481): 950-3.
[http://dx.doi.org/10.1126/science.289.5481.950] [PMID: 10937998]

[44] Coonar AS, Protonotarios N, Tsatsopoulou A, *et al.* Gene for arrhythmogenic right ventricular cardiomyopathy with diffuse nonepidermolytic palmoplantar keratoderma and woolly hair (Naxos disease) maps to 17q21. Circulation 1998; 97(20): 2049-58.
[http://dx.doi.org/10.1161/01.CIR.97.20.2049] [PMID: 9610536]

[45] Protonotarios N, Tsatsopoulou A. Arrhythmogenic right ventricular cardiomyopathy: Clinical forms of the disease. Hellenic J Cardiol 1998; 39 (Suppl. A): 78-80.

[46] Protonotarios N, Tsatsopoulou A, Anastasakis A, *et al.* Genotype-phenotype assessment in autosomal recessive arrhythmogenic right ventricular cardiomyopathy (Naxos disease) caused by a deletion in plakoglobin. J Am Coll Cardiol 2001; 38(5): 1477-84.
[http://dx.doi.org/10.1016/S0735-1097(01)01568-6] [PMID: 11691526]

[47] Rao BH, Reddy IS, Chandra KS. Familial occurrence of a rare combination of dilated cardiomyopathy with palmoplantar keratoderma and curly hair. Indian Heart J 1996; 48(2): 161-2.
[PMID: 8682558]

[48] De Pasquale CG, Heddle WF. Left sided arrhythmogenic ventricular dysplasia in siblings. Heart 2001; 86(2): 128-30.
[http://dx.doi.org/10.1136/heart.86.2.128] [PMID: 11454821]

[49] Sen-Chowdhry S, Syrris P, Prasad SK, *et al.* Left-dominant arrhythmogenic cardiomyopathy: an under-recognized clinical entity. J Am Coll Cardiol 2008; 52(25): 2175-87.
[http://dx.doi.org/10.1016/j.jacc. 2008.09.019]

[50] Pawel BR, de Chadarévian JP, Wolk JH, Donner RM, Vogel RL, Braverman P. Sudden death in childhood due to right ventricular dysplasia: Report of two cases. Pediatr Pathol 1994; 14(6): 987-95.
[http://dx.doi.org/10.3109/15513819409037695] [PMID: 7855018]

[51] Hamid MS, Norman M, Quraishi A, *et al.* Prospective evaluation of relatives for familial arrhythmogenic right ventricular cardiomyopathy/dysplasia reveals a need to broaden diagnostic criteria. J Am Coll Cardiol 2002; 40(8): 1445-50.
[http://dx.doi.org/10.1016/S0735-1097(02)02307-0] [PMID: 12392835]

[52] Nava A, Bauce B, Basso C, *et al.* Clinical profile and long-term follow-up of 37 families with arrhythmogenic right ventricular cardiomyopathy. J Am Coll Cardiol 2000; 36(7): 2226-33.
[http://dx.doi.org/10.1016/S0735-1097(00)00997-9] [PMID: 11127465]

[53] Heidbüchel H, Hoogsteen J, Fagard R, *et al.* High prevalence of right ventricular involvement in endurance athletes with ventricular arrhythmias. Role of an electrophysiologic study in risk stratification. Eur Heart J 2003; 24(16): 1473-80.
[http://dx.doi.org/10.1016/S0195-668X(03)00282-3] [PMID: 12919770]

[54] Henriksen E, Kangro T, Jonason T, *et al.* An echocardiographic study of right ventricular adaptation to physical exercise in elite male orienteers. Clin Physiol 1998; 18(6): 498-503.
[http://dx.doi.org/10.1046/j.1365-2281.1998.00130.x] [PMID: 9818154]

[55] d'Amati G, di Gioia CR, Giordano C, Gallo P. Myocyte transdifferentiation: a possible pathogenetic mechanism for arrhythmogenic right ventricular cardiomyopathy. Arch Pathol Lab Med 2000; 124(2): 287-90.
[http://dx.doi.org/10.1043/0003-9985(2000)124<0287:MT>2.0.CO;2] [PMID: 10656741]

[56] Huber O. Structure and function of desmosomal proteins and their role in development and disease. Cell Mol Life Sci 2003; 60(9): 1872-90.
[http://dx.doi.org/10.1007/s00018-003-3050-7] [PMID: 14523549]

[57] Garrod D, Chidgey M. Desmosome structure, composition and function. Biochim Biophys Acta 2008; 1778(3): 572-87.
[http://dx.doi.org/10.1016/j.bbamem.2007.07.014] [PMID: 17854763]

[58] Garcia-Gras E, Lombardi R, Giocondo MJ, *et al.* Suppression of canonical Wnt/beta-catenin signaling by nuclear plakoglobin recapitulates phenotype of arrhythmogenic right ventricular cardiomyopathy. J Clin Invest 2006; 116(7): 2012-21.
[http://dx.doi.org/10.1172/JCI27751] [PMID: 16823493]

[59] Basso C, Bauce B, Corrado D, Thiene G. Pathophysiology of arrhythmogenic cardiomyopathy. Nat Rev Cardiol 2011; 9(4): 223-33.
[http://dx.doi.org/10.1038/nrcardio.2011.173] [PMID: 22124316]

[60] Basso C, Corrado D, Marcus FI, Nava A, Thiene G. Arrhythmogenic right ventricular cardiomyopathy. Lancet 2009; 373(9671): 1289-300.
[http://dx.doi.org/10.1016/S0140-6736(09)60256-7] [PMID: 19362677]

[61] Mertens C, Kuhn C, Franke WW. Plakophilins 2a and 2b: Constitutive proteins of dual location in the karyoplasm and the desmosomal plaque. J Cell Biol 1996; 135(4): 1009-25.
[http://dx.doi.org/10.1083/jcb.135.4.1009] [PMID: 8922383]

[62] Antoniades L, Tsatsopoulou A, Anastasakis A, *et al.* Arrhythmogenic right ventricular cardiomyopathy caused by deletions in plakophilin-2 and plakoglobin (Naxos disease) in families from Greece and Cyprus: genotype-phenotype relations, diagnostic features and prognosis. Eur Heart J 2006; 27(18): 2208-16.
[http://dx.doi.org/10.1093/eurheartj/ehl184] [PMID: 16893920]

[63] Al-Ghamdi B, Alhassnan Z, Al-Fayyadh M, *et al.* Clinical and genetic characteristics of arrhythmogenic right ventricular cardiomyopathy/dysplasia patients in Saudi Arabia: A single centre experience. Cardiostim-EHRA Europace. Nice, France: Europace. 2016; 2016: pp. (Supp 1)8-11.

[64] Bornslaeger EA, Corcoran CM, Stappenbeck TS, Green KJ. Breaking the connection: displacement of the desmosomal plaque protein desmoplakin from cell-cell interfaces disrupts anchorage of intermediate filament bundles and alters intercellular junction assembly. J Cell Biol 1996; 134(4): 985-1001.
[http://dx.doi.org/10.1083/jcb.134.4.985] [PMID: 8769422]

[65] van der Zwaag PA, Jongbloed JD, van den Berg MP, *et al.* A genetic variants database for arrhythmogenic right ventricular dysplasia/cardiomyopathy. Hum Mutat 2009; 30(9): 1278-83.
[http://dx.doi.org/10.1002/humu.21064] [PMID: 19569224]

[66] Al-Jassar C, Knowles T, Jeeves M, *et al.* The nonlinear structure of the desmoplakin plakin domain and the effects of cardiomyopathy-linked mutations. J Mol Biol 2011; 411(5): 1049-61.
[http://dx.doi.org/10.1016/j.jmb.2011.06.047] [PMID: 21756917]

[67] Arnemann J, Spurr NK, Magee AI, Buxton RS. The human gene (DSG2) coding for HDGC, a second member of the desmoglein subfamily of the desmosomal cadherins, is, like DSG1 coding for desmoglein DGI, assigned to chromosome 18. Genomics 1992; 13(2): 484-6.
[http://dx.doi.org/10.1016/0888-7543(92)90280-6] [PMID: 1612610]

[68] McNally E, MacLeod H, Dellefave-Castillo L. Arrhythmogenic right ventricular dysplasia/cardiomyopathy. Pagon RA, Adam MP, Ardinger HH, Wallace SE, Amemiya A, Bean LJH,

Bird TD, Fong CT, Mefford HC, Smith RJH, Stephens K, editors GeneReviews® [Internet] Seattle, WA: University of Washington, Seattle 2005.http://www.ncbi.nlm.nih.gov/books/ NBK1131/

[69] Posch MG, Posch MJ, Geier C, *et al.* A missense variant in desmoglein□2 predisposes to dilated cardiomyopathy. Mol Genet Metab 2008; 95(1-2): 74-80. [http://dx.doi.org/10.1016/j.ymgme.2008.06.005]

[70] Amagai M, Wang Y, Minoshima S, *et al.* Assignment of the human genes for desmocollin 3 (DSC3) and desmocollin 4 (DSC4) to chromosome 18q12. Genomics 1995; 25(1): 330-2. [http://dx.doi.org/10.1016/0888-7543(95)80154-E] [PMID: 7774948]

[71] Asimaki A, Syrris P, Wichter T, Matthias P, Saffitz JE, McKenna WJ. A novel dominant mutation in plakoglobin causes arrhythmogenic right ventricular cardiomyopathy. Am J Hum Genet 2007; 81(5): 964-73. [http://dx.doi.org/10.1086/521633] [PMID: 17924338]

[72] Leask A, Abraham DJ. TGF-beta signaling and the fibrotic response. FASEB J 2004; 18(7): 816-27. [http://dx.doi.org/10.1096/fj.03-1273rev] [PMID: 15117886]

[73] Rampazzo A. Genetic bases of arrhythmogenic right ventricular Cardiomyopathy. Heart Int 2006; 2(1): 17. [http://dx.doi.org/10.4081/hi.2006.17] [PMID: 21977247]

[74] Laitinen PJ, Swan H, Kontula K. Molecular genetics of exercise-induced polymorphic ventricular tachycardia: Identification of three novel cardiac ryanodine receptor mutations and two common calsequestrin 2 amino-acid polymorphisms. Eur J Hum Genet 2003; 11(11): 888-91. [http://dx.doi.org/10.1038/sj.ejhg.5201061] [PMID: 14571276]

[75] Priori SG, Napolitano C, Memmi M, *et al.* Clinical and molecular characterization of patients with catecholaminergic polymorphic ventricular tachycardia. Circulation 2002; 106(1): 69-74. [http://dx.doi.org/10.1161/01.CIR. 0000020013.73106.D8]

[76] Bauce B, Rampazzo A, Basso C, *et al.* Screening for ryanodine receptor type 2 mutations in families with effort-induced polymorphic ventricular arrhythmias and sudden death: early diagnosis of asymptomatic carriers. J Am Coll Cardiol 2002; 40(2): 341-9. [http://dx.doi.org/10.1016/S0735-1097(02)01946-0] [PMID: 12106942]

[77] Wiemann S, Weil B, Wellenreuther R, *et al.* Toward a catalog of human genes and proteins: sequencing and analysis of 500 novel complete protein coding human cDNAs. Genome Res 2001; 11(3): 422-35. [http://dx.doi.org/10.1101/gr.154701] [PMID: 11230166]

[78] Merner ND, Hodgkinson KA, Haywood AF, *et al.* Arrhythmogenic right ventricular cardiomyopathy type 5 is a fully penetrant, lethal arrhythmic disorder caused by a missense mutation in the TMEM43 gene. Am J Hum Genet 2008; 82(4): 809-21. [http://dx.doi.org/10.1016/j.ajhg.2008.01.010]

[79] Baskin B, Skinner JR, Sanatani S, *et al.* TMEM43 mutations associated with arrhythmogenic right ventricular cardiomyopathy in non-Newfoundland populations. Hum Genet 2013; 132(11): 1245-52. [http://dx.doi.org/10.1007/s00439-013-1323-2] [PMID: 23812740]

[80] Pilichou K, Thiene G, Bauce B, *et al.* Arrhythmogenic cardiomyopathy. Orphanet J Rare Dis 2016; 11: 33. [http://dx.doi.org/10.1186/s13023-016-0407-1] [PMID: 27038780]

[81] Marcus FI, McKenna WJ, Sherrill D, *et al.* Diagnosis of arrhythmogenic right ventricular cardiomyopathy/dysplasia: proposed modification of the task force criteria. Circulation 2010; 121(13): 1533-41. [http://dx.doi.org/10.1161/CIRCULATIONAHA.108.840827] [PMID: 20172911]

[82] Zorzi A, Rigato I, Pilichou K, *et al.* Phenotypic expression is a prerequisite for malignant arrhythmic events and sudden cardiac death in arrhythmogenic right ventricular cardiomyopathy. Europace 2016;

18(7): 1086-94.
[http://dx.doi.org/10.1093/europace/euv205] [PMID: 26138720]

[83] Protonotarios A, Anastasakis A, Panagiotakos DB, *et al.* Arrhythmic risk assessment in genotyped families with arrhythmogenic right ventricular cardiomyopathy. Europace 2016; 18(4): 610-6.
[http://dx.doi.org/10.1093/europace/euv061] [PMID: 25825460]

[84] Corrado D, Basso C, Pavei A, Michieli P, Schiavon M, Thiene G. Trends in sudden cardiovascular death in young competitive athletes after implementation of a preparticipation screening program. JAMA 2006; 296(13): 1593-601.
[http://dx.doi.org/10.1001/jama.296.13.1593] [PMID: 17018804]

[85] Angelini A, Basso C, Nava A, Thiene G. Endomyocardial biopsy in arrhythmogenic right ventricular cardiomyopathy. Am Heart J 1996; 132(1 Pt 1): 203-6.
[http://dx.doi.org/10.1016/S0002-8703(96)90416-0] [PMID: 8701870]

[86] Basso C, Ronco F, Marcus F, *et al.* Quantitative assessment of endomyocardial biopsy in arrhythmogenic right ventricular cardiomyopathy/dysplasia: an *in vitro* validation of diagnostic criteria. Eur Heart J 2008; 29(22): 2760-71.
[http://dx.doi.org/10.1093/eurheartj/ehn415] [PMID: 18819962]

[87] Zorzi A, Migliore F, Elmaghawry M, *et al.* Electrocardiographic predictors of electroanatomic scar size in arrhythmogenic right ventricular cardiomyopathy: implications for arrhythmic risk stratification. J Cardiovasc Electrophysiol 2013; 24(12): 1321-7.
[http://dx.doi.org/10.1111/jce.12246] [PMID: 24016194]

[88] Cox MG, Nelen MR, Wilde AA, *et al.* Activation delay and VT parameters in arrhythmogenic right ventricular dysplasia/cardiomyopathy: toward improvement of diagnostic ECG criteria. J Cardiovasc Electrophysiol 2008; 19(8): 775-81.
[http://dx.doi.org/10.1111/j.1540-8167.2008.01140.x] [PMID: 18373594]

[89] Platonov PG, Calkins H, Hauer RN, *et al.* High interobserver variability in the assessment of epsilon waves: Implications for diagnosis of arrhythmogenic right ventricular cardiomyopathy/dysplasia. Heart Rhythm 2016; 13(1): 208-16.
[http://dx.doi.org/10.1016/j.hrthm.2015.08.031] [PMID: 26304715]

[90] Bluemke DA, Krupinski EA, Ovitt T, *et al.* MR Imaging of arrhythmogenic right ventricular cardiomyopathy: Morphologic findings and interobserver reliability. Cardiology 2003; 99(1): 153-62.

[91] James CA, Bhonsale A, Tichnell C, *et al.* Exercise increases age□related penetrance and arrhythmic risk in arrhythmogenic right ventricular dysplasia/cardiomyopathy□associated desmosomal mutation carriers. J Am Coll Cardiol 2013; 62(14): 1290-7.

[92] Saberniak J, Hasselberg NE, Borgquist R, *et al.* Vigorous physical activity impairs myocardial function in patients with arrhythmogenic right ventricular cardiomyopathy and in mutation positive family members. Eur J Heart Fail 2014; 16(12): 1337-44.
[http://dx.doi.org/10.1002/ejhf.181] [PMID: 25319773]

[93] Corrado D, Wichter T, Link MS, *et al.* Treatment of arrhythmogenic right ventricular cardiomyopathy/dysplasia. Circulation 2015; 132(5): 441-53.
[http://dx.doi.org/10.1161/CIRCULATIONAHA.115.017944] [PMID: 26216213]

[94] Wlodarska EK, Wozniak O, Konka M, Rydlewska-Sadowska W, Biederman A, Hoffman P. Thromboembolic complications in patients with arrhythmogenic right ventricular dysplasia/cardiomyopathy. Europace 2006; 8(8): 596-600.
[http://dx.doi.org/10.1093/europace/ eul053]

[95] Ermakov S, Scheinman M. Arrhythmogenic right ventricular cardiomyopathy – antiarrhythmic therapy. Arrhythm Electrophysiol Rev 2015; 4(2): 86-9.
[http://dx.doi.org/10.15420/AER.2015.04.02.86] [PMID: 26835106]

[96] Bai R, Di Biase L, Shivkumar K, *et al.* Ablation of ventricular arrhythmias in arrhythmogenic right

ventricular dysplasia/cardiomyopathy: Arrhythmia-free survival after endoepicardial substrate based mapping and ablation. Circ Arrhythm Electrophysiol 2011; 4(4): 478-85. [http://dx.doi.org/10.1161/CIRCEP. 111.963066]

[97] Sacher F, Roberts-Thomson K, Maury P, *et al.* Epicardial ventricular tachycardia ablation a multicenter safety study. J Am Coll Cardiol 2010; 55(21): 2366-72. [http://dx.doi.org/10.1016/j.jacc.2009.10.084] [PMID: 20488308]

[98] Corrado D, Calkins H, Link MS, *et al.* Prophylactic implantable defibrillator in patients with arrhythmogenic right ventricular cardiomyopathy/dysplasia and no prior ventricular fibrillation or sustained ventricular tachycardia. Circulation 2010; 122(12): 1144-52. [http://dx.doi.org/10.1161/CIRCULATIONAHA.109.913871] [PMID: 20823389]

[99] Bhonsale A, James CA, Tichnell C, *et al.* Incidence and predictors of implantable cardioverter-defibrillator therapy in patients with arrhythmogenic right ventricular dysplasia/cardiomyopathy undergoing implantable cardioverter-defibrillator implantation for primary prevention. J Am Coll Cardiol 2011; 58(14): 1485-96. [http://dx.doi.org/10.1016/j.jacc.2011.06.043] [PMID: 21939834]

[100] Link MS, Laidlaw D, Polonsky B, *et al.* Ventricular arrhythmias in the North American multidisciplinary study of ARVC: predictors, characteristics, and treatment. J Am Coll Cardiol 2014; 64(2): 119-25. [http://dx.doi.org/10.1016/j.jacc.2014.04.035] [PMID: 25011714]

[101] Wichter T, Paul TM, Eckardt L, *et al.* Arrhythmogenic right ventricular cardiomyopathy. Antiarrhythmic drugs, catheter ablation, or ICD? Herz 2005; 30(2): 91-101. [http://dx.doi.org/10.1007/s00059-005-2677-6] [PMID: 15875097]

[102] Dalal D, Jain R, Tandri H, *et al.* Long-term efficacy of catheter ablation of ventricular tachycardia in patients with arrhythmogenic right ventricular dysplasia/cardiomyopathy. J Am Coll Cardiol 2007; 50(5): 432-40. [http://dx.doi.org/10.1016/j.jacc.2007.03.049] [PMID: 17662396]

[103] te Riele AS, James CA, Groeneweg JA, *et al.* Approach to family screening in arrhythmogenic right ventricular dysplasia/cardiomyopathy. Eur Heart J 2016; 37(9): 755-63. [http://dx.doi.org/10.1093/eurheartj/ehv387] [PMID: 26314686]

[104] Tedford RJ, James C, Judge DP, *et al.* Cardiac transplantation in arrhythmogenic right ventricular dysplasia/cardiomyopathy. J Am Coll Cardiol 2012; 59(3): 289-90. [http://dx.doi.org/10.1016/j.jacc.2011.09.051] [PMID: 22240135]

[105] Bakir I, Brugada P, Sarkozy A, Vandepitte C, Wellens F. A novel treatment strategy for therapy refractory ventricular arrhythmias in the setting of arrhythmogenic right ventricular dysplasia. Europace 2007; 9(5): 267-9. [http://dx.doi.org/10.1093/europace/eum029] [PMID: 17363427]

[106] Chachques JC, Argyriadis PG, Fontaine G, *et al.* Right ventricular cardiomyoplasty: 10-year follow-up. Ann Thorac Surg 2003; 75(5): 1464-8. [http://dx.doi.org/10.1016/S0003-4975(02)04823-3] [PMID: 12735563]

[107] Zacharias J, Forty J, Doig JC, Bourke JP, Hilton CJ. Right ventricular disarticulation. An 18-year single centre experience. Eur J Cardiothorac Surg 2005; 27(6): 1000-4. [http://dx.doi.org/10.1016/j.ejcts.2005.02.020] [PMID: 15896608]

[108] Santangeli P, Pieroni M, Dello Russo A, *et al.* Noninvasive diagnosis of electroanatomic abnormalities in arrhythmogenic right ventricular cardiomyopathy. Circ Arrhythm Electrophysiol 2010; 3(6): 632-8. [http://dx.doi.org/10.1161/CIRCEP.110.958116] [PMID: 20937720]

[109] Menghetti L, Basso C, Nava A, Angelini A, Thiene G. Spin-echo nuclear magnetic resonance for tissue characterisation in arrhythmogenic right ventricular cardiomyopathy. Heart 1996; 76(6): 467-70. [http://dx.doi.org/10.1136/hrt.76.6.467] [PMID: 9014792]

CHAPTER 7

Inherited Cardiac Channelopathies and Sudden Death

Iroegbu Chukwuemeka Daniel[1], **Zhang Hao**[2], **Song Long**[1], **Sheng Tang**[2] and **Jinfu Yang**[1,*]

[1] *Department of Cardiovascular Surgery, The Second Xiangya Hospital, Central South University, Middle Renmin Road 139, 410011 Changsha, China*

[2] *Department of Thoracic and Cardiovascular Surgery, Affiliated Hospital of Xuzhou Medical University, Xuzhou, 99 Huaihai Road West Xuzhou, Jiangsu Province 221000, China*

Abstract: Sudden death is always an unexpected and devastating occurrence. The normal electrophysiological behavior of the human heart is determined by an ordered propagation of excitatory stimuli that result in slow repolarization and a rapid depolarization, thereby, generating action potential in each myocyte. Hence, mutations in or involving cardiac ion channels result in an abnormal propagation or action potential formation, leading to cardiac arrhythmias. Despite the worrisome impact of sudden cardiac death, and sudden infant death syndrome in the society resulting from such arrhythmias, knowledge of the underlying cellular mechanism is poor, and treatment is consequently and continuously limited. This chapter aims to focus on the role of basic science (current diagnostic and therapeutic options) in investigating primary electrical cardiac diseases as a paradigm for cardiac arrhythmias, concentrating on the long-QT syndrome, Brugada syndrome, and catecholaminergic polymorphous ventricular tachycardia. Also, the underlying pathology and physiology of ion channel diseases are described associated with sudden infant death syndrome to provide a clinical perspective of cardiac channelopathies about sudden infant death syndrome. The learning objectives of the chapter would enable practicing physicians/clinicians in the field to:

I. Recognize risk factors, signs, and symptoms that should prompt suspicion of a congenital arrhythmia syndrome,

II. Explain the treatment options, list measures to prevent sudden cardiac death and sudden infant death syndrome, and

III. Finally, describe what can be achieved with molecular genetic diagnostic tests and thereby, comfortably list the difficulties and limitations of interpreting genetic results.

[*] **Corresponding author Jingfu Yang:** Department of Cardiovascular Surgery, The Second Xiangya Hospital, Central South University, Middle Renmin Road 139, 410011 Changsha, China;
E-mail: yjf19682005@csu.edu.cn, Dr.iroegbu_daniel@csu.edu.cn and Dr.iroegbu_daniel@yahoo.com

Jinfu Yang & Iroegbu Chukwuemeka Daniel (Eds.)

Keywords: Arrhythmias, Atrial Fibrillation, Adolescents, Brugada Syndrome, Cardiomyopathy, Cardiology, Channelopathies, Death, Exercise, Genetics, Genetic arrhythmias, Gene-Specific Management, Genetic Testing, Heart, Heart Rhythm Disorders, Infant, Inherited Arrhythmic Disorders, Ion Channel Structure, Ion Channel Function, Ischemic Heart Disease, Pathology of Sudden Cardiac Death, Pathophysiology of Sudden Cardiac Death, Primary Electrical Cardiac Channelopathies, Sudden Death, Sudden Infant Death Syndrome, Susceptibility Genes, Syncope, Ventricular Fibrillation.

INTRODUCTION

Cardiac channelopathies are potentially malignant conditions caused by mutations in channels that affect ion transit across the cardiac myocyte cell membrane. The normal electrophysiological behavior of the heart is regulated by an ordered propagation of excitatory stimuli resulting in rapid depolarization, and slow repolarization, thereby, generating action potentials (AP) in individual myocytes. At the most generic level, abnormalities in the configuration and duration of each single cardiac APs, or propagation, and impulse generation form the basis of a disordered cardiac rhythm (hereditary arrhythmias). Although hereditary arrhythmic syndromes are rare, an early diagnosis would markedly reduce the risk of sudden cardiac death SCD in infants, children, and in the adult population, which are all otherwise healthy people. But a clear distinction for hereditary arrhythmic syndromes should be made by a group of physicians (multidisciplinary team not to be left to cardiologist alone) between primary arrhythmic syndromes caused by dysfunctions in ion channels of cardiac muscles (ion channel disease) and primary structural heart diseases with increased arrhythmia risk [1 - 4]. The most common ion channel diseases are long-QT syndrome (LQTS), short-QT syndrome (SQTS), Brugada syndrome (BrS), and catecholaminergic polymorphous ventricular tachycardia (CPVT) which all have highly variable clinical presentations and risk factors. However, the overall risk factors can be divided into extrinsic factors such as mild infections, bedding material (soft), bed-sharing, and the sleeping position (supine position), and intrinsic factors such as genetic variants (both mutations and polymorphisms), race (*e.g.* African Americans and Maoris from New Zealand), sex (male predominance), develop-mental (prematurity), and environmental factors (smoking both pre- and postnatal and socioeconomic status) [5]. Be it as it may, apart from hereditary arrhythmias and SCD (an unexpected death which occurs within a short period of time due to heart problems or any related heart symptoms), another challenging issue is sudden infant death syndrome (SIDS) victims, seemingly healthy children below the age of one, who die suddenly [6]. However, cases of SIDS are generally accepted to require a complete postmortem examination, including a negative autopsy [7]. Several possible explanations of SIDS have been proposed: infections [8], variants in the genes underlying the AP of the heart [9], fatty acid oxidation disorders [10], and serotonergic brainstem abnormalities [11].

This chapter aims to focus on the role of basic science (current diagnostic and therapeutic options) in investigating primary electrical cardiac diseases as a paradigm for cardiac arrhythmias, concentrating on LQTS, BrS, and CPVT. It will also, describe the underlying pathology and physiology of ion channel diseases associated with SIDS and also provide a clinical perspective of cardiac channelopathies about SIDS. The learning objectives of the chapter would enable practicing physician's/clinicians in the field to:

I. Recognize risk factors, signs, and symptoms that should prompt suspicion of a congenital arrhythmia syndrome.
II. Explain the treatment options, list measures to prevent SCD and SIDS and
III. Finally, describe what can be achieved with molecular genetic diagnostic tests and thereby comfortably list the difficulties and limitations of interpreting genetic results.

CONCEPT (Table 1)

Table 1. Clinical red flags for the presence of a cardiac arrhythmia syndrome*.

Syncope or seizure triggered by I. Exercise (especially swimming) II. Emotion or anxiety III. Sudden auditory stimuli (phone, alarm clock)
Seizures not responsive to antiepileptic medications
Family history of I. Sudden death before age 30 years (including drowning, single person car accident, or sudden infant death syndrome) II. Recurrent syncope
Electrocardiogram abnormalities I. Prolongation of the QT interval II. Notched T waves on >2 precordial leads

* Patients with one or more of these features may benefit from an expedited pediatric cardiology evaluation to assess for an underlying cardiac channelopathy.

- Channelopathies are diseases caused by the disturbed function of ion channel subunits or the proteins that regulate them. These diseases may be either acquired (often resulting from an autoimmune attack on an ion channel) or congenital/inherited (usually resulting from a mutation or mutations in the encoding genes).
- Sudden death (SD) is death that unexpectedly occurs within one hour of symptoms' onset or unwitnessed within 24 h of the deceased being seen alive

and in a reasonable state of health, before the discovery of the body. Though some patients die instantly, the majority of them do have some prodrome.

- SCD is an unexpected death which occurs within a short period due to heart problems or any related heart symptoms, which can also be witnessed or unwitnessed. The time frame usually varies, especially in out-of-clinic settings observed or unwitnessed.
- Sudden infant death syndrome (SIDS) also called "crib death" as many babies who die of SIDS are found in their cribs is the sudden, unexplained death of an infant younger than one-year-old.

HISTORICAL PERSPECTIVE

In general, SD has been known for thousands of years [12]. More than 4000 years ago in Egypt, SD was associated with myocardial ischemia. The Ebers papyrus states that: "If a patient has pain in the arm and left the side of the chest, there is a threat of death." However, 2500 years ago in China, Chio associated SD with an arrhythmia when he said, "An intermittent pulse is a predictor of imminent death". Although around the same time, Hippocrates stated that: "Intense chest pain that radiates to the clavicle and back is a sign of poor prognosis". He was, however, the first writer to introduce the concept of risk factors when he wrote: "Obese individuals are more likely to die suddenly than thin ones ".

Nevertheless, these concepts persist up to date as many publications have drawn the attention of the scientist towards centuries of shock and fear caused by SD [13, 14]. In the 14th century, Count Gaston de Foix (Fig. **1**) who died suddenly after returning from a hunting trip during which he had been in contact with icy water. He had a strong feeling of chest tightness and said: "I am a dead man; may God have mercy on me" [14].

Later on, in the 18th century, a book written by Lancisi [15] on the numerous cases of SD occurring in Rome was published by the order of Pope Clement XI. Also, Heberden in the late 18th century published the first description of "angina pectoris as further clinical and autopsy studies continuously show the association between chest pain and SD with anatomopathological signs of heart disease. Herrick [16] in the 20th century described the clinical features of myocardial infarction (MI) although, Von Bezold in the 19th century carried out an experiment where he described the occlusion of the coronary arteries caused cardiac arrest. As cases of SD increased throughout the 20th century, interest in SD increased, as well as its association with coronary artery disease [17]. Moreover, the importance of deterioration in heart failure (HF) (ventricular function) and its presentation became much clearer regardless of whether it was associated with ischemia or not. Finally, during the latter half of the 20th century, though ischemic heart diseases (IHD) was continually shown to be the cause of SD in 85% of the cases [18], a group of inherited structural alteration diseases (cardiomyopathy) or without apparent organic reason (channelopathies) explained many cases of SD in younger individuals without IHD, whether SD was associated with effort or not [12].

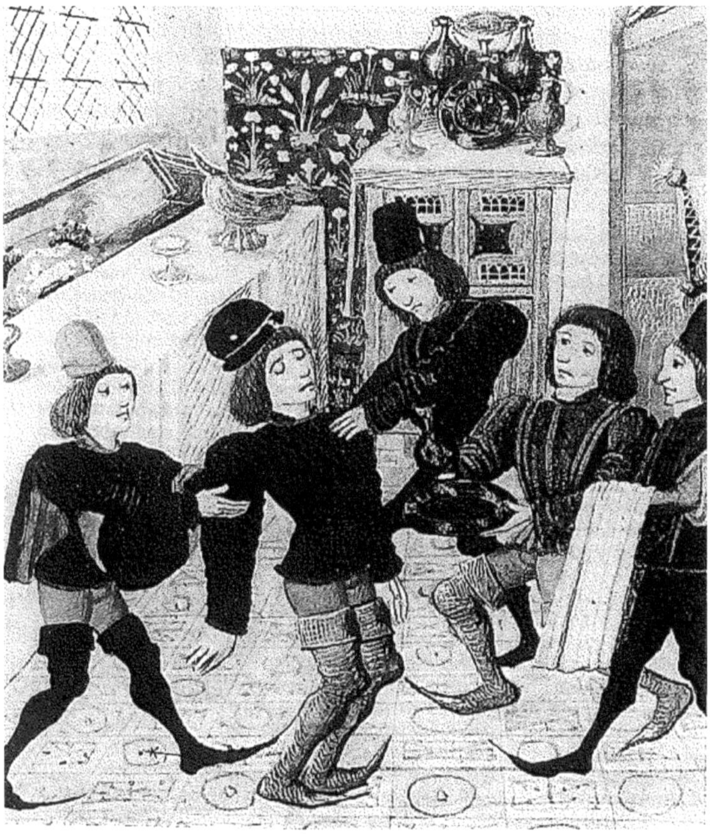

Fig. (1). Death of Count Gaston de Foix.

EPIDEMIOLOGY

Cardiac channelopathies and SD are one of the most significant challenges in modern cardiology due to the enormous number of cases (more than 200,000 per year in the United States alone) and its considerable social impact. Although its incidence rates are lower in some Mediterranean countries, such as Spain [19], and SD can be seen in infants, it is usually rare in the first decades of life due to its association with abnormalities in the autonomic nervous system, increased vagal tone, and impaired repolarization. Channelopathies and SD sometimes appear during sports activities and in the presence of genetic heart diseases such as arrhythmogenic right ventricular cardiomyopathy (ARVC) and hypertrophic cardiomyopathy (HCM). However, the incidence of SD gradually increases with age, particularly from 30-40 years onwards, and is particularly high with associated MI (acute phase) and HF.

MECHANISMS OF VENTRICULAR ARRHYTHMOGENESIS

Cardiac excitability is based on the healthy balance between repolarizing and depolarizing ion currents. Therefore, gene mutations of any form involved in the regulation of cardiac ion channels would potentially result in arrhythmias classified as either abnormal AP propagation or formation. Each ionic current is further distinguished by its time course and ionic selectivity; properties that are conferred by specific ion channels.

Abnormal AP Propagation (Re-Entrant Arrhythmias)

The normal ventricular mammalian myocardium has a highly regulated activation sequence of AP. It occurs when the depolarization wave-front fails to extinguish entirely right after normal activation; therefore, leading to the continuous re-excitation of regions with recovered excitability.

Re-Entrant Arrhythmias Principal Requirements for Initiation

I. An obstacle around which the AP can circulate.
II. Sufficiently slow conduction velocity such that before the wave returns, each region recovers excitability.
III. An existence of unidirectional conduction block, preventing the wave from self-extinguishing.

Abnormal AP Formation

Abnormal AP formation occurs as a result of enhanced automaticity (accelerated depolarization of pacemaker tissue, leading to an increased sympathetic activity), and parasystole (activation of two or more pacemaker regions) or triggered event (generation of extrasystoles originating in areas other than the primary pacemaker).

PATHOPHYSIOLOGY OF SUDDEN DEATH AND SUDDEN INFANT DEATH SYNDROME

SD is the final stage of a chain of events leading to cardiac arrest; these are usually ventricular fibrillation (VF) or, less often, severe bradyarrhythmia [20]. In all cases, there are, however, series of triggering or modulating factors that, by acting on vulnerable myocardium, precipitate SD. Briefly, in the presence of vulnerable myocardium, VF is usually precipitated by the action of various triggering and modulating factors. For example, in a specific environmental or genetic context, and increased sympathetic activity associated with psychological or physical stress that although, not offensive under normal circumstances, can precipitate SD in ion channelopathies and other cardiomyopathies (hereditary diseases), and particular settings like acute ischemia. In SIDS however, a combination of physical and sleep environmental factors makes an infant more vulnerable such as; physical factors (low birth weight [LBW], brain defects, and respiratory infection), and environmental factors (items in the baby's crib, and his or her sleeping position combined with the baby's physical problems).

RISK FACTORS IN SUDDEN INFANT DEATH SYNDROME

Though SIDS can strike any infant, the identified below factors increase the infant's risk. These include:

Maternal Risk Factors

I. Use of drugs or alcohol
II. The use of tobacco (cigarette smoking)
III. Inadequate prenatal care and
IV. Mothers younger than 20 years of age.

Infants Risk Factors

I. Sex (SIDS mostly affect male infants).
II. Premature infants (either born early or as LBW).
III. Infants living with smokers or as passive smokers.
IV. Age (between the second and fourth months of life).
V. Family history (siblings or cousins who died of SIDS).
VI. Race (nonwhite infants mostly develop SIDS though, reasons still not well-understood).

CHANNELOPATHIES AND ION CHANNELS ASSOCIATED WITH SUDDEN INFANT DEATH SYNDROME (TABLE 2)

Brugada Syndrome

Clinical Characteristics: BrS is characterized clinically by VF and episodes of polymorphic ventricular tachycardia (PVT), and electrocardiographically by right bundle branch block (RBBB) and persistent ST-segment elevation in right precordial leads, right ventricle (RV) delay, and negative T-waves which are all associated with a high risk of SCD [21] (Figs. **2** & **3**). Patients suffer from syncope or SCD secondary to VF/ PVT. However, most patients remain completely asymptomatic. It occurs (arrhythmia) after large meals, during rest, or while the patient is fast asleep, which are all due to an increase in vagal tone [22]. Symptoms usually appear between thirty to forty years of age; however, reports of patients affected between ages of one to twenty, and fifty to eighty exist. Males are often symptomatic than females, probably due to the influence of hormones and gender distribution of ion channels across the heart.

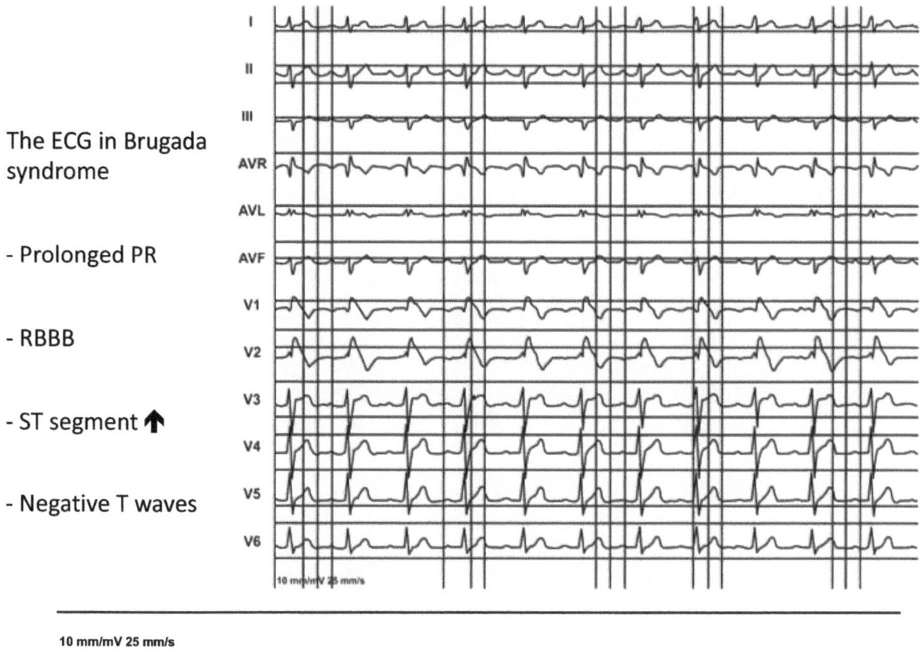

Fig. (2). Typical electrocardiogram of Brugada syndrome.

Pathophysiology and The Molecular Mechanisms of BrS

The proposed mechanism which initially appeared to receive the most comprehensive support both from experimental studies [23] and other related clinical studies [24] ascribes BrS as a primary repolarization disorder. The most common and best studied of these is the loss-of-function mutation of the SCN5A gene, encoding the a-subunit of the voltage-gated Na^+ channel [25]. While many genetic mutations have been associated with BrS [26], they all, however, result in a general imbalance of currents in favor of repolarization over depolarization. Furthermore, the pathophysiological mechanisms responsible for ST-segment changes must operate during the cardiac repolarization phase, and these mechanisms must be based on INa reduction. The deep phase 1 notch in the epicardial AP [26], renders it susceptible to the effects of a reduction in the Na^+ current. However, the decrease in Na^+ current establishes a steep voltage gradient across the RV wall due to short-circuiting of the epicardial AP resulting in extreme shortening [27]. This imbalance in current flow allows for the reactivation of the RV epicardium by neighboring regions of the myocardium, with longer APs producing functional re-entry, referred to as phase 2 re-entry. Nevertheless, even after the recognition of genetic abnormalities in the SCN5A gene, the intense controversy surrounding the underlying mechanisms leading to the ECG abnormalities, arrhythmias, and sudden death [25 - 27] still exist as twelve other genetic variants have been identified [21].

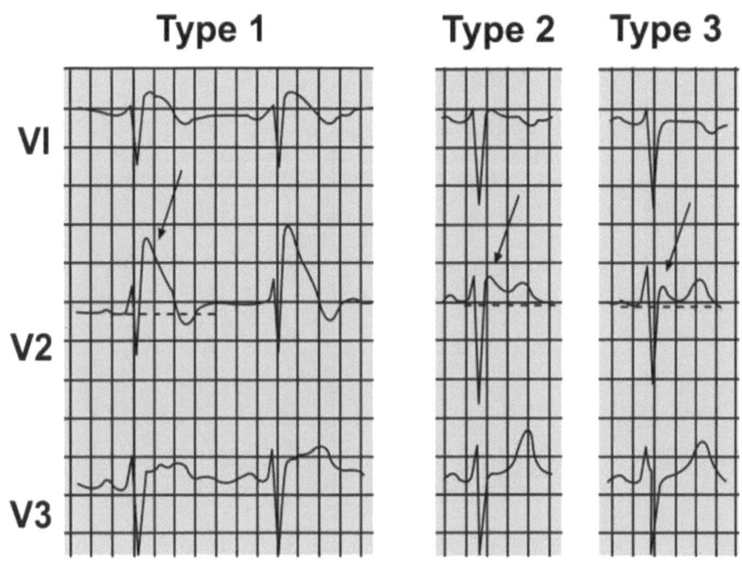

Fig. (3). Brugada type 1, 2, and 3 ECGs: Type 1 ECG: Coved-type ST elevation ≥2 mm with T-wave inversion in at least two of leads V1 to V3. Type 2 ECG: Saddle-back ST elevation with increased descent ≥2 mm and at least 1 mm, elevation of the ST segment. Type 3 ECG: Saddle-back or coved-type ST elevation <1 mm.

Current theories related to BrS:

a. The depolarization theory involves slow preferential conduction in the RV outflow tract, leading to ST-segment elevation in the right precordial leads [25],
b. The repolarization theory focuses on the presence of transmural voltage gradients due to heterogeneity in AP duration between the RV endocardium and epicardium (disequilibrium between INa and Ito) [26], and
c. The neural crest theory provides a potential explanation for the 60% of patients with BrS and the 40% isolated, non-familial cases where mutations in the germinal cells do not appear to play a role [27] (Fig. **4**).

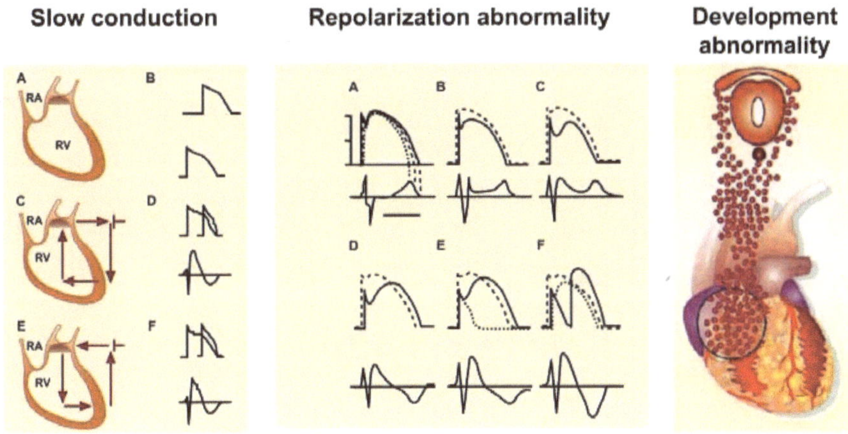

Fig. (4). The three theories about the pathophysiological mechanisms involved in Brugada syndrome.

Genetics: After the first pathogenic mutation in the SCN5A gene encoding, the alpha subunit of the cardiac sodium channel in 1998 was identified [28], several genes have since then been published (SCN1B, RAN GRF, KCNE 3, GPD1L, KCND 3, CACNB2B, CACNA 2D1, SCN2B, SCN5A, SCN3B, TR PM4, KCNJ8, HCN4, KCNE 5, CACNA 1C, and SL MAP) [29]. These genes encode subunits of cardiac sodium, calcium, and potassium channels as well as genes involved in the regulation of trafficking of these channels. Despite the increase in the number of gene mutations, only about 30-35% of BrS patients have been determined to have a genetic cause with 20% of them carrying a pathogenetic mutation in SCN5A [30]. All other genes together are responsible for about 5% of all BrS cases. Therefore, 65% of cases do not have a genetic origin due to the fact that; (i) various copies of number of variations have already been reported in the SCN5A gene [31], (ii) pathogenic mutations associated with BrS can be localized in unknown genes or either (iii) related to epigenetic factors, mainly post-translational modifications, DNA methylation, and RNA mechanisms [32, 33]. All these factors explain in part, the variable expressivity characteristics, and incomplete penetrance in BrS families [34].

Long QT Syndrome

Clinical Characteristics: LQTS prevalence is about 1 in 5000 individuals, relatively making it a common cause of SCD among children and young adults with structurally healthy hearts [35]. It forms a genetically heterogeneous group of conditions, caused by a genetic mutation in either the cardiac sodium or potassium channel or one of their associated regulatory proteins characterized by an increased risk of ventricular arrhythmias, particularly torsade de pointes and prolonged ventricular repolarization. In contrast to BrS, the mutations in LQTS result in favor of depolarizing currents over repolarizing ones (Fig. **5**).

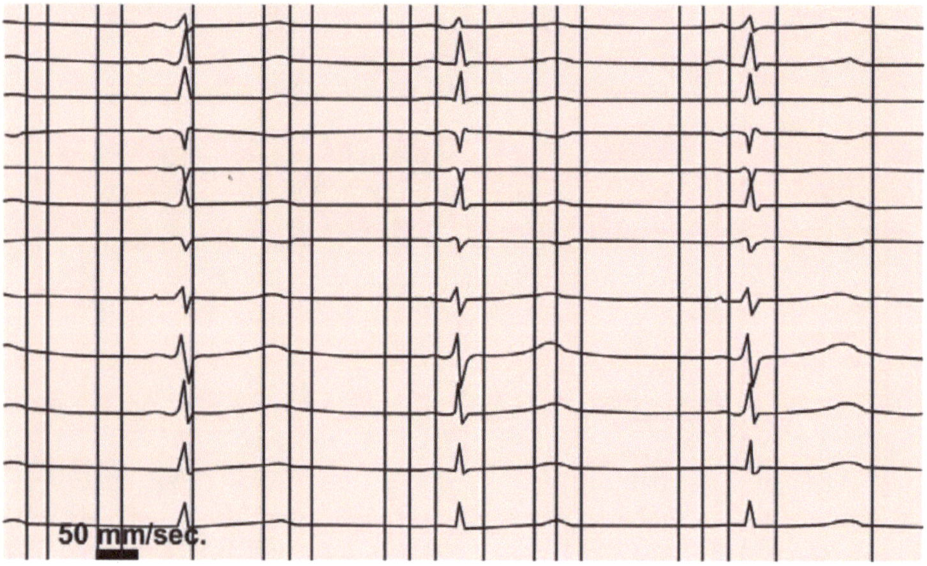

Fig. (5). Long QT syndrome, type 1: prolonged QTc (485 ms), broad-based T waves.

Pathophysiology and The Molecular Mechanism of LQTS: LQTS is typically inherited in an autosomal dominant fashion with variable penetrance, although spontaneous mutations are relatively frequent. Genetic mutations caused in either sodium channel or potassium channel or one of their associated regulatory proteins result in the prolongation of cardiac repolarization and an increased vulnerability to ventricular arrhythmias. The extension of AP duration (APD) generates an arrhythmic substrate resulting in either:

a. An increased refractory period from channels that remain depolarized for more considerable periods creating pockets of the functional block, which may act as the focus for re-entry or
b. Differences in the dispersion of repolarization across the myocardium, creating a functional re-entry phase acting as a trigger for torsade de pointes [36].

Genetics: Approximately 70% of patients with specific clinical LQTS diagnosis have mutations in one of the three dominant LQTS-susceptibility genes and approximately 5-10% of the minor LQTS genotypes that encode for ion channel α subunits and are critically responsible for the orchestration of the cardiac AP.

The Major Three LQTS Genotypes: (KCNQ1-encoded IKs (Kv7.1) potassium channel, KCNH2-encoded IKr (Kv11.1) potassium channel, and SCN5A-encoded INa (Nav1.5) sodium channel) [37 - 39]: Loss-of-function mutations in KCNQ1 cause about 30% of LQTS type 1 (LQT1), while loss-of-function KCNH2 mutations contribute approximately 20% of LQTS (LQT2). Gain-of-function SCN5A mutations underlie roughly 10% of LQTS (LQT3). About 5% of LQTS patients host multiple mutations in these genes and often seen at a much younger age with a more severe phenotype [37]. The vast majority of mutations are small insertion/deletions or single nucleotide substitutions [37 - 39].

The Minor Ten LQTS Genotypes: The encoding for additional ion channel α subunits (KCNJ5, CACNA1C), sodium-channel (SNTA1, SCN4B, CAV3), and key cardiac potassium- (KCNE1, AKAP9, KCNE2) calcium-binding messenger proteins (CALM1, CALM2) or interacting proteins. However, because these play a minor role in LQTS genetic basis, only a few limited genotype-phenotype correlations have been generated.

Catecholaminergic Polymorphic Ventricular Tachycardia

Clinical Characteristics: CPVT is a rare but highly inherited malignant arrhythmic condition due to the action of increased catecholamines during stress or exercise, presenting as SCD or syncope, (Fig. **6**) resulting in a bidirectional VT with an estimated prevalence of 1 in 10,000 individuals. Similar to LQTS, CPVT is primarily an autosomal dominant disease, with a variable phenotype due to incomplete penetration. CPVT most commonly presents in children (mean age eight years). However, cases of children younger than four years of age, adolescence, and adults are well described [40]. Although on average, there is a two-year delay from presentation to diagnosis because children are often misdiagnosed with epilepsy, vasovagal syncope, or concealed LQTS [41].

Pathophysiology and The Molecular Mechanism of CPVT: The underlying mechanism of CPVT revolves around abnormal Ca^{2+} release from the sarcoplasmic reticulum (SR), which is often due either to loss of function mutations in calsequestrin (CASQ2), a SR calcium buffering protein [42] or gain-of-function mutations in the gene encoding RyR2, a critical regulator of Ca^{2+} release from the SR for excitation-contraction coupling [43]. The mutations in CASQ2 or RyR2 result in an increased propensity for ventricular arrhythmias and an intracellular calcium overload at elevated heart rates [44]. This mechanism release is similar to digitalis toxicity, where baseline Ca^{2+} is also elevated, resulting in an arrhythmic trigger [42].

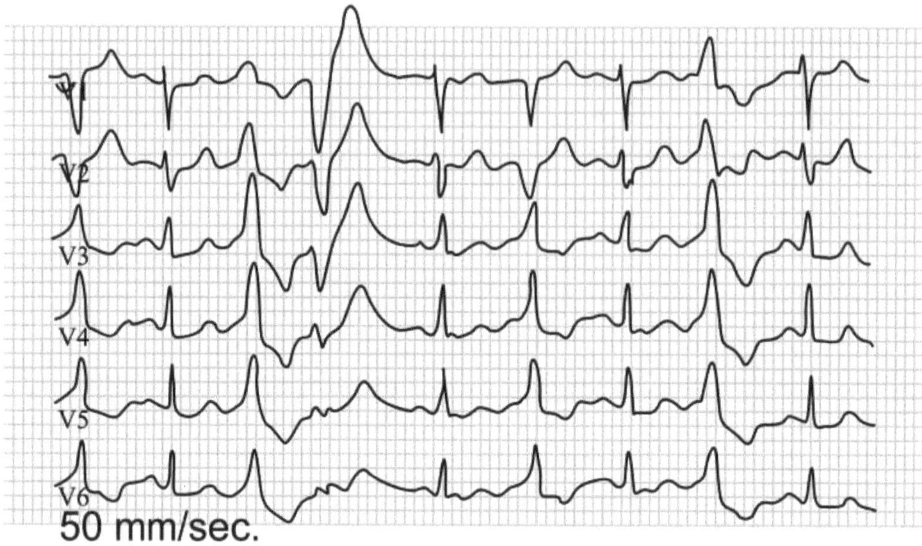

Fig. (6). Catecholaminergic polymorphous ventricular tachycardia. Frequent ventricular extrasystoles during exercise.

Genetics : It transmits in an autosomal dominant fashion, generally affecting boys and girls equally. Apart from the most commonly identified genetic mutation in CPVT (CASQ2 and the RYR2 gene), other genes associated with CPVT include CALM1 encoding Calmodulin, TECRL encoding Trans-2,3-enoyl-CoA reductase-like protein, and TRDN encoding Triadin [45]. However, autosomal recessive pattern inheritance of the disease has been documented though much less common. Also, sometimes, CPVT arises from a sporadic (spontaneous) mutation. In this case, the parents and the siblings are negative for the CPVT-causing gene and at no increased risk.

Other Syndromes

While vast cases of SCD in the absence of structural heart defects are caused by the syndromes mentioned above, other few related syndromes have come to light so far. Short QT syndrome, phenotypically characterized by short APDs and hence QT intervals, can be caused by either a loss of function mutations in Ca^{2+} channels [46] or gain-of-function mutations in K^+ channels [47]. However, progressive cardiac conduction diseases (PCCD) encompass another group of conditions that, while most commonly manifesting as bradycardia, may also cause SCD with SCN5A known as the first gene to be associated with PCCD [48].

Sodium Channel Mutations Involved in SIDS

The sodium channel protein Nav 1.5 is solely responsible for the primary conduction of cardiac sodium current. It is however regulated by four membrane-spanning accessory subunits Nav 1–4, cytosolic proteins (accountable for stabilization and targeting of the cell surface of the channel) as well as, modifying the kinetics and surface density of the channel [49, 50]. Of the approximate 20% of SIDS cases established as being caused by channelopathies, cardiac sodium channel mutations and malformations constitute the majority as mutations/malformation in the channel leads to a late, sustained or increased sodium current, prolonging QT intervals.

Table 2. Genes encoding cardiac ion channel α and β subunits.

α Subunits			**β subunits**	
current	Gene	Human Chromosomal location	Gene	Human Chromosomal location
Inward currents			β1 (SCN1B)	19q13.1-q13.2
• I_{Na}	SCN5A	3p21	β2 (SCN2B)	11q23
• I_{Ca-L}	α 1C (CACNL1A1)	12pter-p13.2	β2 (SCN2B)	11q23
• I_{Ca-T}	α 1H (CACNA1H)	16p13.3	β2 (CACNB2)	10p12
			α2δ (CACNA2D1)	7q21-22
Outward currents			minK/IsK (KCNE1)	21q22.12
• I_{Ks}	KvLQT1 (KCNQ1)	11p15.5	minK/IsK (KCNE1)	21q22.12
• I_{Kr}	HERG (KCNH2)	7q36-q36	MiRP1 (KCNE2)	21q22.12
• I_{Kur}	Kv1.5 (KCNA5)		Kvβ1 (KCNAB1)	3q26.1
• I_{K1}	Kir2.1 (KCNJ2)	17q	Kvβ2 (KCNAB2)	1p36.3
	Kir2.2 (KCNJ12)	17p11.1	SUR2 (ABCC9)	12p12.1
• I_{K-Ach}	GIRK1, Kir3.1 (KCNJ3)	2q24.1	MiRP1 (KCNE2)	21q22.12
	C GIRK4, Kir3.4 (KCNJ5)	11q24		
• I_{K-ATP}	Kir6.2, BIR (KCNJ11)	11p15.1		
• I_{TO}	Kv4.3 (KCND3)	1p13.2		
	Kv1.4 (KCNA4)	11p14		
• I_f, I_h	BCNG2, HCN2	19p13.3		
(P.C)	HCN4	15q24-q25		
• I_{Kp}	TWIK1(KCNK1)	1q42-q43		
	CFTR (ABCC7)	7q31.2		
	KvLQT1 (KCNQ1)	11p15.5		
Common names (usually first assigned) are given first, with the currently designated gene name in parentheses. P.C; Peacemaker current.				

Potassium Channel Mutations Involved in SIDS

The prominent role Na^+ channels play in SID is, however, not the same with cardiac K^+ channel mutations. Although K^+ channels are primarily involved in repolarization in situations with increased sympathetic drive [51], K^+ channel mutations associated with SIDS can be identified in K v 7.1, with the loss and gain of function in K^+ channels in SIDS since SIDS is usually primarily associated with sleep.

Ryanodine Receptor Mutations Involved in SIDS

Ryanodine is a Ca^{2+} -activated Ca^+ release channel receptor, located in the SR in close proximity to the T tubules. This calcium release from SR is termed as calcium-induced calcium release. Ryanodine receptors are usually quiescent during the diastolic interval, but the gain of function mutations in RYR2 results in a leaky Ca^+ release into the cytosol from the receptors, especially under an increased sympathetic tone [51]. The diastolic Ca^{2+} release from SR increases the propensity for delay after depolarizations, which in turn, propagates ventricular arrhythmias.

CHANNELOPATHIES ASSOCIATED WITH SWIMMING-RELATED EVENTS

The combination of activities involved in swimming, including cold-water exposure, facial immersion, and exertion leads to a dominance of sympathetic drive over usual parasympathetic dominance seen in the resting state. Although LQT1 and CPVT are the ion channelopathies most significantly associated with swimming-related events, others have been described, such as LQT216 and LQT7 [52]. Triggers specific for arrhythmia have been associated with particular genotypes (noise and LQT2, sleep, and LQT3) with some clinical reports [53] backing the swimming-triggered cardiac events seen which are pathognomonic for LQT1. However, Choi *et al.* [54] also further evaluated CPVT and swimming-related events, although from a mechanical point of view. Furthermore, premature ventricular contractions are usually identified with individuals who swim [55], and lengthened QT interval with facial immersion (in cold water) occurring during the vulnerable part of repolarization initiating ventricular arrhythmia. However, the reason why some individuals are more at risk than others despite comparable QT intervals is solely based on genetic heterogeneity in autonomic responses [56].

PHYSICAL ACTIVITY, SPORTS, EXERCISE, AND CHILDRENS PHYSIOLOGY

Physical activity is considered as any body movement which requires energy expenditure, thereby, increasing resting metabolic rate, (cleaning up, walking, and/or gardening). However, physical activity include all activities that are either planned, structured, and adapted to specific characteristics of people, to maintain, readjust, and to improve health through physical skills. Although physical activity and *sports* are most of the time performed interchangeably, sports denote any physical activity represented by a sports federation with its own rules including activities performed as an amateur sport, and elite professional sport.

On the other hand, *children's physiology* is unique: slow acclimatization to heat, higher metabolic demand relative to body mass during weight-bearing exercise, greater body surface area to mass ratio, and a reduced cardiac output at a given metabolic rate as compared to adults. Children's cardiac size is generally small, making maximum heart rate higher, which decreases linearly with age. During maximal exercise, stroke volume is limited and, in consequence, improvement will be observed. Therefore, any task, physical activity, and sport performed at maximum effort situations imply acute or chronic adjustments that can either be beneficial (reduced clustering of cardiovascular disease risk factors, reduced risk of obesity, and higher bone density) or harmful to health, depending on the intensity of the activity frequency, and duration. Be it as it may, the author's advice to children of ages 5 to 15 is to indulge in only moderate-to-severe intensity activities 3-5 times per week for 60 minutes.

BASIC ELECTROPHYSIOLOGICAL STUDIES AND METHODS EMPLOYED IN INHERITED CARDIAC ARRHYTHMIAS

As commonly practiced in many fields of medicine, investigation of inherited cardiac arrhythmias has relied on the translational cycle of describing clinical problems via a genetic approach. It also involves studying its genotype at the bench level, and using familial studies to classify the distinguishing features, refining its analytical techniques and characterizing the underlying mechanism(s), which is then further followed by a move back into the hospital in the form of drug trials and risk stratification.

Initial Diagnostic Procedure

Necessary and initial diagnostic steps should include: (i) 12-lead resting ECG (ii) a long-term ECG, and (iii) an echocardiographic examination. They should all be followed through a family history of two to three generations if possible. The patient should be asked explicitly about incidents of syncope, or seizures, and any case(s) of SD in the family.

Indications for Further Diagnostic Procedures

I. Documented arrhythmias
II. Young age SCD among relatives
III. Epilepsy (atypical) in the context of specific triggers

The clinical evaluation of any hereditary arrhythmic syndrome should be determined. Confirmation with genetic testing should be carried out to determine if there is any reason to suspect. If a pathogenic mutation is documented in the patient, it should be used for predictive or diagnostic genetic testing of relatives [57, 58].

Genetic Diagnostic Testing

Molecular genetic testing should be carried out for all suspected diagnosis, especially for genes most often involved, and are worth investigating. Although, the molecular genetic investigation should be carried out on an individual case basis at specialist laboratories. Once the causative genotype is identified in a patient, an option to carry out predictive or diagnostic genetic testing in at-risk persons among the patient's relatives in a step-wise manner (autosomal-dominant inheritance) or cascade pattern (autosomal recessive) should be considered.

Problems in Interpreting Test Results: It should be noted that a "negative" search result for a mutation never rules out a probable clinical diagnosis. Plausibility in "positive" results should be double-checked, since it may be that the mutation identified is not the cause or not the sole cause of the disease [49]. A general genetic test should not be carried out as there is no point without a suspected/definite diagnosis. Such screening often easily results in a misdiagnosis, which leads to false worry in other relatives. Sometimes, a result cannot be correctly interpreted without the genetic and clinical testing of relatives, especially if the mutation in question is unknown even where there is a very definite suspected diagnosis.

PHARMACOTHERAPY

We (the authors) recommend the use of beta-blockers for both CPVT and LQTS. It should also be prescribed for both asymptomatic mutation carriers (primary prevention) and symptomatic mutation carriers (secondary prevention) [59]. As for BrS, flecainide, propafenone, and ajmaline should be used for unmasking its features [22] with the use of an implantable cardioverter defibrillator for the prevention of SCD in these patients [60] (Table **3**).

LIFESTYLE

In all cases, the recommendations about the patient's lifestyle are of central importance with concrete preventive measures taken to avoid specific triggers, and patients must be informed about these. As for asymptomatic persons, however, the general recommendation is to avoid physical activities, exceptionally competitive ones due to the risk that cardiac arrhythmias will occur and will have a negative influence on the disease course. Specific, genotype-related preventive measures are:

I. Avoid sudden loud noises (LQTS2).
II. No competitive sports (valid for all arrhythmia syndromes).
III. Avoid potential QT-prolonging medications (all forms of LQTS).
IV. Avoid medications that are contraindicated for Brugada syndrome.
V. Avoid swimming alone and don't jump into cold water (especially CPVT and LQTS1).

Table 3. Management of LQTS.

Syndrome and Lifestyle Changes	Pharmacotherapy	ICD for High-risk Patients
LQTS – Avoid certain drugs – No competitive sports – Bring down fever early – Avoid electrolyte disturbances (hypokalemia, hypomagnesemia) – Carry an emergency card – Consider changes to work-life if appropriate	– Beta-blockers – In patients with prolonged QTc. – In patients with normal QTc. In some individual cases: – Mexiletine plus beta-blockers for LQTS 3 – (In some particular cases ranolazine or flecainide plus beta-blockers)	(With beta-blockers) – Patients who have survived sudden cardiac death. Symptoms are persisting despite therapy.
CPVT – Avoid certain drugs – No competitive sports – Bring down fever early – Avoid electrolyte disturbances (hypokalemia, hypomagnesemia) – Carry an emergency card – Consider changes to work-life if appropriate	– Beta-blockers, in some individual cases flecainide (plus beta-blockers)	(With beta-blockers) – Patients who have survived sudden cardiac death.
BrS – Avoid certain drugs – No competitive sports – Bring down fever early – Avoid electrolyte disturbances (hypokalemia, hypomagnesemia) – Carry an emergency card – Consider changes to work-life if appropriate	– Quinidine in patients with an electrical storm – Quinidine may also be given prophylactically in the context of clinical studies	– Patients who have survived sudden cardiac death – In patients with type 1 ECG and unexplained syncope – In patients with type 1 ECG and ventricular tachycardia

ICD; Implantable cardioverter defibrillator, ECG; Electrocardiography.
LQTS Long QT syndrome, CPVT; Catecholaminergic polymorphous ventricular tachycardia, and BrS; Brugada arrhythmic syndromes.

GENETIC TESTING ISSUES IN CHANNELOPATHIES

Progress aimed at deciphering the molecular basis for heritable cardiac arrhythmia susceptibility, has reshaped both the clinical management and diagnostic paradigm of these three cardiac channelopathies to include genetic testing, increased awareness of the need to assess disease risk in family members, and gene-specific considerations in therapy. Although successful advances have been made, there still remain unresolved pressing issues in both the genetic, and legal implications with these familial arrhythmic syndromes.

Pitfalls and Limitations of Genetic Testing

The methods used in the genetic identification of mutations are not 100% sensitive, and therefore, a negative genetic test cannot exclude the disorder by itself. Also, specific detectable DNA sequence variants may not have a clear causal role in a patient's condition because they are rare polymorphisms [61] or located in regions of the channel protein that have unknown functional importance. Over time, however, both commercial and the academic sectors have come to understand that most mutations occur in a single family (missense mutations) due to uncertain pathophysiological or functional consequences [62]. In the long run, the likelihood that a particular variant predisposes to arrhythmia or whether the change is merely a rare benign variant [63] leads to difficulties in accurately interpreting the genetic result. However, only a small fraction of all identified genetic variants in the multiple genes associated with CPVT, LQTS, and BrS have been investigated functionally to elucidate a biologically plausible contribution to pathogenesis.

Furthermore, the lack of biological or functional validation of mutation effects in the cardiac channelopathies remains the most severe limitation of genetic test interpretation. Also, the description of a negative genetic test result in an asymptomatic person is a challenge. Also, the possible case of either a false-negative or true-negative test result despite achievements in the genetic discovery of cardiac channelopathies remains a crucial issue common pathology.

Genetics and Medico-Legal Implications

The lack of screening of autosomal recessive patients (cascade screening) is said to pose medico-legal implications on physicians knowingly or unknowingly. For instance, any physician who does not however clinically attempt genotyping, the proband affected by one channelopathy is said to have willfully decided to ignore whether some of the family members are carriers of the disease and thereby are exposed to the risk of life-threatening arrhythmias. Likewise, a physician who after having obtained positive genotyping, does not propose to initiate a family screening of the proband is said to have similarly willfully decided to leave the affected family members, approximately one-half of the first-degree relatives, uninformed about their status and unprotected.

CONCLUSION AND FUTURE DIRECTIONS

A clearer understanding of inherited channelopathies and its underlying molecular biology has arisen as a result of basic research, progressing at a mind-boggling speed due to advances in engineered mice modeling genetic abnormalities. A considerable percentage of inherited cardiac arrhythmias that can lead to SCD at a young age can be recognized, and adequately treated provided physicians pick up warning signs early with the help of family history and ECG readings (Box **1**). It should, however, be apparent to clinicians in general medicine and cardiology that the clinical management and the genetics of these diseases are tied together and it is seldom possible to treat the affected patients effectively without taking into account what has been learned from genetic testing nowadays. Therefore, family physicians, cardiologists, pediatricians, forensic medical specialists, neurologists, pathologists, and anesthetists all play vital roles in the identification of at-risk patients and families. Also, the evaluation of children with seizures is essential as potential cardiac channelopathies can be misdiagnosed as refractory epilepsy, leaving the patient at risk for SD.

Furthermore, drowning can also be seen as a common cause of SD in childhood; however, some cases may not be accidental and occur secondary to cardiac abnormalities. To avoid further misdiagnosis, greater awareness of these cardiac conditions, particularly the ion channelopathies strongly associated with swimming-related events would lead to prompt appropriate treatment followed by identification of other family members which would help identify high-risk SCD family members. Adequate counseling of affected families, continual adjustment of therapy, and rigorous evaluation at regular intervals of cardiac risk patients, all contribute to reduce the incidence of SCD and/or SD in these families. Mothers should also be counseled on the maternal and infantile risk factors of SIDS. Finally, recognizing the fundamental defects in channelopathies would go a long way in providing new treatment strategies, including tailored pharmacotherapy and gene therapy.

Future research should be directed towards next-generation sequencing so that in theory, large numbers of genes can be investigated simultaneously. Although, this will not make recommendations for therapy any more comfortable, as genetic test results are becoming increasingly complex with variants and mutations significance often found to be unclear. Thus, wise use and even more careful interpretation of test results will prove useful [64].

- The following are grounds to suspect long-QT syndrome if structural causes have been ruled out:
  – Prolonged QT interval (♂ ≥440 ms; ♀ ≥460 ms)
  – (Standardized, extensive!) family history positive for syncope incidents, seizures, sudden cardiac death
  – Abnormal T wave morphology (notched, widened, flattened, biphasic, negative)
  – Documented torsade's de pointes
  – Index patient's history: syncope, seizures, palpitations
  – Pathological QTc during stress or exercise
  – Arrhythmias in the context of specific triggers (e.g., swimming, loud noises, medical drugs)
- The following are grounds to suspect Brugada syndrome if structural causes have been ruled out:
  – Brugada type 1, 2, or 3 ECG
  – Family history positive for syncope incidents, seizures, sudden cardiac death
  – Index patient's history: syncope, seizures, palpitations
  – Arrhythmias in the context of specific triggers (pyrexia, after a large meal, after drinking alcohol)
- The following are grounds to suspect catecholaminergic polymorphous ventricular tachycardia if structural causes have been ruled out:
  – Index patient's history: syncope, seizures, palpitations in response to adrenergic stimulation
  – Normal resting ECG, or there may be marked bradycardia
  – Family history positive for syncope incidents, seizures, sudden cardiac death
  – Occurrence of frequent polymorphous ventricular extrasystoles in stress ECG

Box 1 | Grounds for suspicion of LQTS, BrS, and CPVT

LIST OF ABBREVIATIONS

AP	Action Potential
[ARVC	Arrhythmogenic right ventricular cardiomyopathy
APD	Action potential duration
BrS	Brugada syndrome
CPVT	Catecholaminergic polymorphous ventricular tachycardia
HF	Heart failure
HCM	Hypertrophic cardiomyopathy
IHD	Ischemic heart disease
LQTS	Long QT syndrome

MI	Myocardial infarction
LBW	Low birth weight
RV	Right ventricle
RBBB	Right bundle branch block
SR	Sarcoplasmic reticulum
SQTS	Short QT syndrome
SCD	Sudden cardiac death
SIDS	Sudden infant death syndrome
SD	Sudden death
VT	Ventricular tachycardia
VF	Ventricular fibrillation

CONSENT FOR PUBLICATION

Not applicable.

FUNDING

Declared none.

CONFLICT OF INTEREST

The authors confirm that this chapter contents have no conflict of interest.

ACKNOWLEDGEMENTS

Declared none.

REFERENCE

[1] Kauferstein S, Kiehne N, Neumann T, Pitschner HF, Bratzke H. Cardiac gene defects can cause sudden cardiac death in young people. Dtsch Arztebl Int 2009; 106(4): 41-7. [http://dx.doi.org/10.3238/arztebl.2009.0041] [PMID: 19564966]

[2] Behr ER, Dalageorgou C, Christiansen M, *et al.* Sudden arrhythmic death syndrome: familial evaluation identifies inheritable heart disease in the majority of families. Eur Heart J 2008; 29(13): 1670-80. [http://dx.doi.org/10.1093/eurheartj/ehn219] [PMID: 18508782]

[3] Tan HL, Hofman N, van Langen IM, van der Wal AC, Wilde AA. Sudden unexplained death: heritability and diagnostic yield of cardiological and genetic examination in surviving relatives. Circulation 2005; 112(2): 207-13. [http://dx.doi.org/10.1161/CIRCULATIONAHA.104.522581] [PMID: 15998675]

[4] Basso C, Burke M, Fornes P, *et al.* Guidelines for autopsy investigation of sudden cardiac death. Virchows Arch 2008; 452(1): 11-8. [http://dx.doi.org/10.1007/s00428-007-0505-5] [PMID: 17952460]

[5] Kinney HC, Thach BT. The sudden infant death syndrome. N Engl J Med 2009; 361(8): 795-805. [http://dx.doi.org/10.1056/NEJMra0803836] [PMID: 19692691]

[6] Krous HF, Beckwith JB, Byard RW, *et al.* Sudden infant death syndrome and unclassified sudden infant deaths: a definitional and diagnostic approach. Pediatrics 2004; 114(1): 234-8. [http://dx.doi.org/10.1542/peds.114.1.234] [PMID: 15231934]

[7] Willinger M, James LS, Catz C. Defining the sudden infant death syndrome (SIDS): deliberations of an expert panel convened by the National Institute of Child Health and Human Development. Pediatr Pathol 1991; 11(5): 677-84. [http://dx.doi.org/10.3109/15513819109065465] [PMID: 1745639]

[8] Weber MA, Klein NJ, Hartley JC, Lock PE, Malone M, Sebire NJ. Infection and sudden unexpected death in infancy: a systematic retrospective case review. Lancet 2008; 371(9627): 1848-53. [http://dx.doi.org/10.1016/S0140-6736(08)60798-9] [PMID: 18514728]

[9] Schwartz PJ, Priori SG, Bloise R, *et al.* Molecular diagnosis in a child with sudden infant death syndrome. Lancet 2001; 358(9290): 1342-3. [http://dx.doi.org/10.1016/S0140-6736(01)06450-9] [PMID: 11684219]

[10] Boles RG, Buck EA, Blitzer MG, *et al.* Retrospective biochemical screening of fatty acid oxidation disorders in postmortem livers of 418 cases of sudden death in the first year of life. J Pediatr 1998; 132(6): 924-33. [http://dx.doi.org/10.1016/S0022-3476(98)70385-3] [PMID: 9627580]

[11] Paterson DS, Trachtenberg FL, Thompson EG, *et al.* Multiple serotonergic brainstem abnormalities in sudden infant death syndrome. JAMA 2006; 296(17): 2124-32. [http://dx.doi.org/10.1001/jama.296.17.2124] [PMID: 17077377]

[12] Goldstein S. Baye´ s de Luna A, Guindo J Sudden cardiac death. New York: Futura 1994.

[13] Diversus PS. De febre pestilente tractatus et curations quorumdam particularium morborum etc Frankfurt: Heiss of A Wechel 1586.

[14] Froissart J, Trans JT. Chronicles of England, France, Spain and adjoining countries. London: Henry G. Bohn 1849.

[15] Lancisi GM. De Subitaneis Mortibus. Roma: Giovanni Francisco Buagni 1706.

[16] Herrick JB. Clinical features of sudden obstruction of the coronary arteries. JAMA 1912; 59: 2015-22. [http://dx.doi.org/10.1001/jama.1912.04270120001001] [PMID: 6350634]

[17] Kuller L, Lilienfeld A, Fisher R. An epidemiological study of sudden and unexpected deaths in adults. Medicine (Baltimore) 1967; 46(4): 341-61. [http://dx.doi.org/10.1097/00005792-196707000-00003] [PMID: 6043997]

[18] Myerburg RJ, Junttila MJ. Sudden cardiac death caused by coronary heart disease. Circulation 2012; 125(8): 1043-52. [http://dx.doi.org/10.1161/CIRCULATIONAHA.111.023846] [PMID: 22371442]

[19] Sans S, Puigdefábregas A, Paluzie G, Monterde D, Balaguer-Vintró I. Increasing trends of acute myocardial infarction in Spain: the MONICA-Catalonia Study. Eur Heart J 2005; 26(5): 505-15. [http://dx.doi.org/10.1093/eurheartj/ehi068] [PMID: 15618037]

[20] Baye´ s-Genı's A, Vin˜olas X, Guindo J, Fiol M, Baye´ s de Luna A. Electrocardiographic and clinical precursors of ventricular fibrillation: chain of events. J Cardiovasc Electrophysiol 1995; 6: 410-7. [http://dx.doi.org/10.1111/j.1540-8167.1995.tb00415.x]

[21] Brugada P, Brugada J. Right bundle branch block, persistent ST segment elevation and sudden cardiac death: a distinct clinical and electrocardiographic syndrome. A multicenter report. J Am Coll Cardiol 1992; 20(6): 1391-6. [http://dx.doi.org/10.1016/0735-1097(92)90253-J] [PMID: 1309182]

[22] Berne P, Brugada J. Brugada syndrome 2012. Circ J 2012; 76(7): 1563-71. [http://dx.doi.org/10.1253/circj.CJ-12-0717] [PMID: 22789973]

[23] Yan GX, Antzelevitch C. Cellular basis for the Brugada syndrome and other mechanisms of arrhythmogenesis associated with ST-segment elevation. Circulation 1999;100:1660e6.

[24] Shimizu W, Aiba T, Kurita T, et al. Paradoxic abbreviation of repolarization in epicardium of the right ventricular outflow tract during augmentation of Brugada-type ST segment elevation. J Cardiovasc Electrophysiol 2001;12:1418e21.

[25] Coronel R, Casini S, Koopmann TT, *et al.* Right ventricular fibrosis and conduction delay in a patient with clinical signs of Brugada syndrome: a combined electrophysiological, genetic, histopathologic, and computational study. Circulation 2005; 112(18): 2769-77. [http://dx.doi.org/10.1161/CIRCULATIONAHA.105.532614] [PMID: 16267250]

[26] Antzelevitch C. The Brugada syndrome: ionic basis and arrhythmia mechanisms. J Cardiovasc Electrophysiol 2001; 12(2): 268-72. [http://dx.doi.org/10.1046/j.1540-8167.2001.00268.x] [PMID: 11232628]

[27] Elizari MV, Levi R, Acunzo RS, *et al.* Abnormal expression of cardiac neural crest cells in heart development: a different hypothesis for the etiopathogenesis of Brugada syndrome. Heart Rhythm 2007; 4(3): 359-65. [http://dx.doi.org/10.1016/j.hrthm.2006.10.026] [PMID: 17341404]

[28] Chen Q, Kirsch GE, Zhang D, *et al.* Genetic basis and molecular mechanism for idiopathic ventricular fibrillation. Nature 1998; 392(6673): 293-6. [http://dx.doi.org/10.1038/32675] [PMID: 9521325]

[29] Nielsen MW, Holst AG, Olesen SP, Olesen MS. The genetic component of Brugada syndrome. Front Physiol 2013; 4: 179. [http://dx.doi.org/10.3389/fphys.2013.00179] [PMID: 23874304]

[30] Kapplinger JD, Tester DJ, Alders M, *et al.* An international compendium of mutations in the SCN5A-encoded cardiac sodium channel in patients referred for Brugada syndrome genetic testing. Heart Rhythm 2010; 7(1): 33-46. [http://dx.doi.org/10.1016/j.hrthm.2009.09.069] [PMID: 20129283]

[31] Eastaugh LJ, James PA, Phelan DG, Davis AM. Brugada syndrome caused by a large deletion in SCN5A only detected by multiplex ligation-dependent probe amplification. J Cardiovasc Electrophysiol 2011; 22(9): 1073-6. [http://dx.doi.org/10.1111/j.1540-8167.2010.02003.x] [PMID: 21288276]

[32] Webster AL, Yan MS, Marsden PA. Epigenetics and cardiovascular disease. Can J Cardiol 2013; 29(1): 46-57. [http://dx.doi.org/10.1016/j.cjca.2012.10.023] [PMID: 23261320]

[33] Kim GH, Ryan JJ, Archer SL. The role of redox signaling in epigenetics and cardiovascular disease. Antioxid Redox Signal 2013; 18(15): 1920-36. [http://dx.doi.org/10.1089/ars.2012.4926] [PMID: 23480168]

[34] Giudicessi JR, Ackerman MJ. Determinants of incomplete penetrance and variable expressivity in heritable cardiac arrhythmia syndromes. Transl Res 2013; 161(1): 1-14. [http://dx.doi.org/10.1016/j.trsl.2012.08.005] [PMID: 22995932]

[35] Goldenberg I, Moss AJ. Long QT syndrome. J Am Coll Cardiol 2008;51(24):2291e300.

[36] Salama G, London B. Mouse models of long QT syndrome. J Physiol 2007;578:43e53.

[37] Tester DJ, Will ML, Haglund CM, Ackerman MJ. Compendium of cardiac channel mutations in 541 consecutive unrelated patients referred for long QT syndrome genetic testing. Heart Rhythm 2005; 2(5): 507-17. [http://dx.doi.org/10.1016/j.hrthm.2005.01.020] [PMID: 15840476]

[38] Splawski I, Shen J, Timothy KW, *et al.* Spectrum of mutations in long-QT syndrome genes. KVLQT1, HERG, SCN5A, KCNE1, and KCNE2. Circulation 2000; 102(10): 1178-85. [http://dx.doi.org/10.1161/01.CIR.102.10.1178] [PMID: 10973849]

[39] Napolitano C, Priori SG, Schwartz PJ, *et al.* Genetic testing in the long QT syndrome: development and validation of an efficient approach to genotyping in clinical practice. JAMA 2005; 294(23): 2975-80. [http://dx.doi.org/10.1001/jama.294.23.2975] [PMID: 16414944]

[40] Priori SG, Napolitano C, Memmi M, *et al.* Clinical and molecular characterization of patients with catecholeminergic polymorphic ventricular tachycardiaCirculation 2002;106(1):69e74

[41] Leenhardt A, Lucet V, Denjoy I, Grau F, Ngoc DD, Coumel P. Catecholaminergic polymorphic ventricular tachycardia in children. A 7-year follow-up of 21 patients. Circulation 1995;91(5):1512e9.

[42] Lahat H, Eldar M, Levy-Nissenbaum E, *et al.* Autosomal recessive catecholamine- or exercise-induced polymorphic ventricular tachycardia: clinical features and assignment of the disease gene to chromosome 1p13-21. Circulation 2001;103:2822e7.

[43] Marks AR, Priori S, Memmi M, *et al.* Involvement of the cardiac ryanodine receptor/ calcium release channel in catecholaminergic polymorphic ventricular tachycardia. J Cell Physiol 2002;190:1e6.

[44] Mines G. On circulating excitations in heart muscles and their possible relation to tachycardia and fibrillation Trans R Soc Can 1914;8:43e52

[45] Lieve KV, van der Werf C, Wilde AA. Catecholaminergic Polymorphic Ventricular Tachycardia. Circ J 2016; 80(6): 1285-91. [http://dx.doi.org/10.1253/circj.CJ-16-0326] [PMID: 27180891]

[46] Antzelevitch C, Pollevick GD, Cordeiro JM, *et al.* Loss-of-function mutations in the cardiac calcium channel underlie a new clinical entity characterized by ST-segment elevation, short QT intervals, and sudden cardiac death. Circulation 2007;115:442e9.

[47] Brugada R, Hong K, Dumaine R, *et al.* Sudden death associated with short-QT syndrome linked to mutations in HERG. Circulation 2004;109:30e5. [http://dx.doi.org/10.1161/01.CIR.0000109482.92774.3A]

[48] Grant AO, Carboni MP, Neplioueva V, *et al.* Long QT syndrome, Brugada syndrome, and conduction system disease are linked to a single sodium channel mutation. J Clin Invest 2002;110:1201e9.

[49] Schwartz PJ, Stramba-Badiale M, Crotti L, *et al.* Prevalence of the congenital long-QT syndrome. Circulation 2009; 120(18): 1761-7. [http://dx.doi.org/10.1161/CIRCULATIONAHA.109.863209] [PMID: 19841298]

[50] Tomás M, Napolitano C, De Giuli L, *et al.* Polymorphisms in the NOS1AP gene modulate QT interval duration and risk of arrhythmias in the long QT syndrome. J Am Coll Cardiol 2010; 55(24): 2745-52. [http://dx.doi.org/10.1016/j.jacc.2009.12.065] [PMID: 20538168]

[51] Jost N, Virág L, Bitay M, *et al.* Restricting excessive cardiac action potential and QT prolongation: a vital role for IKs in human ventricular muscle. Circulation 2005; 112(10): 1392-9. [http://dx.doi.org/10.1161/CIRCULATIONAHA.105.550111] [PMID: 16129791]

[52] Efremidis M, Pappas LK, Sideris A, Letsas KP, Gavrielatos GD, Kardaras F. Swimming-triggered aborted sudden cardiac death in a patient with Andersen-Tawil syndrome. Int J Cardiol 2006; 112(2): e45-7. [http://dx.doi.org/10.1016/j.ijcard.2006.02.028] [PMID: 16859779]

[53] Ackerman MJ, Tester DJ, Porter CJ. Swimming, a gene-specific arrhythmogenic trigger for inherited long QT syndrome. Mayo Clin Proc 1999; 74(11): 1088-94. [http://dx.doi.org/10.4065/74.11.1088] [PMID: 10560595]

[54] Choi G, Kopplin LJ, Tester DJ, Will ML, Haglund CM, Ackerman MJ. Spectrum and frequency of cardiac channel defects in swimming-triggered arrhythmia syndromes. Circulation 2004; 110(15):

2119-24.
[http://dx.doi.org/10.1161/01.CIR.0000144471.98080.CA] [PMID: 15466642]

[55] Ishikawa H, Matsushima M, Nagashima M, Osuga A. Screening of children with arrhythmias for arrhythmia development during diving and swimming--face immersion as a substitute for diving and exercise stress testing as a substitute for swimming. Jpn Circ J 1992; 56(9): 881-90.
[http://dx.doi.org/10.1253/jcj.56.881] [PMID: 1404843]

[56] Schwartz PJ, Vanoli E, Crotti L, *et al.* Neural control of heart rate is an arrhythmia risk modifier in long QT syndrome. J Am Coll Cardiol 2008; 51(9): 920-9.
[http://dx.doi.org/10.1016/j.jacc.2007.09.069] [PMID: 18308161]

[57] Lu CW, Lin JH, Rajawat YS, *et al.* Functional and clinical characterization of a mutation in KCNJ2 associated with Andersen-Tawil syndrome. J Med Genet 2006; 43(8): 653-9.
[http://dx.doi.org/10.1136/jmg.2006.040816] [PMID: 16571646]

[58] Hofman N, Wilde AA, Tan HL. Diagnostic criteria for congenital long QT syndrome in the era of molecular genetics: do we need a scoring system? Eur Heart J 2007; 28(11): 1399.
[http://dx.doi.org/10.1093/eurheartj/ehm118] [PMID: 17483524]

[59] Zipes DP, Camm AJ, Borggrefe M, *et al.* ACC/AHA/ESC 2006 Guidelines for Management of Patients With Ventricular Arrhythmias and the Prevention of Sudden Cardiac Death: A report of the American College of Cardiology/American Heart Association Task Force and the European Society of Cardiology Committee for Practice Guidelines (writing committee to develop Guidelines for Management of Patients With Ventricular Arrhythmias and the Prevention of Sudden Cardiac Death): developed in collaboration with the European Heart Rhythm Association and the Heart Rhythm Society. Circulation 2006; 114(10): e385-484.
[http://dx.doi.org/10.1161/CIRCULATIONAHA.106.178233] [PMID: 16935995]

[60] Benito B, Brugada R, Brugada J, Brugada P. Brugada syndrome. Prog Cardiovasc Dis 2008; 51(1): 1-22.
[http://dx.doi.org/10.1016/j.pcad.2008.05.002] [PMID: 18634914]

[61] Ackerman MJ, Splawski I, Makielski JC, *et al.* Spectrum and prevalence of cardiac sodium channel variants among black, white, Asian, and Hispanic individuals: implications for arrhythmogenic susceptibility and Brugada/long QT syndrome genetic testing. Heart Rhythm 2004; 1(5): 600-7.
[http://dx.doi.org/10.1016/j.hrthm.2004.07.013] [PMID: 15851227]

[62] Kapplinger JD, Tester DJ, Salisbury BA, *et al.* Spectrum and prevalence of mutations from the first 2,500 consecutive unrelated patients referred for the FAMILION long QT syndrome genetic test. Heart Rhythm 2009; 6(9): 1297-303.
[http://dx.doi.org/10.1016/j.hrthm.2009.05.021] [PMID: 19716085]

[63] Kapa S, Tester DJ, Salisbury BA, *et al.* Genetic testing for long-QT syndrome: distinguishing pathogenic mutations from benign variants. Circulation 2009; 120(18): 1752-60.
[http://dx.doi.org/10.1161/CIRCULATIONAHA.109.863076] [PMID: 19841300]

[64] Tester DJ, Ackerman MJ. Genetic testing for potentially lethal, highly treatable inherited cardiomyopathies/channelopathies in clinical practice. Circulation 2011; 123(9): 1021-37.
[http://dx.doi.org/10.1161/CIRCULATIONAHA.109.914838] [PMID: 21382904]

CHAPTER 8

Chagas Cardiomyopathy: The Fate of Newborns, Pregnant Mothers, and Their Unborn Child

Iroegbu Chukwuemeka Daniel* and **Jinfu Yang**

Department of Cardiovascular Surgery, The Second Xiangya Hospital, Central South University, Middle Renmin Road 139, 410011 Changsha, China

Abstract: Congenital Chagas disease known as a neglected tropical disease can, however, be considered as an ecological model of multiple and complex interactions between parasites, the pregnant woman, placenta, and the unborn child. Indeed, congenital infection is a rather rare event, it can, however, occur and be found in any part of the world and the lack of a well-established surveillance program means that the diagnosis can probably be easily missed putting both the pregnant mother and the fetus, with the newborn at risk. In this era of globalization with the ongoing European immigration policies, Congenital Chagas disease would no longer become confined to only poor rural areas and endemic countries, eventually becoming a significant public health concern. Bearing this in mind, the possibility of Chagasic disease, in general, becoming the new human immunodeficiency virus in third world African countries and developing African nations in the foreseeable future is inevitable. The simple fact that both the policymakers, and the health care providers are ignorant of the disease and also lack both the technical knowledge and understanding of the disease modes of transmission, progression, pathology, and its pathophysiology make it futuristically possible. This chapter aims to discuss the presenting global challenge of this neglected tropical disease, its ecological interactions and also try to better understand the mechanisms sequentially associated with the transmission of live parasites from maternal blood and the development of congenital infection (asymptomatic) or congenital Chagas disease (symptomatic) in the fetus and newborns (in both endemic and non-endemic areas).

Keywords: Acute trypanosomal cruzi infection, Acute repair, Benznidazole, Chagas disease, Cardiomyopathy, Congenital Chagas disease, Congenital infection, Cardiac surgery, Co-infection, Cardiac arrhythmia, Dilated cardio-myopathy, Heart failure, Heart transplantation, Immune response, Immunosup-pression, Left ventricular aneurysm, Left ventricle, Magnetic resonance imaging, Maternal and fetal transmission, Microhematocrit, Maternal residence, Neglected

* **Corresponding author Iroegbu Chukwuemeka Daniel**: Department of Cardiovascular Surgery, The Second Xiangya Hospital, Central South University, Middle Renmin Road 139, 410011 Changsha, China;
E-mails: yjf19682005@csu.edu.cn, Dr.iroegbu_daniel@yahoo.comDr.iroegbu_daniel@csu.edu.cn

tropical disease, Nifurtimox, Organ transplantation, Placenta, Prognosis, PCR, Parasitemia, Risk factors, *Trypanosoma cruzi*.

INTRODUCTION

Chagas cardiomyopathy is the most frequent presenting type of Chagas disease caused by the protozoan *Trypanosoma cruzi* (*T. cruzi*) (Heteroptera, Reduviidae, Hemiptera, and Triatominae), transmitted to humans when these blood-sucking vector bugs faeces come in contact with the patient's lacerated skin or eye mucosa which was first described in 1909 by Carlo Chagas [1, 2]. This anthropozoonosis, also termed American trypanosomiasis, represents the fourth largest tropical disease after malaria, TB, and schistosomiasis [3]. However, apart from congenital route of infection (from infected mother to their offspring during pregnancy or at birth) [4] (main focus described in this chapter), other known routes of infection include oral transmission of infected food [5] and/or drinks contaminated with triatomine bug feces [6 - 8], blood transfusion [9], organ transplantation [10], and accidental transmission through contaminated laboratory materials [11]. Although described more than hundred years ago [12], Chagas cardiomyopathy has continued to be a significant cause of morbidity and mortality in Latin America [13, 14] affecting about 6 million people with approximately over 30 000 new cases detected every year [15, 16]. According to WHO recent estimation [17], about 1,125,000 women in fertile age are infected with *T. cruzi* in Latin America, with the incidence of congenital infection being 8668 cases per year, with nearly 50% of cases grouped in Colombia, Argentina, and Mexico. Although maternal-fetal transmission varies among different countries based on the results obtained from national registries [18]. The disease onset is divided into two stages: an acute phase, with high levels of T., cruzi in the bloodstream, and a chronic phase where the symptoms are nearly observed 8-10 years after the infection. Cardiac manifestations seen include but not restricted to cardiac arrhythmias, left and right cardiac chamber hypertrophy, and heart failure [19]. However, the changes in heart are connected to a set of molecular and cellular changes in cardiac tissue such as collagen deposition [20], reduced cellular contractility [21] oxidative stress [22], increased myocyte apoptosis [23], altered cellular metabolism [24], and disturbance of electrical properties of the heart [25, 26].

Considered as a neglected tropical disease (NTD) by World Health Organization (WHO), congenital route of infection is gradually becoming a significant public health problem as the infection can arise in both acute and chronic phases of the disease, be repeated at each pregnancy, and observed from one generation to another (vertical transmission). The occurrence of congenital Chagas diseases; however, results from complex interactions between the parasite, the mother, and the fetus in the specific context of pregnancy. Several strains of *T. cruzi* (displaying specific features) interact with:

I. The immune system of the pregnant woman (showing responses modulated by genetic and environmental factors)
II. The placenta (fetal organ) and finally,
III. The immune system of her fetus (showing reactions also susceptible to be modulated by maternal and environmental factors, and depending on the fetus own genetic background).

This chapter aims to discuss the presenting global challenge of this neglected tropical disease (NTD) [13], its ecological interactions and also tries to better understand the mechanisms sequentially associated with the transmission of live parasites from maternal blood and the development of congenital infection (asymptomatic) or congenital Chagas disease (symptomatic) in the fetus and newborns (in both endemic and non-endemic areas).

DEFINITIONS

Chagas disease is a term used for the disease itself in general. However, the term Chagas cardiomyopathy encompasses all cases of Chagas disease with cardiac involvement, which is defined by the presence of at least a typical abnormal electrocardiographic reading in patients who test positive serologically against *T cruzi*. Chagas cardiomyopathy could also have some characteristical features similar to that of Dilated cardiomyopathy hence termed Dilated Chagas cardiomyopathy which refers to the hemodynamic pattern of the Chagas cardiomyopathy that is characterized by left ventricular (LV) enlargement with global or segmental systolic function impairment, regardless of electrocardiographic findings.

NATURAL HISTORY

Chagas disease is a complex condition with a long, varied clinical course and prognosis (Fig. **1**). The majority (65-75%) of infected individuals remain asymptomatic throughout life.

Although some patients develop mild-moderate segmental wall motion abnormalities, conduction defects only while others may develop severe symptoms of heart failure, life-threatening ventricular arrhythmias, and thromboembolic phenomena (See **Appendix**). However, it is of importance to note that sudden cardiac death (SCD) can be seen even in the absence of previous significant signs or symptoms of chronic Chagas cardiomyopathy (CCC) [27]. Be it as it may, Chagas disease evolves in two stages (acute and chronic phases). Acute Chagas disease occurs with a primary infection, while chronic Chagas disease is further clinically subdivided into four, namely:

I. Indeterminate
II. Cardiac
III. Digestive, and
IV. Mixed type (both cardiac and gastrointestinal).

They are all staged on the basis of the severity of involvement according to the American College of Cardiology (ACC) and American Heart Association (AHA) guidelines for the diagnosis and management of heart failures in adults [28 - 30].

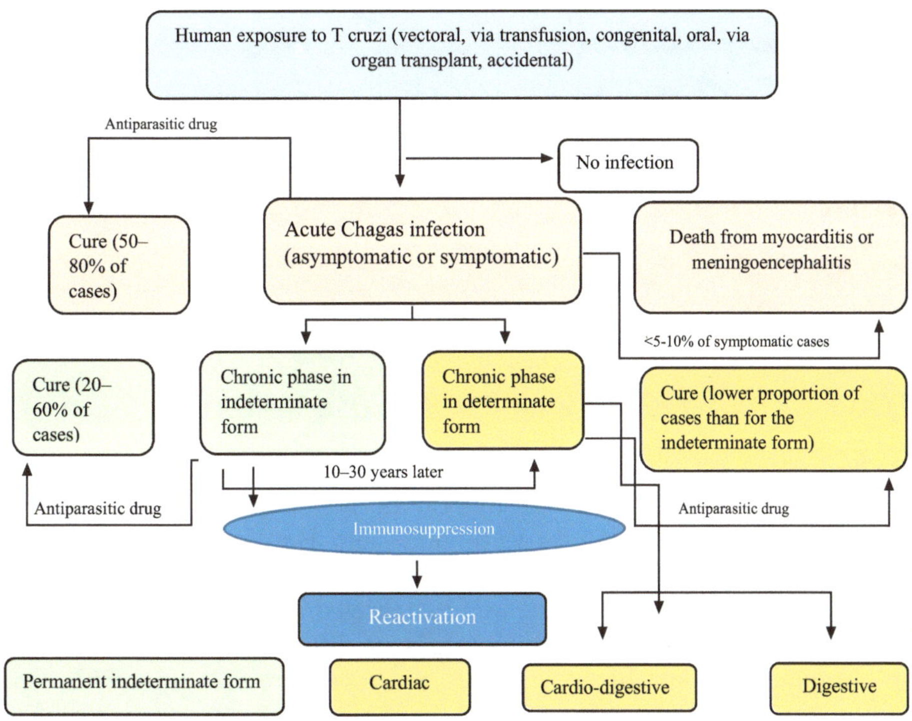

Fig. (1). Natural history of Chagas disease in humans.

EPIDEMIOLOGY

In the Americas, Chagas disease is responsible for approximately 7.5 times as many disability-adjusted life-years lost as compared to malaria [31] (See **Appendix**). The global epidemiologic profile of Chagas disease is as a result of two significant forces: large scale rural-to-urban migration and domestic vector-borne transmission over a lifetime [16, 32]. Despite improvements and an incidence decline in endemic countries (Argentina, Bolivia, Paraguay, Uruguay, Chile, Brazil, and Mexico) due to massive vector-eradication campaigns, Chagas disease is currently worldwide on the rise again even in Europe [33 - 37], as a result of congenital transmission as a dominant route of infection (Fig. **2**).

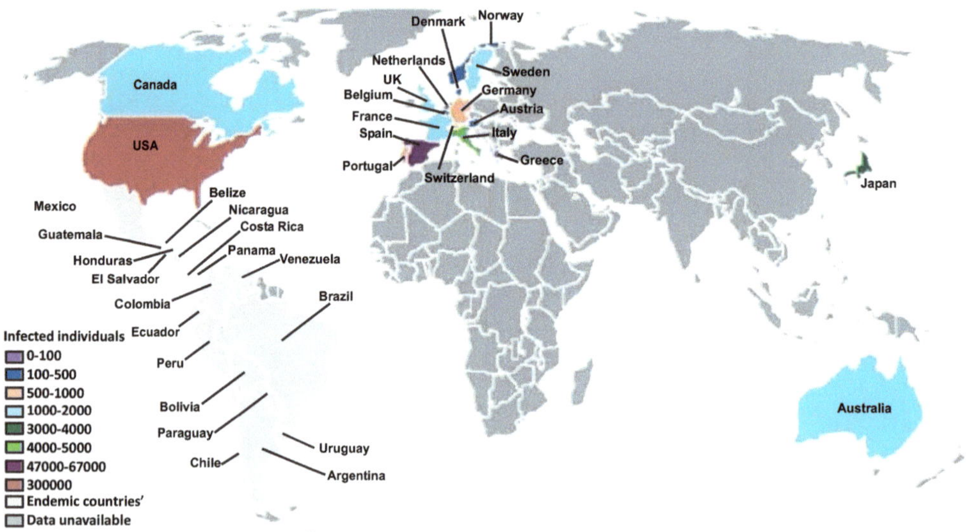

Fig. (2). Estimated number of immigrants with *Trypanosoma cruzi* infection living in non-endemic countries.

BIOLOGY AND LIFE CYCLE OF *TRYPANOSOMA CRUZI*

T. cruzi biological life cycle of the invertebrate host begins when these "assassin" bugs infected with *T. cruzi* feed and suck on the vertebrate host blood (Fig. **3A, B & C**). The invertebrate hosts are Reduvidae and Hemiptera such as Triatoma infestans, Panstrongylus megistus, Rhodnius prolixus, and others. After the blood meal, the gastrointestinal tract of the bug increases due to pressure, as a result, the bug defecates on the skin near the puncture wound transmitting the parasite to the host by scrapping around the area during feeding before escaping. This aspect is vital for it to act as a transmitter for *T. cruzi* since infective stages of *T. cruzi* reach the stab wound when the bug defecates during food intake. When the victim rubs the pathogen-contained feces into the fresh puncture wound or when the pathogen-contained bugs defecate and penetrate intact mucosa, mainly those of the eyes, highly contagious and very ambulatory metacyclic trypomastigotes of *T. cruzi* are transmitted into the blood flow of the host [38, 39]. The trypomastigotes are then successively disseminated into the organism of the host and preferably infect cells of the mononuclear phagocytic and reticuloendothelial system [40]. Briefly, intracellular parasites augment in the cytoplasm of the host cell by binary division while the parasitophorous vacuole is then formed during the life cycle of *T. cruzi* [41]. Nucleated cells can be infected by *T. cruzi*. However, *T. cruzi* predominantly replicates in intestinal mucosa as well as cardiac muscle cells, cells of the nervous system, gonads, and the placenta [42, 43]. The metacyclic trypomastigotes morphology changes to intracellular amastigotes with a diameter of 3–5 µm right after its penetration into the host cell cytoplasm when they lose their undulating membrane which is a characteristic feature of mobile trypomastigotes [44]. Intracellular amastigotes are transformed into trypomastigotes after undergoing several rounds of division approximately 20-µm long [45].

Unlike *T. brucei* caused by African sleeping sickness, intracellular replication of *T. cruzi* in host cells is mandatory, since the pathogenic agent is not able to divide in the blood. For this reason, the intracellular amastigote form of *T. cruzi* is always present and can be histopathologically detected in tissue samples from liver, brain heart muscle, and spleen. The life cycle of *T. cruzi* persists when the bug feast on infected host blood and the parasites transform in the bug´s midgut to

A

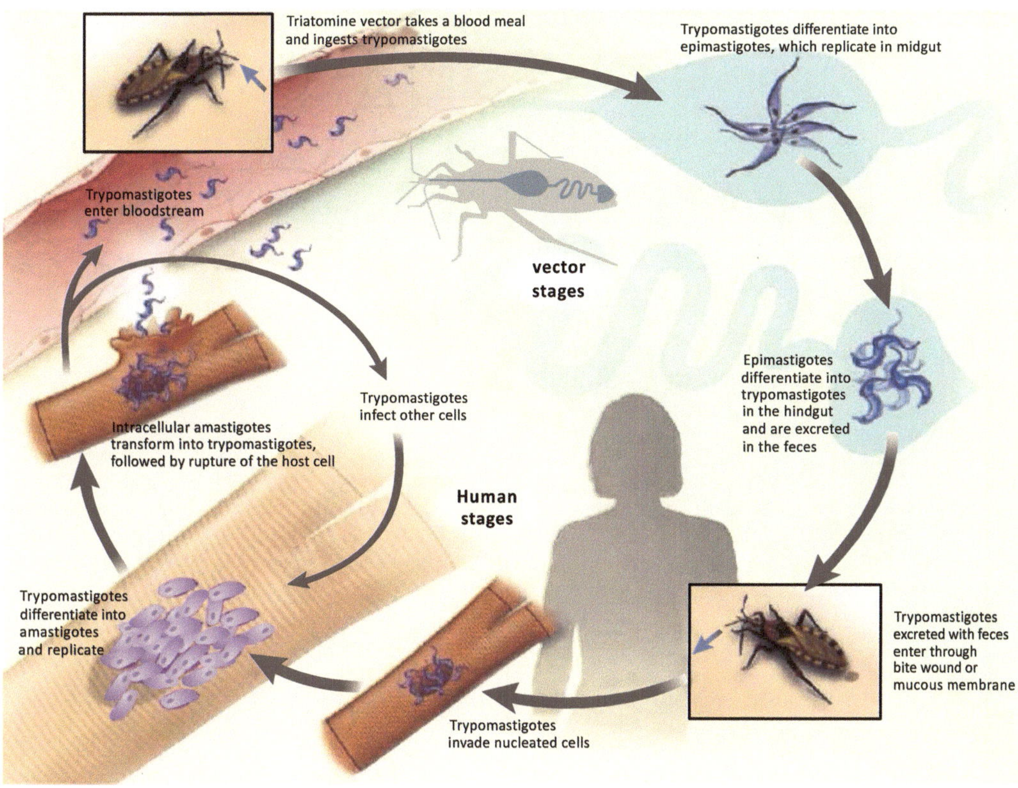

Fig. 3 cont.....

B

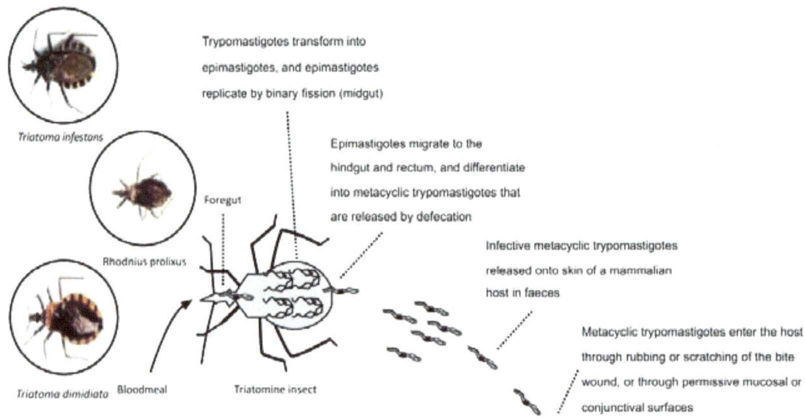

C

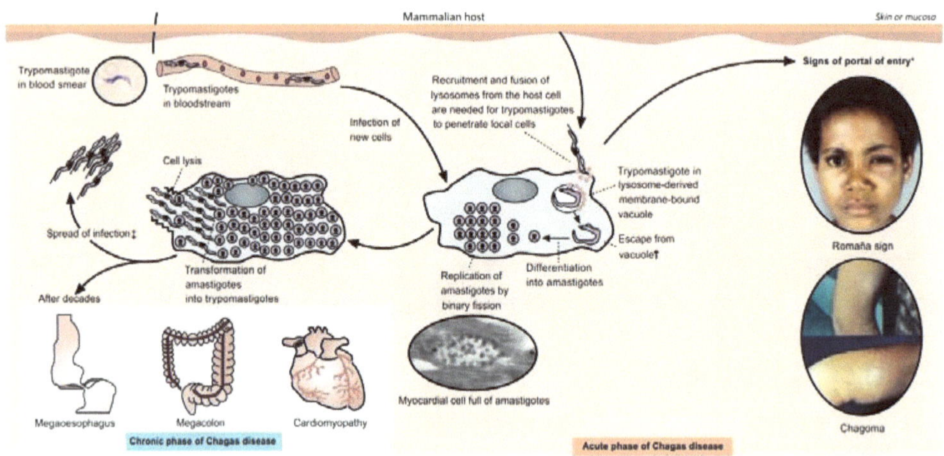

Fig. (3A, B & C). [A]. Life Cycle of *Trypanosoma cruzi* [B]. Vector-borne transmission of *Trypanosoma cruzi* [C]. *Penetration of the intact mucous membrane of the eye by infective trypomastigotes leads to a painless reaction of the conjunctiva, with unilateral edema of both eyelids and lymphadenitis of the preauricular ganglia (Romaña sign). †Trypomastigotes in the host cell escape from the parasitophorous vacuole and are released into the cytoplasm by a unique mechanism. ‡Trypomastigotes lyse infected cells, invade adjacent tissues, and spread *via* the lymphatics and bloodstream to distant sites, mainly muscle cells (cardiac, smooth, and skeletal) and ganglion cells, where they undergo further cycles of intracellular multiplication.

epimastigote forms and multiply by binary fission. Finally, the highly infectious metacyclic trypomastigotes develop in the rectum of the bug and will be passed again with the feces during a subsequent second blood meal [46].

ACUTE PHASE

T. cruzi incubation period ranges from about 1 to 2 weeks just right after the vector-borne transmission [16] and typically lasts for about 8 to 12 weeks (Fig. **4**). Most cases usually go undiagnosed as the majority of carriers are either asymptomatic or manifest mild to nonspecific symptoms such as malaise, fever, and splenomegaly. However, a small percentage of patients in the acute phase is marked by inflammation at the site of inoculation: Romaña sign (unilateral conjunctivitis and painless swelling of the upper and lower eyelids) or the pathognomonic chagoma sign (*T cruzi* skin abscess). When detected, mild cardiac anomalies such as tachycardia and fever (temperature of about 36.8°C to 39°C) are often noted. Although, few patients present with a fulminant type phase (pericardial effusion and myocarditis) [32] which might be misleading and confusing to diagnose at first. However, an advanced ECG finding, such as atrial fibrillation, ventricular arrhythmias, and right bundle-branch block, signals a worse prognosis [47].

INDETERMINATE PHASE

After the acute phase, most patients pass into an indeterminate phase [47] which is defined by the absence of any physical signs and symptoms of the disease, normal ECG and chest radiographs [48] (Fig. **4**). The indeterminate period is quite challenging most especially as it is quite tricky also to distinguish the acute fulminant type, which can be seen in some few patients. Although an extensive evaluation is highly needed to fulfill the strict criteria and adequately diagnose this phase, not all patients are subjected to this complete evaluation as it could be expensive, discomforting and in most cases, of little to no clinical value in the long run [49]. However, the current recommendation for evaluation for suspected or newly diagnosed Chagas disease in the United States includes a serological examination based on two different assays for anti-*T. cruzi* immunoglobulin G, proper history taking, a physical exam, an ECG, and a 30-second rhythm strip. Serological confirmation remains the current recommendation for the evaluation of patients in the States with suspected or newly diagnosed Chagas disease which is based on two different assays for anti–*T cruzi* immunoglobulin G and also includes; a thorough history, a proper physical examination, an ECG, and a 30-second rhythm strip. An additional workup for the cardiovascular system is only needed when this first evaluation raises clinical suspicion of a more advanced disease from [29]. It is also imperative to note that, even if an advance clinical assessment does not reveal myocarditis, it is still possible for patients to meet the criteria for the indeterminate form to have subclinical myocarditis.

EVOLUTION TO CHAGAS HEART DISEASE

Linear progression from acute to chronic phase (chronic Chagas cardiomyopathy) is uncommon and rare (<5-10%) even in hyperendemic regions [50]. However, it is still very much possible, most, especially in untreated cases. More commonly, chronic Chagas cardiomyopathy develops after several decades of the indeterminate form of the disease, which indicates the level of imbalance between the host immune system and the parasite (Fig. **4**). Evolution progressive drivers to Chagas cardiomyopathy include but not limited to the severity of acute infection, male sex, parasite strain, exposure to reinfection, genetic background, environment, alcoholism, and nutritional status (discussed in details elsewhere in the chapter) [47].

PREVALENCE OF *T. CRUZI* AMONG PREGNANT WOMEN IN BOTH ENDEMIC AND NON-ENDEMIC COUNTRIES

There is still a high variance of reported *T. cruzi* seroprevalence cases among pregnant women across the Americas [51, 52]. Although this largely depends on the age of the woman, the setting (urban *vs.* rural), the country, and the laboratory technique used during the screening process [53]. However, congenital route of infection for Chagas disease is rapidly becoming a globalized public health issue mainly due to the rise in immigration recently due to economic hardships from endemic Chagas disease countries to a non-endemic one such as Japan [4, 54].

PATHOLOGY AND PATHOGENESIS OF CHAGAS CARDIO-MYOPATHY

Pathology

Trypanosoma cruzi can parasitize any tissue derived from embryonic mesoderm, endoderm, and neuroectoderm; the intensity of infection is related to the genetics of the host and parasite. Smooth and striated muscles, bone marrow, phagocytic mononuclear system, and gonadal cells can be heavily parasitized [55]. Apart from the widespread immunological reaction, which is characterized by hepatomegaly, splenomegaly, and lymphadenopathy, intense direct tissue parasitism and high-grade parasitemia results in the inflammation of the heart, cardiac enlargement, and pericardial effusions. However, the resultant myocarditis is typically diffused with interstitial edema, vascular dilatation, myocyte necrosis, mononuclear and polymorphonuclear infiltrations. Moreover, the inflammatory processes also extend into the endocardium resulting in mural thrombosis and also involve the conduction systems of the heart representing a lesion of late-onset [56, 57]. In congenitally infected newborns, lesions appear at the very start and in stillborn after autopsy owing to the infant's immature immune system [57].

A histological study of the placenta clearly shows mild and focal placentitis with rare amastigotes or a diffused involvement with heavy parasitism [56].

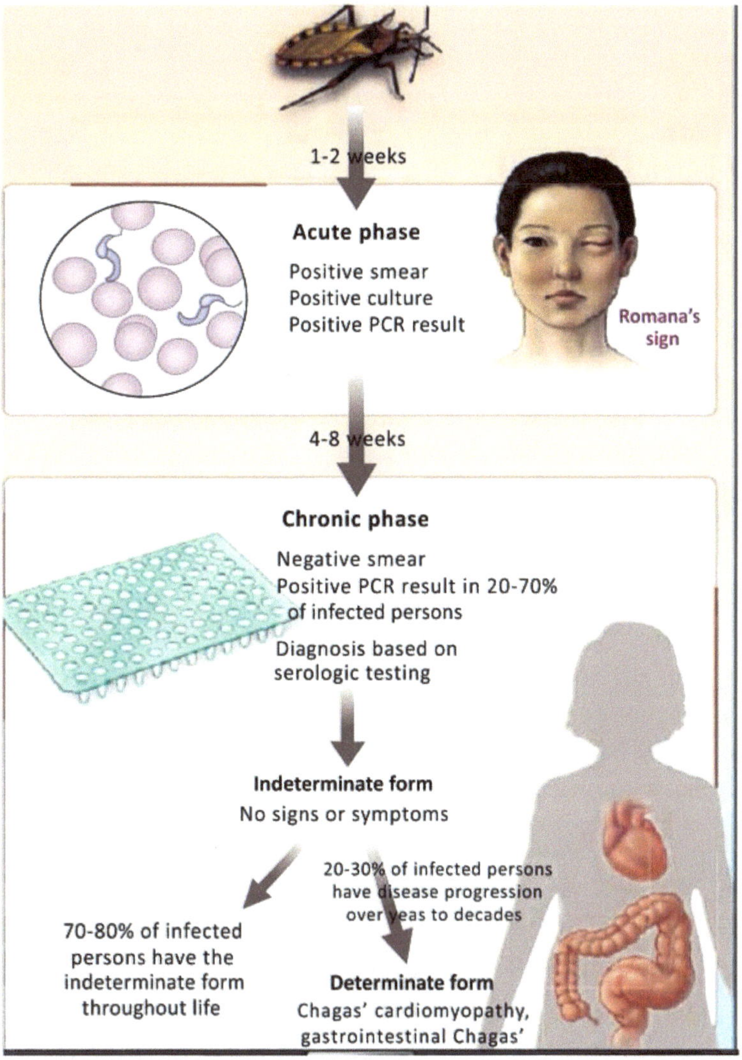

Fig. (4). Phases of *Trypanosoma cruzi* Infection. The acute phase of *T. cruzi* infection is characterized by microscopically detectable parasitemia lasting 8 to 12 weeks. Diagnosis during the chronic phase of infection relies on serologic assays. Persons with chronic *T. cruzi* infection but without signs or symptoms of Chagas' disease are considered to have the indeterminate form of the disease. It is estimated that 20 to 30% of people who initially have the indeterminate form of Chagas' disease have progression over a period of years or decades to clinically evident cardiac heart disease.

Pathogenesis

The pathogenesis of Chagas cardiomyopathy and congenital infection is complicated. Autoreactivity triggered by the disease and a parasite-driven immune response are the two primary mechanisms which instigate and drive both acute and chronic myocarditis, with two secondary mechanisms namely; coronary microvascular derangements and neurogenic disturbances which are responsible for the associated cardiac alterations [19, 58]. However, the host susceptibility and *T. cruzi* strains play a crucial role in the disease severity and the clinical pattern. Infection-triggered autoreactivity and a direct parasite-targeted immune response combine to produce myocytolysis, substantial inflammation, and a superimposed reactive and reparative fibrosis characteristic for the chronic phase [19, 59, 60]. The host immune system response to *T. cruzi* infection is key to determining the disease severity and progress. A relative symbiosis period occurs between the host and their pathogen as clearly evident in the asymptomatic indeterminate clinical phase, which can persist for decades or a lifetime. It is, however, explanatory as patients in the indeterminate phase display a balanced production of inflammatory and anti-inflammatory cytokines, whereas, patients who tend to progress to the chronic phase of the disease appear to lose this coregulation [59, 60].

PHYSIOPATHOLOGY OF CONGENITAL CHAGAS INFECTION

The physiopathology of congenital infection involves the parasite reaching the fetus *via* the hematogenous route, which is further transmitted across the placenta [61]. The maternal-fetal transmission of the parasite mainly occurs through the marginal sinus spreading through the chorionic plate, infecting fibroblasts and macrophages and finally reaching a fetal vessel, inducing a fatal infection through this hematogenous route [61, 62]. Less frequently, congenital *T. cruzi* transmission can also occur *via* the oral route through ingestion of infected amniotic fluid or *via* the hematogenous pathway through placental breaches and tears that may occur during delivery [63, 64].

CLINICAL MANIFESTATIONS OF CHAGAS CARDIOMYOPATHY IN INFANTS, CHILDREN, AND PREGNANT WOMEN (FIG. 5A & B)

Clinical Manifestations in Infants and Children

The clinical events, such as congestive heart failure, respiratory distress syndrome, hepatomegaly, splenomegaly, anasarca, anemia, neurologic signs, petechiae, abnormal ECG findings, and an Apgar score < 7 at 1 min [63, 65], vary enormously from asymptomatic cases to fetal infection in the newborn and children which are more often dependent on the level of parasitemia at birth.

Clinical manifestations can be present at birth or appear within days or weeks after birth [63]. If left untreated, children enter the indeterminate phase of the disease with some of them developing chronic diseases with common cardiac abnormalities [66]. Although, the signs and symptoms observed mainly in newborns are usually not specific and may occur with other congenital infections such as toxoplasma or cytomegalovirus (TORCH syndrome).

Clinical Manifestations in Pregnant Women

In pregnant women and adults in general, Chagas cardiomyopathy has the same striking clinical feature as that of dilated cardiomyopathy. However, the typical involvement of the sinus node, electric conduction system, and the predominant distribution of fibrosis to the apical, and posterior regions of the LV helps distinguish Chagas cardiomyopathy from other cardiomyopathies. Various clinical manifestations encountered include electric conduction abnormalities, myocardial contractile dysfunction, arrhythmias, and or thromboembolism [67].

Arrhythmias: Arrhythmias (atrial and ventricular) and a wide variety of other abnormalities with the conduction system is the center point experienced in pregnant mothers with Chagas cardiomyopathy which also serves as a predictor of the disease severity and outcome [68, 69].

Cardiac arrhythmias mostly can appear to be the sole manifestation of Chagas disease, the purported arrhythmic syndrome, but usually, occur in combination with thromboembolic events or heart failure [70].

Atrial Tachyarrhythmias : Although, atrial fibrillation is typically seen in patients with dilated cardiomyopathy often indicating advanced myocardial damage which is a significant risk factor for stroke, independent of LV function [71] and a predictor of mortality [68, 72]. However, atrial fibrillation is also the most common supraventricular arrhythmia found in Chagas cardiomyopathy, which is further enhanced in pregnancy [16, 31, 33, 71, 73 - 76]. Commonly in atrial fibrillation, intraventricular and atrioventricular conduction delays and concurrent LV systolic dysfunction result in slow ventricular rate response [68, 72, 77].

Ventricular Tachyarrhythmias: The primary ventricular arrhythmogenic substrates in Chagas cardiomyopathy disease are fibrotic and necrotic myocardial lesions [78, 79] as these lesions change the cardiac electric potential and disrupt the intercellular junctions forming the basis of reentrant circuits for ventricular arrhythmias [80].

A

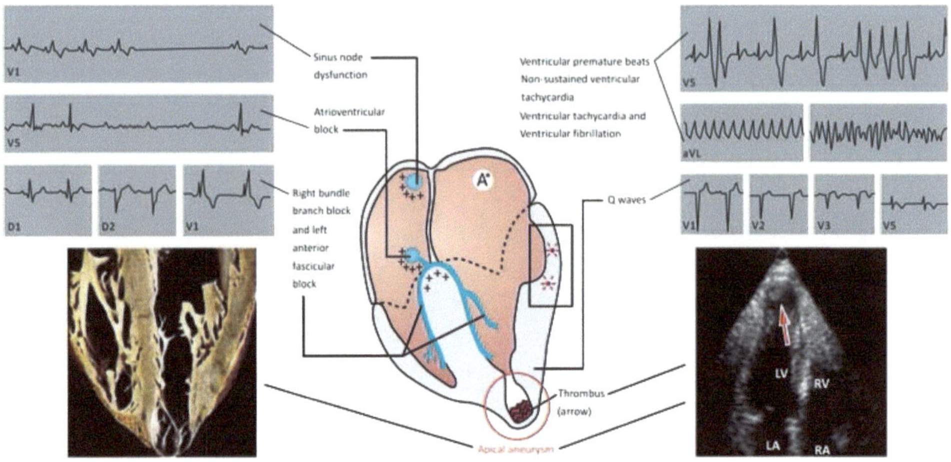

B

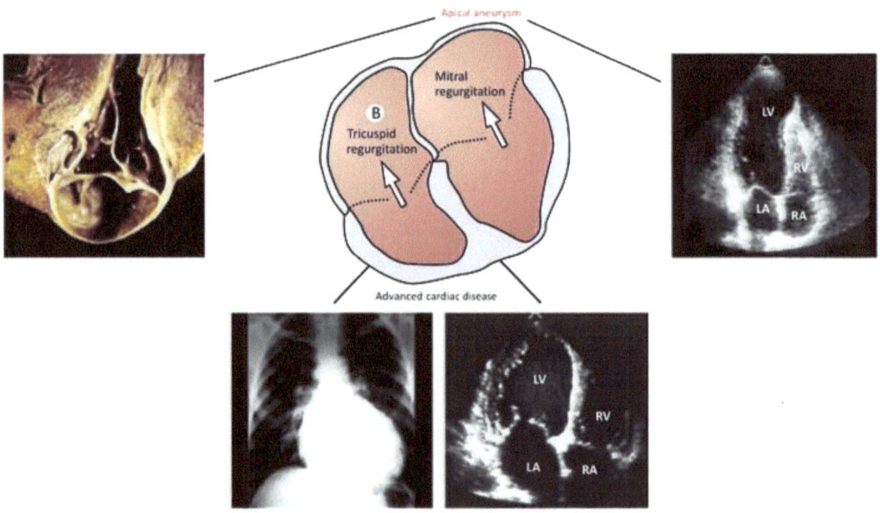

Fig. (5A & B). Common findings in infants, children, and pregnant women with chronic Chagas disease.

Bradyarrhythmia and Conduction System Abnormalities: Chagas heart disease is an essential cause of bradyarrhythmia's and pacemaker implantation [81]. Widespread fibrosis shows a preference for the cardiac conduction system, affecting the sinus node, atrioventricular node, and bundles of his [72]. The combination of the left anterior fascicular block (LBBB) and right bundle branch block (RBBB) is strongly suggestive of Chagas cardiomyopathy and should prompt a search for risk factors and serological evaluation of those at risk. Sick sinus syndrome can manifest as a sinoatrial block, sinus pauses, and bradycardia in severe cases, bradycardia-tachycardia syndrome [68, 82].

Ventricular Aneurysms: Ventricular aneurysms, which is typically apically located as seen echocardiographically [83] vary in size ranging from hollow punch lesions to giant aneurysms hardly distinguishable from those seen with myocardial infarction [84]. The presence of a ventricular aneurysm, however, predicts the development of stroke and mural thrombus [85 - 87] which largely contributes to the substrate for ventricular arrhythmias.

Heart Failure: Heart failure is easily diagnosed in pregnant women with Chagas cardiomyopathy, which is typically caused by the progressive dilated cardiomyopathy, which is commonly associated with Chagas cardiomyopathy. However, abnormalities of systolic and diastolic function coexist as right-sided heart failure can be more prominent in some patients than left-sided systolic failure, a hint for the diagnosis for chronic Chagas cardiomyopathy as the cause for heart failure. Although isolated right-sided heart failure is not frequent, and right ventricular (RV) dysfunction usually is associated with LV dysfunction in advanced stages of Chagas cardiomyopathy [88].

Thromboembolism: Chagas disease is a significant potential cause of stroke commonly diagnosed as Chagas-associated stroke [85, 89]. The classical cause of Chagas-associated stroke is as a result of the cardioembolic intracardiac thrombi, a resultant cause of poor ventricular function and atrial arrhythmias [90] easily misdiagnosed during pregnancy as the presenting signs encountered during clinical evaluations include homonymous hemianopia, motor or sensory deficit involving the face, arm, and leg, and higher cerebral dysfunction such as visuospatial deficit or aphasia [87].

PARASITE DIVERSITY AND THEIR PARASITIC FEATURES

The Current Approach of Molecular Biodiversity of *T. cruzi*

T. cruzi is classified into six phylogenetic lineages, also known as discrete typing units (DTUs) named TcI to TcVI. DTUs differ in an ecological niche, vector and reservoir hosts, and in their geographical distributions. However, TcV and TcVI are hybrids derived from TcII and TcIII. TcV and TcVI are associated with Chagas disease mainly in the central and southern part of America, whereas TcI is the most abundant and widely dispersed of all the *T. cruzi* DTUs in the Americas

[91]. Although closely related to each other, they are not necessarily identical and can also be distinguished from each other using molecular markers like nuclear (SSU rDNA) and mitochondrial (Cytb) genetic markers [92].

Parasitic Features Involved in The Development of Congenital Chagas Disease

The maternal-fetal transmission and the development of congenital Chagas disease solely depend on the capacity and the parasitic features of the infecting *T. cruzi* strains:

I. To invade and multiply rapidly within host cells (virulence), inducing high parasitemia's
II. To limit the pregnant woman's effective immune response, the placenta (trophoblastic in the first line and mesenchymal in the second line of defenses), and the fetus.

TRYPANOSOMA CRUZI INFECTION ON FERTILITY, AND PREGNANCY OUTCOMES

Indeed, the cause of infertility is complex, diverse in endemic and non-endemic areas, and also dependent on the *T. cruzi* infecting strain on the male and female reproductive organs, and even the hormone-producing glands too. Stillbirth and neonatal mortality mostly occur in endemic areas and untreated severe maternal-fetal infection, reactivation or co-infection [93] with high parasitemia levels. However, morbidity and mortality are also experienced at high levels in non-endemic areas due to the little knowledge of the disease by practitioners.

RELATIONSHIP BETWEEN PARASITEMIA, PARASITE INFECTING STRAIN, AND IMMUNE DEFECT IN PREGNANT WOMEN WITH OTHER SUSCEPTIBLE FACTORS MODULATING THEIR IMMUNE STATUS

I. The rapid multiplication in pregnant women leading to congenital infection is dependent on the parasitic strain. The strain virulence and its capacity to limit the efficiency of immune responses create a vicious circle where the parasite-driven immune deficiency and its virulence lead to a high parasitemia level, which in turn reinforce immune deficiency.
II. The host genetic factors result in an immune deficiency in pregnant women, leading to more poor control of parasite multiplication, higher parasitemias, and the occurrence of congenital infection although maternal predisposition to the transmission of the parasite is also a possible variable [94].
III. The physiological immune environment of pregnancy also plays a crucial role

in the congenital infection of the unborn fetus. More so, primiparity is also another contributing factor to parasite transmission as lower levels of prolactin, and a higher level of cortisol are produced in primiparas compared to multiparas [94].

IV. Maternal gut microbiome of a pregnant woman plays an essential immune modulating role in the disease transmission like the leakage of bacterial lipopolysaccharide which is a Toll-Like Receptor (TLR) 4 ligand from which the gut microbiome upregulates the production of IL-10 (an immunosuppressive cytokine) by *T. cruzi*-infected dendritic cell [95].

V. Malnutrition and poverty are always associated with *T. cruzi* infection quickly favoring congenital transmission by worsening the immune system of the pregnant woman [96] which also plays a vital role in the differences observed between transmission rates in endemic and non-endemic countries [97].

INTERACTION BETWEEN *TRYPANOSOMA CRUZI* AND THE PLACENTA

The relationship found between parasite and the placenta is clinically based on the importance of placental lesions and the possible transmission occurrence including the parasitic level, strain and other susceptible factors involved in pregnancy (Fig. **6**). Possible interactions, eventually leading to the congenital transmission of the infection include:

I. The overflow of the placental defense system by the massive load in the intervillous space, leads to the rupture of the trophoblastic barrier, the transmission of large quantities of free trypomastigotes and amastigote-infected cells. These processes eventually result in placentitis and the activation of other pathological mechanisms; therefore, overriding the protective nature of the placenta [98].

II. The presence of mild to moderate amount of parasite in the intervillous space aids its transmission through the marginal zone. Other possible interactions leading to the congenital transmission involve an alternate route deprived of trophoblast, which consists of the non-trophoblastic epithelium, and smooth muscle cells embedded in the extracellular matrix [99]. Additionally, the placental second line of defense (mesenchymal defense), fibroblast, and the macrophages within the chorion are also involved. Over time, the parasite eventually infects the endothelial cells and myocytes lining fetal vessels embedded in a chorionic plate or umbilical cord, and gains access to the fetal circulation. They ultimately affect myocytes, and endothelial cells lining fetal vessels embedded in a chorionic plate or umbilical cord and gain access to the fetal circulation [62], eventually leading to premature rupture, and premature birth as the infection spreads through the membranes surrounding the fetus, inducing their embrittlement [65].

III. The parasite transmission of both trypomastigotes and amastigote-infected cells through placental tears/breaches, which occurs naturally with labor contractions during delivery allowing micro transfusions. Although, it is slightly possible for this to be avoided through a planned cesarean section.

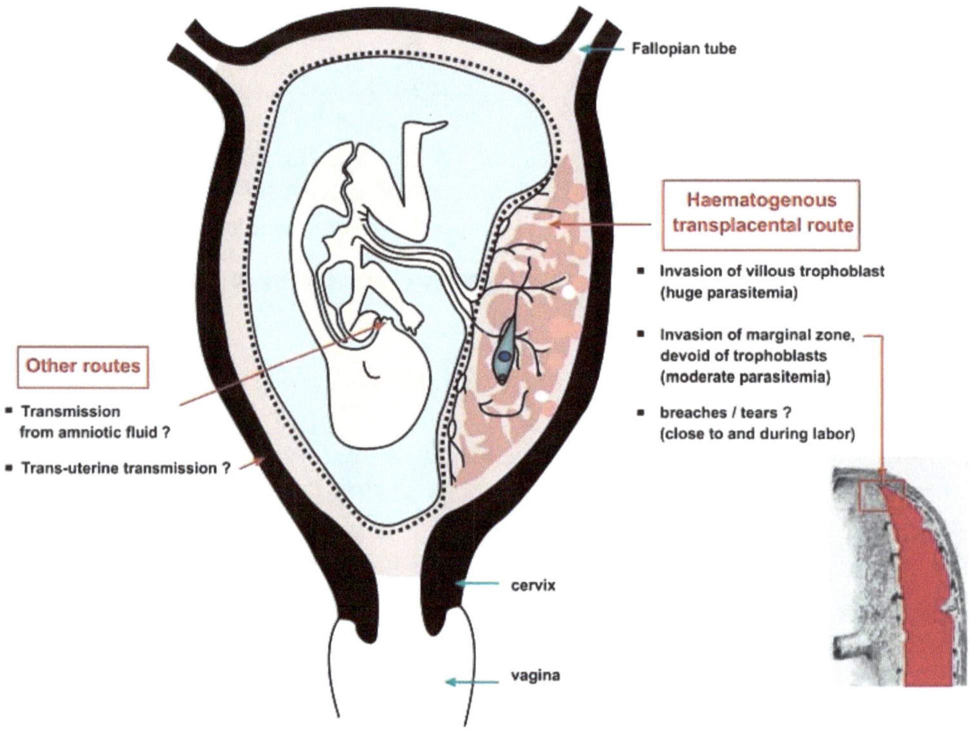

Fig. (6). Possible routes of maternal-fetal transmission of *Trypanosoma cruzi*.

BASIC DEPENDANTS OF PARASITIC AMOUNTS, INTERACTIONS, SEVERITY AND THE DEVELOPMENT OF CONGENITAL CHAGAS DISEASE IN FETUS AND NEWBORNS

I. The number of parasites transmitted from their mothers.

II. The ability for the infecting parasite strain(s) to invade and multiply into cells/tissues and/or to hinder the efficiency of immune responses in the fetus or newborn.

III. The time needed for the parasite to multiply right from the time of transmission during pregnancy [100] and finally,

IV. The extent of the own individual fetal/neonatal innate and adaptive immune responses against parasites modulated according to the maternal imprinting.

RISK FACTORS FOR CONGENITAL TRANSMISSION

Maternal Factors

I. Obstetrical history.
II. Immunological status.
III. The maternal phase of the disease.
IV. Mothers with detectable parasitemia.
V. The precedent of siblings with congenital infection.
VI. Mothers living or migrating from endemic areas.
VII. Mothers living or migrating from areas with a high rate of transmission.
VIII. Mothers with decreased T-cell-mediated responses to *T. cruzi*, coinfection with Malaria or HIV.

Parasitic Factors

I. The type of *Trypanosoma cruzi* strain.
II. The parasitic load.

RISK STRATIFICATION FOR CHRONIC CHAGAS CARDIOMYOPATHY AND RELATED STROKE

It is essential to carry out risk stratification scores early in the cardiac course when possible for both chronic Chagas cardiomyopathy and related stroke in pregnant mothers (Fig. **7**). The Rassi score is a vital risk stratification score for patients with an already established cardiomyopathy which uses six factors (a combination of clinical symptoms, demographics, and test results) with weighted values to classify patients by risk of ten-year mortality: low (10%), medium (44%), and high (84%) [101] (Fig. **8**). However, the Sousa score, published more recently, uses four factors (LV function, syncope, QT dispersion, and premature ventricular contractions) to predict the risk of SCD as low (0–2 points), intermediate (3–4 points), and high (>5 points) [102]. As for risk stratification for stroke [103], four variables are included: systolic dysfunction (2 points), apical aneurysm (1 point), abnormal ventricular repolarization (1 point), and age >48 years (1 point).

DIAGNOSIS AND MONITORING

For a proper treatment of the disease, and a better understanding of its progress and mode transmissions, a complete diagnostic test must be carried out starting with a thorough clinical history taking of the pregnant mother. It is also essential to carry out laboratory diagnostical test (Molecular and serological) in newborns from women leaving and from endemic regions. It should be done as soon as possible right after the birth to best explain to the mother the necessity to treat the newborn without delay to avoid situations where contact is lost once the mother leaves the health care facility [104] (Fig. **9**). According to the Technical Group on "Prevention and Control of Congenital Transmission and Case Management of Congenital Infections" (IVa) of WHO Program on Control of Chagas disease, the gold standard for diagnosis of congenital infection is the detection of blood parasites at any time after birth. Also, according to the working group, a positive *T. cruzi* specific serology in infants aged >8months is diagnostically certain when the previous transmission by vectors and blood transfusion has been ruled out [105].

	Risk factor			**Treatment**
	NHYA class III or IV	Left ventricular systolic dysfunction (echocardiography) or cardiomegaly (chest radiography), or both	Non-sustained ventricular tachycardia (24-h Holter monitoring)	
Very high	Present*	Present	Present	ACE inhibitor, spironolactone, amiodarone, diuretics, digitalis, β blocker†, cardiac transplant‡, possibly treat with an implantable cardioverter defibrillator
High	Absent	Present	Present	ACE inhibitor, amiodarone, diuretic‡, β blocker†, possibly treat with an implantable cardioverter defibrillator
Intermediate	Absent	Present	Absent	ACE inhibitor, β blocker, diuretic‡, possibly treat with an antiparasitic drug
Intermediate	Absent	Absent	Present	Possibly treat with amiodarone and an antiparasitic drug
Low	Absent	Absent	Absent	Possibly treat with an antiparasitic drug

Fig. (7). Stratification of risk of death associated with Chagas heart disease and recommended treatment. NYHA=New York Heart Association. ACE=angiotensin-converting enzyme. *Nearly all patients with Chagas heart disease in NYHA class III or IV also have left ventricular systolic dysfunction on echocardiogram and non-sustained ventricular tachycardia on 24-h Holter monitoring. †If clinically tolerated. ‡ For selected patients.

Molecular Diagnosis

The identification of parasite antigens or DNA in blood can suggest the presence of infection. Also, the detection of *T. cruzi* antigens in urines and serum by capture ELISA assays is diagnostic, especially in congenital cases from pregnant mothers in endemic regions.

Risk factor	Points
NYHA class III or IV	5
Cardiomegaly (chest radiograph)	5
Segmental or global wall motion abnormality (2D echocardiogram)	3
Non-sustained ventricular tachycardia (24-h Holter)	3
Low QRS voltage (ECG)	2
Male sex	2

Total points	Total mortality Five years	Ten years	Risk
0-6	2%	10%	Low
7-11	18%	44%	Intermediate
12-20	63%	84%	High

Fig. (8). Prognostic factors in Chagas heart disease. Rassi score.

However, the molecular amplification of parasite nuclear or kinetoplast DNA helps improve the detection of low-level parasitemia's in both the mother and child as results can be obtained in a short time although, still currently under evaluation by WHO [105]. Be it as it may, the test should be confirmed with subsequent samples at approximately three, and nine months after birth [100].

Serological Diagnosis

Although, in the first months of life, conventional serology might not be useful due to the transference of maternal antibodies through the placenta. However, the use of shed acute-phase antigen (SAPA) detects acute or congenital infection [106]. In newborns, precise definitive diagnosis is only made nine months after the maternal antibodies have disappeared and the presence of anti-*T. cruzi* antibodies with the standard serological test is confirmed. As with chronic cases, the use of two different serological tests is recommended.

Antenatal Screening

According to the recommendations of the Technical Group IVa on "Prevention and Control of Congenital Transmission and Case Management of Congenital Infections," prenatal serological testing is recommended for pregnant women:

I. Living in disease-endemic areas
II. Residing in disease nonendemic areas and have occasionally received a blood transfusion in disease-endemic areas, and
III. Who are living in disease nonendemic areas and are born or have lived previously in disease-endemic areas or whose mothers were born in such areas [105].

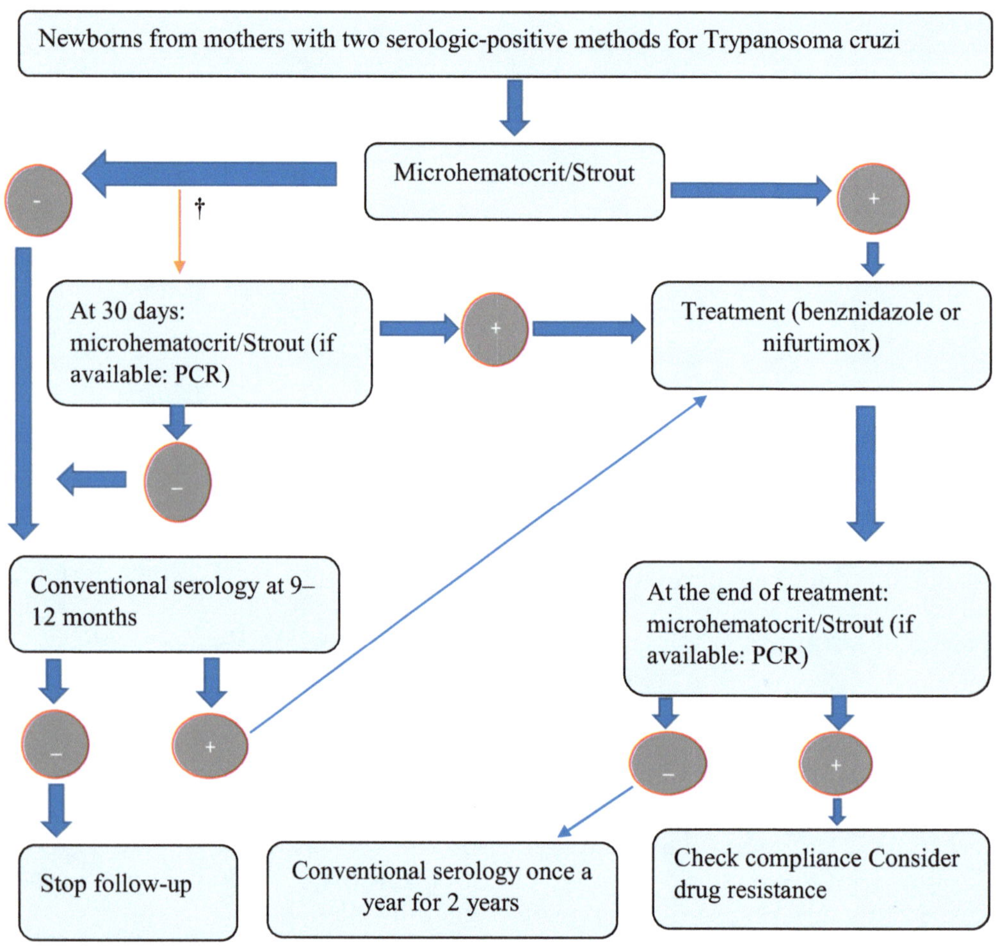

Fig. (9). Algorithm for the screening of newborns from *Trypanosoma cruzi*-infected women.

Electrocardiogram

ECG is one of the most important initial evaluation of pregnant women with definite or suspected Chagas disease (Table **1**). Patients coming from endemic regions without a known infection, the existence of common electrocardiographic abnormalities on the ECG should raise the clinical suspicion and an additional reason to order a serological test. Furthermore, for patients with a confirmed serological diagnosis of chronic Chagas disease, an ECG can identify those with established cardiomyopathy, in whom typical ECG findings will occur or, if normal, can draw the physician's attention to the presence of a chronic indeterminate form, which should be established by normal radiological tests and absence of any clinical manifestation. Electrocardiographic abnormalities such as atrial fibrillation and atrioventricular blocks should be treated swiftly as such electrocardiographic abnormalities are related to high risk of death [107]. Repeated ECG test is mandatory as it determines the cardiomyopathies progress [108]. However, for patients with symptoms of cardiac arrhythmias, such as syncope and palpitations, after an obligatory ECG test, a further Holter monitoring and stress testing are essential.

Electrocardiographic Stress Test Monitoring

Chronic Chagas heart disease patients typically have a relatively preserved exercise capacity, even in the face of a depressed ventricular function and marked ECG changes. Therefore, cardiac stress goes beyond assessing exercise abilities but instead accessing exercise chronotropic responses, which can be decreased as a result of previously described autonomic impairment. It is also useful in uncovering complex ventricular arrhythmias, in particular when Holter monitoring is unavailable. Finally, any patient with Chagas heart disease and advanced heart failure for whom cardiac transplantation has been considered, cardiac stress testing is recommended.

Be it as it may, we do not, however, support its use in pregnant women. If necessary, it should be applied with caution and at the physician's discretion.

Holter Monitoring

Holter monitoring is useful in patients with presyncope or syncope as these symptoms are caused by tachyarrhythmia or bradyarrhythmia [16]. Pregnant women at the chronic phase of Chagas cardiomyopathy irrespective of severity, require 24-hour Holter monitoring to assess the density and presence of complex ventricular arrhythmia, atrioventricular conduction, and sinus node disease [27]. Nonsustained ventricular tachycardia [VT] on Holter monitoring is an independent marker of higher risk of death [101].

Chest X-Ray

It is of vital importance to note that, chest X-rays should be avoided in pregnant women be it that it facilitates the assessment of atrial and ventricular size.

Although, the appropriate timing to carry out this investigation varies, in our experience, we the authors suggest that it is safe to carry out chest X-rays 5 to 6 weeks after delivery bearing in mind that the mammary gland is susceptible to trapping X-ray films at a high rate due to lactation early on especially at the very first 4 weeks after delivery. However, the enlargement of all four cardiac chambers without pulmonary congestion suggests Chagas cardiomyopathy and should prompt additional imaging and serological assessment in patients without a confirmed diagnosis of Chagas disease. Chest X-rays help to provide useful information on the presence and extent of pericardial effusion and also, signs and symptoms of patients with heart failure. Asymptomatic patients with a normal ECG should have a chest x-ray to confirm indeterminate Chagas disease [58].

Table 1. Cardiac Rhythm Abnormalities More Commonly Detected in Chagas Cardiomyopathy.

More Typical Findings	Less Commonly Seen
Bradyarrhythmia's and conduction system abnormalities	
RBBB ± left anterior fascicular block	Incomplete RBBB left bundle branch block
First-degree atrioventricular block	Isolated left anterior fascicular block
Second- and third-degree atrioventricular block	Sinus bradycardia with HR ≤40 bpm
Sinus bradycardia with HR >40 bpm	Sinus node dysfunction
Atrial tachyarrhythmias	
Atrial fibrillation	
Ventricular tachyarrhythmias	
Frequent PVCs, often polymorphic	Isolated monomorphic PVCs
Nonsustained VT	
Other	
Primary ST- and T-wave abnormalities	Nonspecific ST- and T-wave abnormalities
Pathological Q waves or electric inactive areas	Low limb lead voltage

HR-heart rate; PVC, premature ventricular contraction; RBBB, right bundle-branch block; and VT, ventricular tachycardia.

Echocardiography

The early use of echocardiography helps improve the understanding of early cardiac involvement in pregnant women, which is essentially a myopericarditis as the use of X-ray is detrimental to the unborn child. Common findings include pericardial effusion (40%-50%), regional wall motion abnormalities (0%- 20%), and a global decreased left ventricular ejection fraction (0%-30%) [109] (Table **2**).

Nuclear Medicine Test

Although, an expensive test, it provides helpful complementary information and also elucidates some vital aspects in the pathogenesis and pathophysiology of Chagas cardiomyopathy. It is, however, useful in patients with poor acoustic windows or when additional information about myocardial perfusion, myocardial sympathetic innervation or RV function is required [110].

Table 2. Most Common Echocardiographic Findings in Chronic Chagas Disease.

Segmental wall motion abnormalities: akinesis, hypokinesis, or dyskinesia.
Mitral and tricuspid regurgitation
A mural thrombus, mainly at LV apex
RV dysfunction
Dilated cardiomyopathy
LV diastolic dysfunction
LV aneurysm
Inferior-inferolateral wall, usually basal segments

LV- left ventricular; and RV- right ventricular.

Single-Photon Emission Computed Tomography: This helps identify patients who have both regional wall abnormality and a fixed perfusion defect typically associated with areas of fibrosis [111, 112] despite normal epicardial coronary on angiography [113]. Over time, however, the perfusion defects worsen as fibrosis increases with fewer reversible and more fixed areas of inadequate perfusion [114]. Single-photon emission computed tomography imaging also helps to correlate Chagasic chest pain syndrome with microvascular perfusion defects, a potential cause of myocardial damage [113].

Radionuclide Ventriculography (Multigated Acquisition): Its scans provide a more precise ventricular function information [85 - 87] as it, however, doesn't depend on geometrical assumptions for left ventricular ejection fraction (LVEF), averaging hundreds of cardiac cycles, identifying aneurysms, and also not affected by the spherical shape. It is, however, typically seen in dilated cardiomyopathy unlike M-mode and 2-dimensional echocardiography where ejection (EF) is reliant on a formula that assumes a standard ventricular geometry. Furthermore, this Multigated scans are also useful for quantification of RV function (qualitative by echocardiography) and add valuable information to myocardial perfusion assessment, allowing correlation between regional wall motion abnormalities and perfusion defects [115].

Cardiac Catheterization: Cardiac catheterization is indicated in patients with advanced heart failure to assess the feasibility of cardiac transplantation, providing a direct measurement of pulmonary vascular resistance. It also helps to distinguish organ rejection and reactivation of *T cruzi* infection after cardiac transplantation. However, cardiac catheterization also helps to identify Chagasic symptoms mimicking coronary artery disease.

Cardiac Magnetic Resonance: Cardiac Magnetic Resonance (CMR) imaging provides a superior image for the anatomic and functional evaluation of all cardiac chambers, detecting mural thrombosis, tissue characterization and also providing a direct measurement of both RVEF and LVEF. CMR also has a strong potential for improving the prognostic evaluation of patients in the chronic phase of Chagas cardiomyopathy beyond that of Rassi score. Moreover, CMR imaging helps in identifying patients who develop malignant arrhythmia in the absence of global ventricular systolic dysfunction but showing regional areas of fibrotic myocardium [110, 116, 117].

THERAPEUTIC MANAGEMENT

The non-operative treatment of Chagas cardiomyopathic patients consists of four main approaches: (i) elimination of *Trypanosoma cruzi*; (ii) management of heart failure; (iii) prevention of thromboembolic events; and (iv) device management of conduction disorders.

Anti-Trypanosomal Treatment

Both Benznidazole and Nifurtimox shorten the clinical course of illness, reduce symptoms severity, and the duration of parasitemia in congenital transmission with high success rate [118] when therapy is initiated early (Table **3**). Benznidazole and Nifurtimox are the only drugs with proven efficacy against *T. cruzi* infection. As of 14th May 2018, benznidazole (manufactured by Exeltis and distributed by Foundation Care) became commercially available and approved by the Food and Drug Administration in the United States. Benznidazole, a nitroimidazole derivative, is considered to be the first-line treatment, based on a better side-effect profile than nifurtimox, as well as a more extensive evidence base for efficacy [29]. However, the most frequently observed adverse effects are dermatologic, usually mild rashes that respond to antihistamines [119, 120]. In case of severe or exfoliative dermatitis associated with fever and lymphadenopathy, treatment should immediately be interrupted.

Heart Failure

The management of heart failure in routine clinical practice includes a combination of β-blockers, angiotensin receptor blockers, or angiotensin-converting enzyme (ACE), anticoagulation, digoxin, and diuretics. ACE inhibitors are our first-line treatment for the chronic phase, reduced LVEF and, segmental wall motion impairment despite preserved global LV function. We also recommend the addition of aldosterone receptor antagonist for patients in class II to IV New York Heart Association heart failure and an LVEF ≤35% as these medications also improve the general quality of life in patients with LV dysfunction among the general population with dilated cardiomyopathy [16, 31, 76]. However, unless specifically contraindicated, β-blocker therapy is recommended for all symptomatic or previously symptomatic patients in the chronic phase and a reduced EF as it also improves the patient's clinical status [121].

Table 3. Anti-Trypanosomal Treatment.

	Benznidazole	**Nifurtimox**	**Comments**
Total daily dose (mg/kg)	5–8	8–10	--
Times per day	Twice	Three times	--
Administration	Oral	Oral	--
Treatment duration (days)	60	60–120	--
Metabolism	Hepatic	Hepatic—NADPH P450 reductase	--
Mechanism of action	Inhibition of protein and RNA synthesis in *Trypanosoma cruzi*	Free oxygen radical formation	--
Metabolic pathway	Renal excretion 60–70%	Renal excretion of metabolites	--
Anorexia, weight loss	++	++	--
Nausea, vomiting	++	++	--
Fatigue, headache, insomnia, vertigo, seizures	++	+++	No need to discontinue/Sometimes need to discontinue
Peripheral neuropathy, polyneuropathy	+++ (late in the course of treatment	+++ (early in the course of treatment	Discontinuation
Dermatitis, rash	++	++	Not necessary to stop treatment unless there is a purpuric rash
Bone marrow suppression	+++	+++	Leukopenia, thrombocytopenia Discontinuation

(Table 2) cont.....

Interactions with immunosuppressive drugs	Possible with drugs that interact with cytochrome P450	Not known	Close monitoring of adverse events
Interactions with antiretrovirals	Possible with drugs that interact with cytochrome P450	Not known	Close monitoring of adverse events
Warnings	Alcohol, aspirin, anticoagulants Mutagenicity in experimental animals	Alcohol, aspirin	--
Contraindications	Pregnancy, severe kidney and liver insufficiency	Pregnancy, acute kidney, and liver insufficiency	--

Furthermore, these medications provide protection against the development of ventricular arrhythmia and sudden death due to the autonomic imbalance resulting from an incomplete denervated myocardium and predominant parasympathetic dysautonomia. Finally, we recommend the use of anticoagulants for patients who have a previous thromboembolic event or the presence of a cardiac thrombus detected by echocardiography [30]. We also recommend the use of anticoagulants in patients with apical aneurysm, especially small aneurysms with a narrow neck that are at high risk for thrombus formation.

Treatment of Arrhythmia and Prevention of Sudden Cardiac Death

Antiarrhythmic Drugs: Isolated ventricular premature complexes are the most common arrhythmia phased and it, however, requires no treatment in patients with preserved ventricular function. Also, treatment is similarly not routinely recommended for patients with asymptomatic non-sustained VT and complex ventricular extrasystoles. Although, Amiodarone the drug of choice which is still not yet proven to decrease the risk of SCD is empirically prescribed for patients thus, improving symptoms and reducing the density of ventricular arrhythmia [19, 122]. Amiodarone should be considered in high-risk patients with LV dysfunction and non-sustained VT associated with symptoms, and in patients with delayed enhancement by CMR [123], late signal potentials on ECGs, T-wave variability [124], T-wave micro-alternans [125], ventricular ectopic beats, and Nonsustained VT by 24-hour Holter monitoring.

Implantable Cardiac Defibrillator: Clinically, patients with Chagas heart disease experience a higher rate of malignant ventricular arrhythmia and resultant SCD [78] than other cardiomyopathic population. However, until the CHAGASICS trial (Amiodarone Against ICD Therapy in Chagas Cardiomyopathy for Primary Prevention of Death) [126] which is currently underway to establish the benefit of implantable cardioverter defibrillator (ICD) therapy for the primary prevention of death in patients, there are no data to support recommendations for the primary prevention of death in patients.

Ablation Therapy: Although not routinely used clinically to treat ventricular tachycardic Chagasic pregnant cardiomyopathic women, if necessary, we recommend the use of catheter-based technique (only in centers with vast experience in such cases) if medication fails, or intolerable side effects develops [127, 128] as the goal of ablation is to pinpoint and disrupt the circuit through ablation of critical isthmuses. Furthermore, indication for VT ablation includes:

I. Antiarrhythmic drugs not tolerated or are not desired. Sustained symptomatic monomorphic VT, including VT, terminated by ICDs recur despite antiarrhythmic drug therapy;
II. Control of incessant sustained monomorphic VT or VT storm that is not the result of a transient reversible cause;
III. Bundle-branch reentrant or interfascicular VT; and
IV. Ventricular fibrillation that is refractory to antiarrhythmic therapy or recurrent sustained polymorphic VT and when there is a suspected trigger that can be targeted for ablation.

Pacemaker Implantation: Sick sinus syndrome and an advance atrioventricular block are the main indications for pacemaker implantation in a pregnant woman with Chagas cardiomyopathy. Its recommendations are the same as the international guidelines for other conditions. However, we recommend that this procedure should be individualized and done only in experienced centers with such high case volume. Careful measures should also be taken to avoid adverse outcomes and, or complications, which would be detrimental to the pregnant mother and her unborn child.

HOW TO MONITOR THERAPEUTIC TREATMENT EFFICACY

The definition for a complete cure for Chagas cardiomyopathy and a congenitally infected child is established based on the disappearance of antibodies once conventional serology becomes persistently negative [31, 129]. Therapeutic failure is defined as the persistence of parasites after completing treatment using PCR or parasitological methods. In cases of persistent parasitemia, it is vital to consider parasite resistance in addition to verification of the correct drug use and its application too.

SURGICAL TREATMENT

Preoperative Considerations

Although, we do not recommend the surgical treatment of pregnant mothers with confirmed Chagas cardiomyopathy instead we recommend a further therapeutic antitrypanosomal treatment with Benznidazole which is useful if treatment regimen is strictly adhered to by the patient coupled with a follow-up clinic visit to monitor the treatment efficacy. Bearing this in mind, the management of patients with Chagasic disease, in general, is a collaborative team effort from cardiac surgery to electrophysiology, heart failure, and infectious disease department. If, however, surgical treatment of the pregnant mother is mandatory, we advise that a comprehensive discussion with a heart failure specialist (cardiological team) is made regarding the need for volume optimization, beta-blockers, and even circulatory support for the bridge to surgery. The infectious disease team assesses the pregnant woman and provides recommendations regarding the need for antitrypanosomal therapy while the electrophysiology team manages the anti-arrhythmic medication therapy and cardiac resynchronization devices if required. In our experience, antibiotic treatment is not needed unless if the patient is immunocompromised and develops reactivation of the infection due to immunosuppression. Heart transplant, in general, is a well-planned surgery be it a pregnant woman or not which also requires a well-structured preoperative workup such as electrocardiogram, echocardiography, right and left heart catheterization (depending on the biventricular function), cardiac MRI, and the assessment of other systems if necessary. We recommend a pre-transplant evaluation of donors whether they are in endemic or non-endemic regions [130, 131].

Indications

• Aneurysm with or without thrombus formation (**See Fig. 10 A & B**) and.

• Advanced heart failure (disease progression despite optimal medical therapy) (Table **4**).

Surgery

Heart transplantation is now accepted as the treatment of choice for chronic Chagasic cardiomyopathy, in spite of the risk of infection reactivation [132] (Fig. **11**). Selection criteria with that of the general transplantation are quite similar. However, compared to the general population, transplant with Chagas cardiomyopathic patient is better where transplantation at one month is (80%), one year (70%), and ten years (42%) [133]. Despite the risk of *T cruzi* reactivation after transplantation and immunosuppression, prophylactic antitrypanosomal therapy is not recommended [134, 135]. Quantitative *T cruzi* PCR provides sufficient sensitivity to detect a reactivation before complications such as allograft dysfunction develop [134].

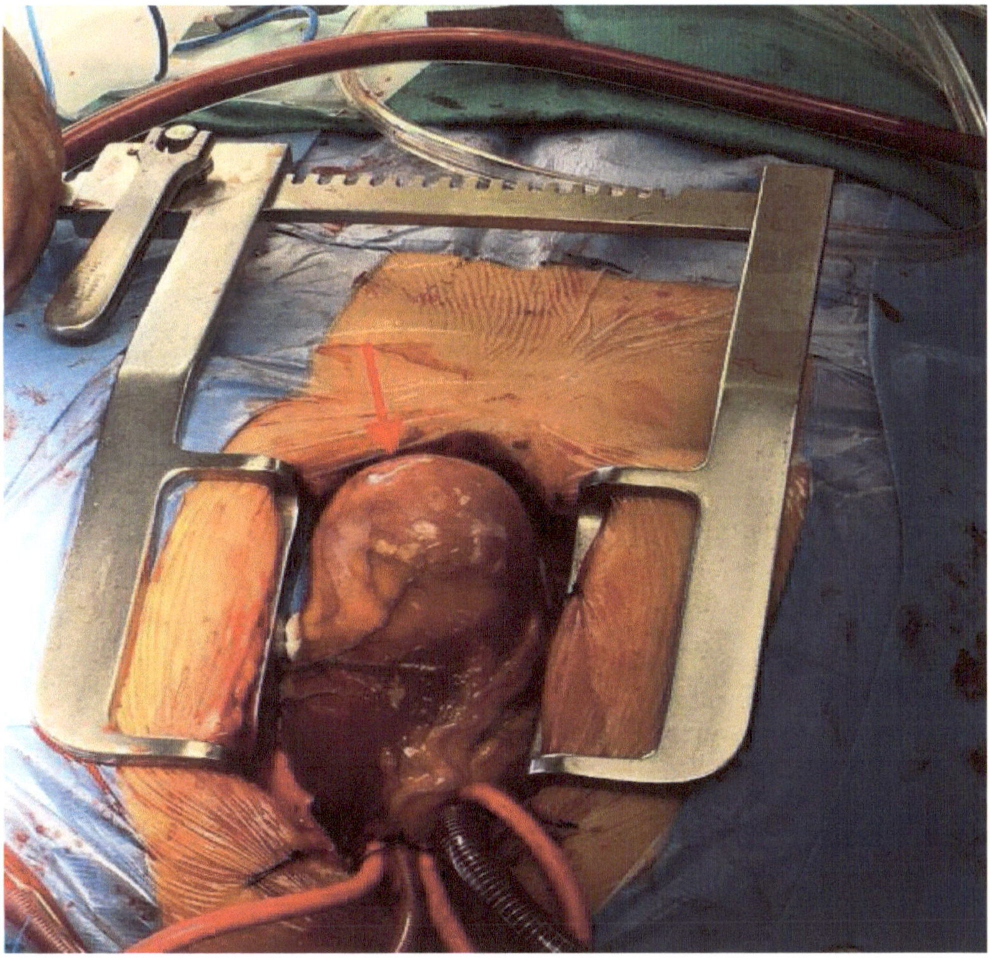

Fig. (10A). An apical thin-walled portion of the left ventricle resembling a true aneurysm shown post-median sternotomy (red arrow).

CONTINUING CHALLENGES AND THE FUTURE OF CHAGAS CARDIOMYOPATHY

Although considered as an NTD by WHO, any progress made in the field still faces challenges and setbacks because:

I. Majority of the patients are asymptomatic until they progress into the predominant type of the disease (cardiac type) with severe symptoms and irreversible complications requiring surgery [136].
II. In the chronic phase, parasites are thus, rooted deep into the tissues, with only low-level transient circulating parasites which are undetectable by traditional parasitological methods.
III. The gold-standard tool of certificate cure is conventional serology, but negative seroconversion can lag the treatment years behind [137].

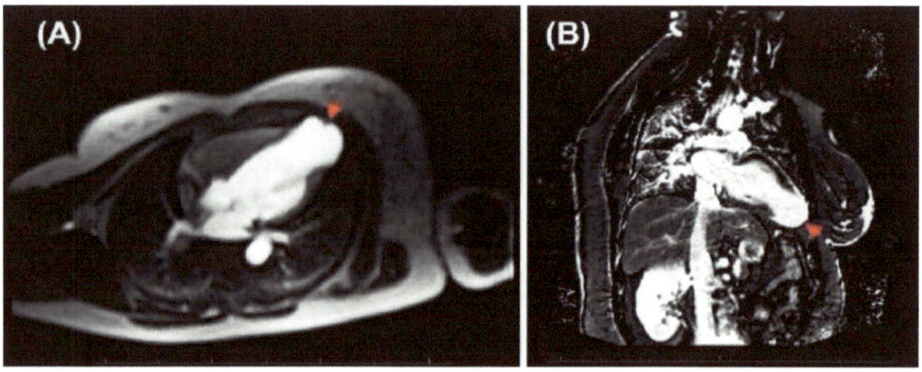

Fig. (10B). Transverse section view of cardiac magnetic resonance imaging elaborating further the anatomy of the aneurysm (red arrowhead). [B]. Sagittal view of the same study (red arrowhead).

Table 4. Potential Indications for Heart Transplantation in End-Stage Chagas' Heart Disease (1-year Survival Probability).

Predictors of Mortality	Annual Survival Estimate
Persistent NYHA Class IV	20%
LVEF <30%	20%
Patients on inotropic support	0%
lack of b-blocker use and hyponatremia, LVEF <31%, NYHA Class IV, and digoxin use	23%
Maximal oxygen consumption rate <10 mL. kg. min -1 at cardio-spirometry	0%
Patients receiving ICD therapy with clustering of 4 or more shocks by day 30	19%

NHA, New York Heart Association; LVEF, left ventricular ejection fraction; ICD, implantable cardioverter-defibrillator.

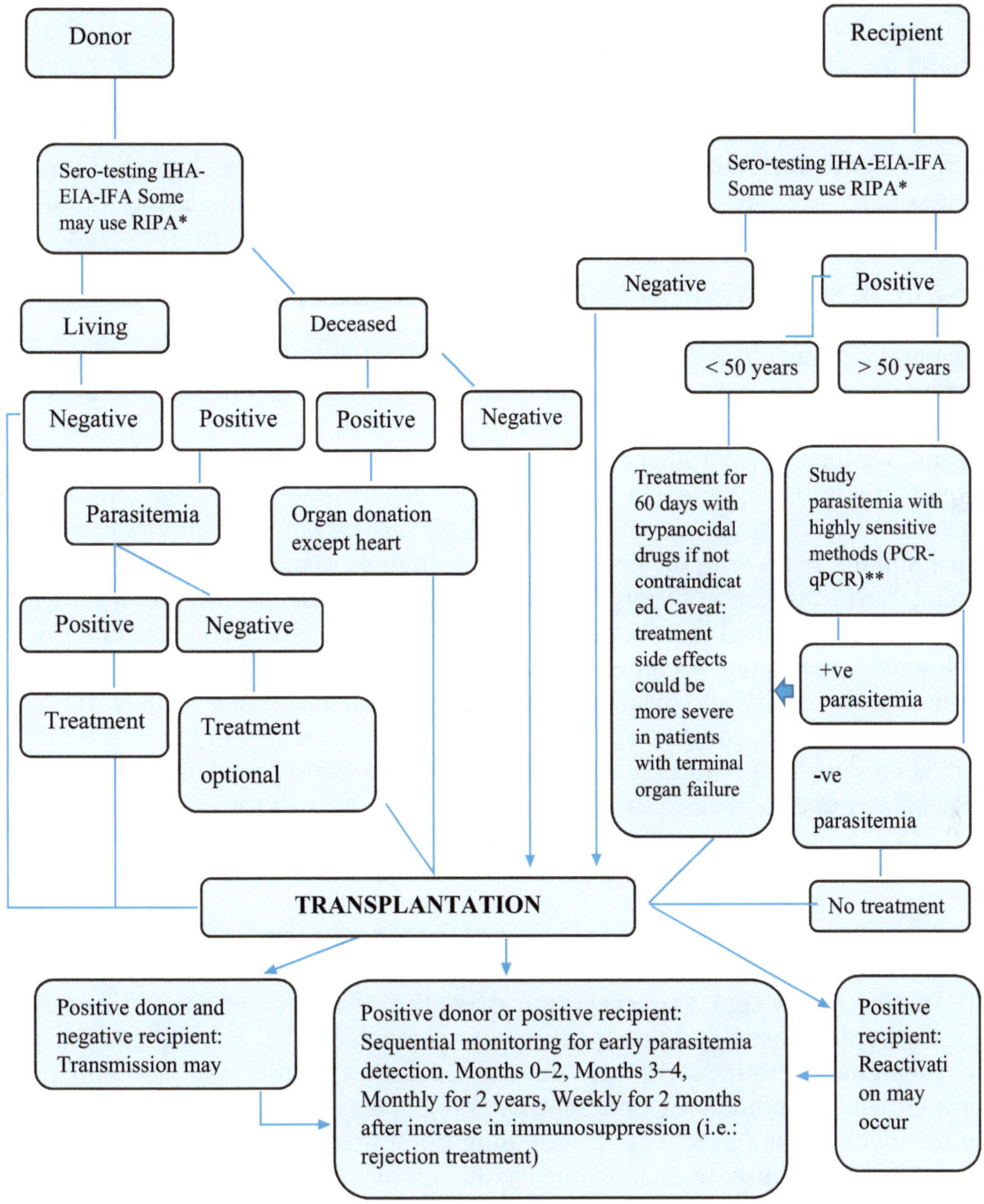

Fig. (11). Authors recommended algorithm for Chagas disease management in patients with solid organ transplantation. EIA, enzyme immunoassay; IFA, indirect immunofluorescence assay; IHA, indirect hemagglutination assay; qPCR, quantitative PCR; RIPA, radioimmunoprecipitation assay.

Therefore, the development of an effective vaccine and improved new therapeutic method is crucial and also an essential step in tackling the disease for their potential use during pregnancy and the prevention of congenital transmission also protecting against further cardiac complications. Be it as it may, there is still hope for the future in the field as the number of groups are currently in the advanced stages of developing novel therapies, including both DNA- and antigen-based vaccines [138 - 142] as well as other anti-trypanosomal drugs including chemical agents that competitively inhibit the function of critical *T. cruzi* enzymes [143].

CONCLUDING REMARKS AND FUTURE DIRECTIONS

Congenital Chagas disease is also known as a neglected tropical disease, however, it can be considered as an ecological model of multiple and complex interactions between parasites, the pregnant woman, placenta, and the unborn child. Indeed, congenital infection is a rather rare event, it can, however, occur and be found in any part of the world, and the lack of a well-established surveillance program means that the diagnosis can probably be easily missed putting both the pregnant mother and the fetus, with the newborn at risk. In this era of globalization with the ongoing European immigration policies, Congenital Chagas disease would no longer become confined to only poor rural areas or regions and endemic countries which would eventually become a significant public health concern. Bearing this in mind, the possibility of Chagasic disease, in general, becoming the new HIV in third world African countries and developing African nations in the foreseeable future is inevitable. It is futuristically possible due to the simple fact that both the policymakers and the health care providers are ignorant of the disease and also lack both the technical knowledge and understanding of the disease modes of transmission, progression, pathology, and its pathophysiology.

Nevertheless, the most significant challenges faced so far remain the development of new and accessible treatment options with fewer adverse effects, and a platform for the design and execution of multicenter studies to validate and improve the diagnostic and therapeutic options available. Therefore, it is crucial that researchers familiar with the disease in both endemic and non-endemic countries establish bilateral and multilateral Chagas disease collaboration. It would, however, go a long way in providing other health care professionals (not competent in the disease management) the ample opportunity to learn from decades of experience from these scientists thus, ensuring both collaborative platform and unlimited resources to advance the search for better ways to diagnose, treat and prevent the disease.

Appendix

Epidemiology, clinical manifestations, and diagnosis of acute or reactivated Chagas disease by the mechanism of disease acquisition. *Refers to symptomatic cases; since 95% of acute infections from the vectorial transmission are asymptomatic, and 5–10% of patients with severe symptoms die, estimated mortality in this phase of infection is between one in 200 and one in 400 — †depends on the underlying disease and the patients' clinical condition.

	Geographical Distribution	Predominant Population	Incubation Time	Clinical Presentation	Diagnosis	Mortality
Vectoral	Endemic countries	Children and adolescents	1–2 weeks	Asymptomatic; fever, malaise, lymphadenopathy, hepatosplenomegaly, subcutaneous edema; signs of the portal of entry (Romaña sign, chagoma); myocarditis, meningoencephalitis	Diagnosis	Low (<5–10%) *
Transfusion-based	Endemic and non-endemic countries	Adults	8–120 days	Same as for vectorial but excluding signs of the portal of entry	Diagnosis	Variable†
Congenital	Endemic and Nonendemic countries	Neonates and children younger than one year	Up to a few weeks	Asymptomatic; abortion, neonatal death, prematurity, low birth weight, low Apgar score; hypotonicity, fever, hepatosplenomegaly, respiratory distress, anemia; myocarditis, meningoencephalitis, mega viscera, edema	Diagnosis	Unknown
Oral	Amazon basin, and regional outbreaks	Individuals of any age from the same family or community	3–22 days	Same as for transfusion-based plus headache, myalgia, vomiting, abdominal pain, jaundice, diarrhea, and digestive hemorrhage	Diagnosis	High (8–35%)

(Appendix 3) cont.....

Reactivation based	Endemic and non-endemic countries	Patients with associate immunosuppressive states	Variable	Same as for transfusion-based plus panniculitis, subcutaneous parasite-containing nodules, and skin ulcers	Diagnosis	Variable†

LIST OF ABBREVIATIONS

ACC American College of Cardiology

AHA American heart association

ACE Angiotensin-converting enzyme

CMR Cardiac magnetic resonance

CCC Chronic Chagas cardiomyopathy

DTU Discrete typing units

ECG Electrocardiography

EF Ejection fraction

IDC Implantable cardioverter defibrillator

LF Left ventricle

LVEF Left ventricular ejection fraction

NTD Neglected tropical disease

RV Right ventricle

SCD Sudden cardiac death

SAPA Shed acute phase antigen

VT Ventricular tachycardia

WHO World Health Organization

CONSENT FOR PUBLICATION

Not applicable.

CONFLICT OF INTEREST

The authors confirm that this chapter contents have no conflict of interest.

ACKNOWLEDGEMENTS

Declared none.

REFERENCE

[1] Pays JF. Chagas Carlos Justiniano Ribeiro (1879-1934). Bull Soc Pathol Exot 2009; 102(5): 276-9. [PMID: 20131419]

[2] Voelker R. A century after Chagas disease discovery, hurdles to tackling the infection remain. JAMA 2009; 302(10): 1045-7. [http://dx.doi.org/10.1001/jama.2009.1269] [PMID: 19738081]

[3] Sosa-Estani S, Segura EL. Etiological treatment in patients infected by *Trypanosoma cruzi*: experiences in Argentina. Curr Opin Infect Dis 2006; 19(6): 583-7. [http://dx.doi.org/10.1097/01.qco.0000247592.21295.a5] [PMID: 17075335]

[4] Schmunis GA, Yadon ZE. Chagas disease: a Latin American health problem becoming a world health problem. Acta Trop 2010; 115(1-2): 14-21. [http://dx.doi.org/10.1016/j.actatropica.2009.11.003] [PMID: 19932071]

[5] Pereira KS, Schmidt FL, Guaraldo AM, Franco RM, Dias VL, Passos LA. Chagas' disease as a foodborne illness. J Food Prot 2009; 72(2): 441-6. [http://dx.doi.org/10.4315/0362-028X-72.2.441] [PMID: 19350996]

[6] Yoshida N. Molecular mechanisms of *Trypanosoma cruzi* infection by oral route. Mem Inst Oswaldo Cruz 2009; 104 (Suppl. 1): 101-7. [http://dx.doi.org/10.1590/S0074-02762009000900015] [PMID: 19753464]

[7] Beltrão HdeB, Cerroni MdeP, Freitas DR, *et al.* Investigation of two outbreaks of suspected oral transmission of acute Chagas disease in the Amazon region, Para State, Brazil, in 2007. Trop Doct 2009; 39(4): 231-2. [http://dx.doi.org/10.1258/td.2009.090035] [PMID: 19762577]

[8] Valente SA, da Costa Valente V, das Neves Pinto AY, *et al.* Analysis of an acute Chagas disease outbreak in the Brazilian Amazon: human cases, triatomines, reservoir mammals and parasites. Trans R Soc Trop Med Hyg 2009; 103(3): 291-7. [http://dx.doi.org/10.1016/j.trstmh.2008.10.047] [PMID: 19118852]

[9] Wanderley DM, de Carvalho ME, Mantegazza E, Yasumaru S, Barata LC. Transfusional Chagas infection detected in the program for the control of Chagas disease in the state of São Paulo (Brazil). Rev Saude Publica 1992; 26(3): 203-5. [http://dx.doi.org/10.1590/S0034-89101992000300012] [PMID: 1342502]

[10] Kun H, Moore A, Mascola L, *et al.* Transmission of *Trypanosoma cruzi* by heart transplantation. Clin Infect Dis 2009; 48(11): 1534-40. [http://dx.doi.org/10.1086/598931] [PMID: 19400748]

[11] Herwaldt BL. Laboratory-acquired parasitic infections from accidental exposures. Clin Microbiol Rev 2001; 14(4): 659-88. [http://dx.doi.org/10.1128/CMR.14.3.659-688.2001] [PMID: 11585780]

[12] Chagas C. Nova tripanosomíase humana. Mem Inst Oswaldo Cruz 1909; 1: 159-218. [http://dx.doi.org/10.1590/S0074-02761909000200008]

[13] Bern C. Chagas' Disease. N Engl J Med 2015; 373(5): 456-66. [http://dx.doi.org/10.1056/NEJMra1410150] [PMID: 26222561]

[14] World Health Organization. (WHO) Global burden of disease estimates for 2000-2012. Geneva: World Health Organization 2014.

[15] Chagas disease in Latin America: an epidemiological update based on 2010 estimates. Wkly Epidemiol Rec 2015; 90(6): 33-43. [PMID: 25671846]

[16] Rassi A Jr, Rassi A, Marin-Neto JA. Chagas disease. Lancet 2010; 375(9723): 1388-402. [http://dx.doi.org/10.1016/S0140-6736(10)60061-X] [PMID: 20399979]

[17] WHO. Chagas disease in Latin America: an epidemiological update based on 2010 estimates. Wkly Epidemiol Rec 2015; 90(6): 33-43.
[PMID: 25671846]

[18] Howard EJ, Xiong X, Carlier Y, Sosa-Estani S, Buekens P. Frequency of the congenital transmission of *Trypanosoma cruzi*: a systematic review and meta-analysis. BJOG 2014; 121(1): 22-33.
[http://dx.doi.org/10.1111/1471-0528.12396] [PMID: 23924273]

[19] Marin-Neto JA, Cunha-Neto E, Maciel BC, Simões MV. Pathogenesis of chronic Chagas heart disease. Circulation 2007; 115(9): 1109-23.
[http://dx.doi.org/10.1161/CIRCULATIONAHA.106.624296] [PMID: 17339569]

[20] Kumar R, Kline IK, Abelmann WH. Experimental *Trypanosoma cruzi* myocarditis: relative effects upon the right and left ventricles. Am J Pathol 1969; 57(1): 31-48.
[PMID: 4242332]

[21] Roman-Campos D, Duarte HL, Sales PA Jr, *et al.* Changes in cellular contractility and cytokines profile during *Trypanosoma cruzi* infection in mice. Basic Res Cardiol 2009; 104(3): 238-46.
[http://dx.doi.org/10.1007/s00395-009-0776-x] [PMID: 19190953]

[22] Wen JJ, Vyatkina G, Garg N. Oxidative damage during chagasic cardiomyopathy development: role of mitochondrial oxidant release and inefficient antioxidant defense. Free Radic Biol Med 2004; 37(11): 1821-33.
[http://dx.doi.org/10.1016/j.freeradbiomed.2004.08.018] [PMID: 15528041]

[23] Tostes S Jr, Bertulucci Rocha-Rodrigues D, de Araujo Pereira G, Rodrigues V Jr. Myocardiocyte apoptosis in heart failure in chronic Chagas' disease. Int J Cardiol 2005; 99(2): 233-7.
[http://dx.doi.org/10.1016/j.ijcard.2004.01.026] [PMID: 15749181]

[24] Vyatkina G, Bhatia V, Gerstner A, Papaconstantinou J, Garg N. Impaired mitochondrial respiratory chain and bioenergetics during chagasic cardiomyopathy development. Biochim Biophys Acta 2004; 1689(2): 162-73.
[http://dx.doi.org/10.1016/j.bbadis.2004.03.005] [PMID: 15196597]

[25] Roman-Campos D, Sales-Junior P, Duarte HL, *et al.* Novel insights into the development of chagasic cardiomyopathy: role of PI3Kinase/NO axis. Int J Cardiol 2013; 167(6): 3011-20.
[http://dx.doi.org/10.1016/j.ijcard.2012.09.020] [PMID: 23031286]

[26] Roman-Campos D, Sales-Júnior P, Duarte HL, *et al.* Cardiomyocyte dysfunction during the chronic phase of Chagas disease. Mem Inst Oswaldo Cruz 2013; 108(2): 243-5.
[http://dx.doi.org/10.1590/0074-0276108022013019] [PMID: 23579807]

[27] Rassi A Jr, Rassi A, Marin-Neto JA. Chagas heart disease: pathophysiologic mechanisms, prognostic factors and risk stratification. Mem Inst Oswaldo Cruz 2009; 104 (Suppl. 1): 152-8.
[http://dx.doi.org/10.1590/S0074-02762009000900021] [PMID: 19753470]

[28] Yancy CW, Jessup M, Bozkurt B, *et al.* 2013 ACCF/AHA guideline for the management of heart failure: a report of the American College of Cardiology Foundation/American Heart Association Task Force on practice guidelines. Circulation 2013; 128(16): e240-327.
[http://dx.doi.org/10.1161/CIR.0b013e31829e8776] [PMID: 23741058]

[29] Bern C, Montgomery SP, Herwaldt BL, *et al.* Evaluation and treatment of chagas disease in the United States: a systematic review. JAMA 2007; 298(18): 2171-81.
[http://dx.doi.org/10.1001/jama.298.18.2171] [PMID: 18000201]

[30] Andrade JP, Marin Neto JA, Paola AA, *et al.* I Latin American Guidelines for the diagnosis and treatment of Chagas' heart disease: executive summary. Arq Bras Cardiol 2011; 96(6): 434-42.
[http://dx.doi.org/10.1590/S0066-782X2011000600002] [PMID: 21789345]

[31] WHO Expert Committee. Control of Chagas Disease 2002.www.whqlibdoc.who.int/trs/WHO_TRS_905.pdf

[32] Rassi A Jr, Rassi A, Marcondes de Rezende J. American trypanosomiasis (Chagas disease). Infect Dis Clin North Am 2012; 26(2): 275-91. [http://dx.doi.org/10.1016/j.idc.2012.03.002] [PMID: 22632639]

[33] Gascon J, Bern C, Pinazo MJ. Chagas disease in Spain, the United States and other non-endemic countries. Acta Trop 2010; 115(1-2): 22-7. [http://dx.doi.org/10.1016/j.actatropica.2009.07.019] [PMID: 19646412]

[34] Basile L, Jansá JM, Carlier Y, *et al.* Working Group on Chagas Disease. Chagas disease in European countries: the challenge of a surveillance system. Euro Surveill 2011; 16(37): 16. [PMID: 21944556]

[35] Angheben A, Anselmi M, Gobbi F, *et al.* Chagas disease in Italy: breaking an epidemiological silence. Euro Surveill 2011; 16(37): 16. [PMID: 21944554]

[36] Perez-Molina JA, Perez-Ayala A, Parola P, Jackson Y, Odolini S, Lopez-Velez R. and EuroTravNet Network. EuroTravNet: imported Chagas disease in nine European countries, 2008 to 2009. Euro Surveill Bull 2011; 16.

[37] Albajar-Vinas P, Jannin J. The hidden Chagas disease burden in Europe. Euro Surveill 2011; 16(38): 16. [http://dx.doi.org/10.2807/ese.16.38.19975-en] [PMID: 21958529]

[38] Brener Z. Biology of *Trypanosoma cruzi*. Annu Rev Microbiol 1973; 27: 347-82. [http://dx.doi.org/10.1146/annurev.mi.27.100173.002023] [PMID: 4201691]

[39] Vickerman K. Developmental cycles and biology of pathogenic trypanosomes. Br Med Bull 1985; 41(2): 105-14. [http://dx.doi.org/10.1093/oxfordjournals.bmb.a072036] [PMID: 3928017]

[40] De Souza W. Basic cell biology of *Trypanosoma cruzi*. Curr Pharm Des 2002; 8(4): 269-85. [http://dx.doi.org/10.2174/1381612023396276] [PMID: 11860366]

[41] Tan H, Andrews NW. Don't bother to knock-the cell invasion strategy of *Trypanosoma cruzi*. Trends Parasitol 2002; 18(10): 427-8. [http://dx.doi.org/10.1016/S1471-4922(02)02368-1] [PMID: 12377585]

[42] Kollien AH, Schaub GA. The development of *Trypanosoma cruzi* in Triatominae. Parasitol Today 16: 381-7.

[43] Burleigh BA, Andrews NW. The mechanisms of Trypanosoma cruzi invasion of mammalian cells. Annu Rev Microbiol 1995; 49: 175-200.

[44] Tyler KM, Engman DM. The life cycle of *Trypanosoma cruzi* revisited. Int J Parasitol 2001; 31(5-6): 472-81. [http://dx.doi.org/10.1016/S0020-7519(01)00153-9] [PMID: 11334932]

[45] de Souza W. Cell biology of *Trypanosoma cruzi*. Int Rev Cytol 1984; 86: 197-283. [http://dx.doi.org/10.1016/S0074-7696(08)60180-1] [PMID: 6368447]

[46] de Souza W. Cell biology of *Trypanosoma cruzi*. Int Rev Cytol 1984; 86: 197-283. [http://dx.doi.org/10.1016/S0074-7696(08)60180-1] [PMID: 6368447]

[47] Prata A. Clinical and epidemiological aspects of Chagas disease. Lancet Infect Dis 2001; 1: 92–100. [http://dx.doi.org/10.1016/S1473-3099(01)00065-2]

[48] Ministério da Saúde Brasil. Brazilian Consensus on Chagas disease. Rev Soc Bras Med Trop 2005; 38 (Suppl. 3): 7-29. [in Portuguese].

[49] Marin-Neto JA, Almeida Filho OC, Pazin-Filho A, Maciel BC. [Indeterminate form of Chagas' disease. Proposal of new diagnostic criteria and perspectives for early treatment of cardiomyopathy]. Arq Bras Cardiol 2002; 79(6): 623-7. [in Portuguese].

[PMID: 12532246]

[50] Fernandez AB, Nunes MC, Clark EH, *et al.* Electrocardiographic and echocardiographic abnormalities in Chagas disease: findings in residents of rural Bolivian communities hyperendemic for Chagas disease. Glob Heart 2015; 10(3): 159-66. [http://dx.doi.org/10.1016/j.gheart.2015.07.004] [PMID: 26407511]

[51] Sosa-Estani S, Gamboa-León MR, Del Cid-Lemus J, *et al.* Working Group. Use of a rapid test on umbilical cord blood to screen for *Trypanosoma cruzi* infection in pregnant women in Argentina, Bolivia, Honduras, and Mexico. Am J Trop Med Hyg 2008; 79(5): 755-9. [http://dx.doi.org/10.4269/ajtmh.2008.79.755] [PMID: 18981518]

[52] Chippaux JP, Santalla JA, Postigo JR, *et al.* Sensitivity and specificity of Chagas Stat-Pak test in Bolivia. Trop Med Int Health 2009; 14(7): 732-5. [http://dx.doi.org/10.1111/j.1365-3156.2009.02288.x] [PMID: 19392737]

[53] Brutus L, Santalla JA, Salas NA, Schneider D, Chippaux JP. [Screening for congenital infection by *Trypanosoma cruzi* in France]. Bull Soc Pathol Exot 2009; 102(5): 300-9. [PMID: 20131424]

[54] Schmunis GA. Epidemiology of Chagas disease in non-endemic countries: the role of international migration. Mem Inst Oswaldo Cruz 2007; 102 (Suppl. 1): 75-85. [http://dx.doi.org/10.1590/S0074-02762007005000093] [PMID: 17891282]

[55] Teixeira AR, Nascimento RJ, Sturm NR. Evolution and pathology in chagas disease--a review. Mem Inst Oswaldo Cruz 2006; 101(5): 463-91. [http://dx.doi.org/10.1590/S0074-02762006000500001] [PMID: 17072450]

[56] Bittencourt AL, Garcia AG. The placenta in hematogenous infections. Pediatr Pathol Mol Med 2002; 21(4): 401-32. [http://dx.doi.org/10.1080/pdp.21.4.401.432] [PMID: 12092706]

[57] Bittencourt AL, Garcia AG. Pathogenesis and pathology of hematogenous infections of the fetus and newborn. Pediatr Pathol Mol Med 2002; 21(4): 353-99. [http://dx.doi.org/10.1080/pdp.21.4.353.399] [PMID: 12092705]

[58] Marin-Neto JA, Rassi A, Maciel BC, Simoes M, Schmidt A. Chagas heart disease.Evidence- Based Cardiology. 3rd ed. New York, NY: Wiley Blackwell 2010; pp. 823-41.

[59] Machado FS, Dutra WO, Esper L, *et al.* Current understanding of immunity to *Trypanosoma cruzi* infection and pathogenesis of Chagas disease. Semin Immunopathol 2012; 34(6): 753-70. [http://dx.doi.org/10.1007/s00281-012-0351-7] [PMID: 23076807]

[60] Cunha-Neto E, Chevillard C. Chagas disease cardiomyopathy: immunopathology and genetics. Mediators Inflamm 2014; 2014683230 [http://dx.doi.org/10.1155/2014/683230] [PMID: 25210230]

[61] Shippey SH III, Zahn CM, Cisar MM, Wu TJ, Satin AJ. Use of the placental perfusion model to evaluate transplacental passage of *Trypanosoma cruzi.* Am J Obstet Gynecol 2005; 192(2): 586-91. [http://dx.doi.org/10.1016/j.ajog.2004.07.079] [PMID: 15696007]

[62] Fernandez-Aguilar S, Lambot MA, Torrico F, *et al.* [Placental lesions in human *Trypanosoma cruzi* infection]. Rev Soc Bras Med Trop 2005; 38 (Suppl. 2): 84-6. [PMID: 16482822]

[63] Carlier Y, Truyens C. "Maternal-fetal transmission of Trypanosoma cruzi," in American Trypanosomiasis—Chagas Disease One Hundred Years of Research. Elsevier 2010; pp. 539-81.

[64] Carlier Y, Truyens C, Deloron P, Peyron F. Congenital parasitic infections: a review. Acta Trop 2012; 121(2): 55-70. [http://dx.doi.org/10.1016/j.actatropica.2011.10.018] [PMID: 22085916]

[65] Torrico F, Alonso-Vega C, Suarez E, *et al.* Maternal *Trypanosoma cruzi* infection, pregnancy

outcome, morbidity, and mortality of congenitally infected and non-infected newborns in Bolivia. Am J Trop Med Hyg 2004; 70(2): 201-9.
[http://dx.doi.org/10.4269/ajtmh.2004.70.201] [PMID: 14993634]

[66] Schijman AG. "Congenital Chagas disease," in Congenital and Other Related Infectious Diseases of the Newborn. Amsterdam, The Netherlands: Elsevier 2006; Vol. 13: pp. 223-59.
[http://dx.doi.org/10.1016/S0168-7069(06)13012-8]

[67] Rocha MO, Ribeiro AL, Teixeira MM. Clinical management of chronic Chagas cardiomyopathy. Front Biosci 2003; 8: e44-54.
[http://dx.doi.org/10.2741/926] [PMID: 12456332]

[68] Ribeiro AL, Marcolino MS, Prineas RJ, Lima-Costa MF. Electrocardiographic abnormalities in elderly Chagas disease patients: 10-year follow-up of the Bambui Cohort Study of Aging. J Am Heart Assoc 2014; 3(1)e000632
[http://dx.doi.org/10.1161/JAHA.113.000632] [PMID: 24510116]

[69] Pereira LdS. Freitas EC, Fidalgo AS, Andrade MC, Cândido DdS, da Silva Filho JD, Michailowsky V, Oliveira MdF, Queiroz JA. Clinical and epidemiological profile of elderly patients with Chagas disease followed between 2005-2013 by pharmaceutical care service in Ceará State, northeastern Brazil. Rev Inst Med Trop São Paulo 2015; 57: 145-52.
[http://dx.doi.org/10.1590/S0036-46652015000200008]

[70] Ribeiro AL, Nunes MP, Teixeira MM, Rocha MO. Diagnosis and management of Chagas disease and cardiomyopathy. Nat Rev Cardiol 2012; 9(10): 576-89.
[http://dx.doi.org/10.1038/nrcardio.2012.109] [PMID: 22847166]

[71] Lima-Costa MF, Matos DL, Ribeiro AL. Chagas disease predicts 10-year stroke mortality in community-dwelling elderly: the Bambui Cohort Study of Aging. Stroke 2010; 41: 2477–2482.
[http://dx.doi.org/10.1161/STROKEAHA.110.588061]

[72] Nunes MC, Dones W, Morillo CA, Encina JJ, Ribeiro AL. Chagas disease: an overview of clinical and epidemiological aspects. J Am Coll Cardiol 2013; 62(9): 767-76.
[http://dx.doi.org/10.1016/j.jacc.2013.05.046] [PMID: 23770163]

[73] Navarro M, Navaza B, Guionnet A, López-Vélez R. Chagas disease in Spain: need for further public health measures. PLoS Negl Trop Dis 2012; 6(12)e1962
[http://dx.doi.org/10.1371/journal.pntd.0001962] [PMID: 23301105]

[74] Montgomery SP, Starr MC, Cantey PT, Edwards MS, Meymandi SK. Neglected parasitic infections in the United States: Chagas disease. Am J Trop Med Hyg 2014; 90(5): 814-8.
[http://dx.doi.org/10.4269/ajtmh.13-0726] [PMID: 24808250]

[75] Verani JR, Montgomery SP, Schulkin J, Anderson B, Jones JL. Survey of obstetrician-gynecologists in the United States about Chagas disease. Am J Trop Med Hyg 2010; 83(4): 891-5.
[http://dx.doi.org/10.4269/ajtmh.2010.09-0543] [PMID: 20889886]

[76] Jackson Y, Varcher Herrera M, Gascon J. Economic crisis and increased immigrant mobility: new challenges in managing Chagas disease in Europe. Bull World Health Organ 2014; 92(10): 771-2.
[http://dx.doi.org/10.2471/BLT.13.134072] [PMID: 25378732]

[77] Barros ML, Ribeiro A, Nunes MdoC, Rocha MO. [Association between left ventricular wall motion abnormalities and ventricular arrhythmia in the indeterminate form of Chagas disease]. Rev Soc Bras Med Trop 2011; 44(2): 213-6. [in Portuguese].
[http://dx.doi.org/10.1590/S0037-86822011005000020] [PMID: 21503552]

[78] Barbosa MP, Carmo AA, Rocha MO, Ribeiro AL. Ventricular arrhythmias in Chagas disease. Rev Soc Bras Med Trop 2015; 48(1): 4-10.
[http://dx.doi.org/10.1590/0037-8682-0003-2014] [PMID: 25714933]

[79] Rossi MA, Tanowitz HB, Malvestio LM, *et al.* Coronary microvascular disease in chronic Chagas cardiomyopathy including an overview on history, pathology, and other proposed pathogenic

mechanisms. PLoS Negl Trop Dis 2010; 4(8)e674
[http://dx.doi.org/10.1371/journal.pntd.0000674] [PMID: 20824217]

[80] de Paola AA, Horowitz LN, Miyamoto MH, *et al.* Angiographic and electrophysiologic substrates of ventricular tachycardia in chronic Chagasic myocarditis. Am J Cardiol 1990; 65(5): 360-3.
[http://dx.doi.org/10.1016/0002-9149(90)90302-H] [PMID: 2301265]

[81] Rincon LG, Rocha MO, Pires MT, *et al.* [Clinical profile of Chagas and non-Chagas' disease patients with cardiac pacemaker]. Rev Soc Bras Med Trop 2006; 39(3): 245-9. [in Portuguese].
[http://dx.doi.org/10.1590/S0037-86822006000300003] [PMID: 16906246]

[82] Marcolino MS, Palhares DM, Ferreira LR, Ribeiro AL. Electrocardiogram and Chagas disease: a large population database of primary care patients. Glob Heart 2015; 10(3): 167-72.
[http://dx.doi.org/10.1016/j.gheart.2015.07.001] [PMID: 26407512]

[83] Barbosa MM, Costa Rocha MO, Vidigal DF, *et al.* Early detection of left ventricular contractility abnormalities by two-dimensional speckle tracking strain in Chagas' disease. Echocardiography 2014; 31(5): 623-30.
[http://dx.doi.org/10.1111/echo.12426] [PMID: 25232573]

[84] Acquatella H. Echocardiography in Chagas heart disease. Circulation 2007; 115(9): 1124-31.
[http://dx.doi.org/10.1161/CIRCULATIONAHA.106.627323] [PMID: 17339570]

[85] Carod-Artal FJ, Gascon J. Chagas disease and stroke. Lancet Neurol 2010; 9(5): 533-42.
[http://dx.doi.org/10.1016/S1474-4422(10)70042-9] [PMID: 20398860]

[86] Nunes MC, Kreuser LJ, Ribeiro AL, *et al.* Prevalence and risk factors of embolic cerebrovascular events associated with Chagas heart disease. Glob Heart 2015; 10(3): 151-7.
[http://dx.doi.org/10.1016/j.gheart.2015.07.006] [PMID: 26407510]

[87] Dias Junior JO, da Costa Rocha MO, de Souza AC, *et al.* Assessment of the source of ischemic cerebrovascular events in patients with Chagas disease. Int J Cardiol 2014; 176(3): 1352-4.
[http://dx.doi.org/10.1016/j.ijcard.2014.07.266] [PMID: 25131915]

[88] Nunes MdoC, Barbosa MdeM, Brum VA, Rocha MO. Morphofunctional characteristics of the right ventricle in Chagas' dilated cardiomyopathy. Int J Cardiol 2004; 94(1): 79-85.
[http://dx.doi.org/10.1016/j.ijcard.2003.05.003] [PMID: 14996479]

[89] Nunes MC, Barbosa MM, Ribeiro AL, Barbosa FB, Rocha MO. Ischemic cerebrovascular events in patients with Chagas cardiomyopathy: a prospective follow-up study. J Neurol Sci 2009; 278(1-2): 96-101.
[http://dx.doi.org/10.1016/j.jns.2008.12.015] [PMID: 19162278]

[90] Aras R, da Matta JA, Mota G, Gomes I, Melo A. Cerebral infarction in autopsies of chagasic patients with heart failure. Arq Bras Cardiol 2003; 81(4): 414-416, 411-413.
[http://dx.doi.org/10.1590/S0066-782X2003001200008] [PMID: 14666283]

[91] Zingales B, Miles MA, Campbell DA, *et al.* The revised *Trypanosoma cruzi* subspecific nomenclature: rationale, epidemiological relevance and research applications. Infect Genet Evol 2012; 12(2): 240-53.
[http://dx.doi.org/10.1016/j.meegid.2011.12.009] [PMID: 22226704]

[92] Ramírez JD, Duque MC, Montilla M, Cucunubá Z, Guhl F. Natural and emergent *Trypanosoma cruzi* I genotypes revealed by mitochondrial (Cytb) and nuclear (SSU rDNA) genetic markers. Exp Parasitol 2012; 132(4): 487-94.
[http://dx.doi.org/10.1016/j.exppara.2012.09.017] [PMID: 23031800]

[93] Torrico F, Vega CA, Suarez E, *et al.* Are maternal re-infections with *Trypanosoma cruzi* associated with higher morbidity and mortality of congenital Chagas disease? Trop Med Int Health 2006; 11(5): 628-35.
[http://dx.doi.org/10.1111/j.1365-3156.2006.01623.x] [PMID: 16640615]

[94] Hermann E, Truyens C, Alonso-Vega C, *et al.* Congenital transmission of *Trypanosoma cruzi* is associated with maternal enhanced parasitemia and decreased production of interferon- gamma in

response to parasite antigens. J Infect Dis 2004; 189(7): 1274-81.
[http://dx.doi.org/10.1086/382511] [PMID: 15031797]

[95] Poncini CV, Alba Soto CD, Batalla E, Solana ME, González Cappa SM. *Trypanosoma cruzi* induces regulatory dendritic cells *in vitro*. Infect Immun 2008; 76(6): 2633-41.
[http://dx.doi.org/10.1128/IAI.01298-07] [PMID: 18347042]

[96] Rytter MJ, Kolte L, Briend A, Friis H, Christensen VB. The immune system in children with malnutrition--a systematic review. PLoS One 2014; 9(8)e105017
[http://dx.doi.org/10.1371/journal.pone.0105017] [PMID: 25153531]

[97] Azogue. E. Women and congenital Chagas' disease in Santa Cruz, Bolivia: epidemiological and sociocultural aspects. Soc Sci Med 1993; 37: 503-11.

[98] Haider, S., Knofler, M. Human tumour necrosis factor: physiological and pathological roles in placenta and endometrium. Placenta 2009; 30: 111-23.

[99] Nanaev AK, Kosanke G, Kemp B, Frank HG, Huppertz B, Kaufmann P. The human placenta is encircled by a ring of smooth muscle cells. Placenta 2000; 21(1): 122-5.
[http://dx.doi.org/10.1053/plac.1999.0455] [PMID: 10692260]

[100] Bua J, Volta BJ, Perrone AE, *et al.* How to improve the early diagnosis of *Trypanosoma cruzi* infection: relationship between validated conventional diagnosis and quantitative DNA amplification in congenitally infected children. PLoS Negl Trop Dis 2013; 7(10)e2476.
[http://dx.doi.org/10.1371/journal.pntd.0002476] [PMID: 24147166]

[101] Rassi A Jr, Rassi A, Little WC, *et al.* Development and validation of a risk score for predicting death in Chagas' heart disease. N Engl J Med 2006; 355(8): 799-808.
[http://dx.doi.org/10.1056/NEJMoa053241] [PMID: 16928995]

[102] de Souza AC, Salles G, Hasslocher-Moreno AM, *et al.* Development of a risk score to predict sudden death in patients with Chaga's heart disease. Int J Cardiol 2015; 187: 700-4.
[http://dx.doi.org/10.1016/j.ijcard.2015.03.372] [PMID: 25919755]

[103] Sousa AS, Xavier SS, Freitas GR, Hasslocher-Moreno A. Prevention strategies of cardioembolic ischemic stroke in Chagas' disease. Arq Bras Cardiol 2008; 91(5): 306-10.
[http://dx.doi.org/10.1590/S0066-782X2008001700004] [PMID: 19142374]

[104] Bern C, Verastegui M, Gilman RH, *et al.* Congenital *Trypanosoma cruzi* transmission in Santa Cruz, Bolivia. Clin Infect Dis 2009; 49(11): 1667-74.
[http://dx.doi.org/10.1086/648070] [PMID: 19877966]

[105] Carlier Y, Torrico F, Sosa-Estani S, *et al.* Congenital Chagas disease: recommendations for diagnosis, treatment and control of newborns, siblings and pregnant women. PLoS Negl Trop Dis 2011; 5(10)e1250.
[http://dx.doi.org/10.1371/journal.pntd.0001250] [PMID: 22039554]

[106] Mallimaci MC, Sosa-Estani S, Russomando G, *et al.* Early diagnosis of congenital *Trypanosoma cruzi* infection, using shed acute phase antigen, in Ushuaia, Tierra del Fuego, Argentina. Am J Trop Med Hyg 2010; 82(1): 55-9.
[http://dx.doi.org/10.4269/ajtmh.2010.09-0219] [PMID: 20064996]

[107] Covarrubias C, Cortez M, Ferreira D, Yoshida N. Interaction with host factors exacerbates *Trypanosoma cruzi* cell invasion capacity upon oral infection. Int J Parasitol 2007; 37(14): 1609-16.
[http://dx.doi.org/10.1016/j.ijpara.2007.05.013] [PMID: 17640647]

[108] Nascimento BR, Araújo CG, Rocha MO, *et al.* The prognostic significance of electrocardiographic changes in Chagas disease. J Electrocardiol 2012; 45(1): 43-8.
[http://dx.doi.org/10.1016/j.jelectrocard.2011.04.011] [PMID: 21704321]

[109] Pinto AY, Valente SA, Valente Vda C. Emerging acute Chagas disease in Amazonian Brazil: case reports with serious cardiac involvement. J Electrocardiol 2004; 45: 43-48.
[http://dx.doi.org/10.1590/S1413-86702004000600010]

[110] Marin-Neto JA, Romano MMD, Maciel BC, Simões MV, Schmidt A. Cardiac imaging in Latin America: Chagas heart disease. Curr Cardiovasc Imaging Rep 2015; 8: 1-5. [http://dx.doi.org/10.1007/s12410-015-9324-2]

[111] Costa HS, Lima MM, de Sousa GR, *et al.* Functional capacity and risk stratification by the Six-minute Walk Test in Chagas heart disease: comparison with Cardiopulmonary Exercise Testing. Int J Cardiol 2014; 177(2): 661-3. [http://dx.doi.org/10.1016/j.ijcard.2014.09.172] [PMID: 25449475]

[112] Peix A, García R, Sánchez J, *et al.* Myocardial perfusion imaging and cardiac involvement in the indeterminate phase of Chagas disease. Arq Bras Cardiol 2013; 100(2): 114-7. [http://dx.doi.org/10.5935/abc.20130023] [PMID: 23503819]

[113] Hagar JM, Rahimtoola SH. Chagas' heart disease in the United States. N Engl J Med 1991; 325(11): 763-8. [http://dx.doi.org/10.1056/NEJM199109123251103] [PMID: 1870649]

[114] Hiss FC, Lascala TF, Maciel BC, Marin-Neto JA, Simões MV. Changes in myocardial perfusion correlate with deterioration of left ventricular systolic function in chronic Chagas' cardiomyopathy. JACC Cardiovasc Imaging 2009; 2(2): 164-72. [http://dx.doi.org/10.1016/j.jcmg.2008.09.012] [PMID: 19356551]

[115] Simoes MV, Oliveira LF, Hiss FC, *et al.* Characterization of the apical aneurysm of chronic Chagas' heart disease by scintigraphic image co-registration. Arq Bras Cardiol 2007; 89: 131-134.

[116] Rochitte CE, Oliveira PF, Andrade JM, *et al.* Myocardial delayed enhancement by magnetic resonance imaging in patients with Chagas' disease: a marker of disease severity. J Am Coll Cardiol 2005; 46(8): 1553-8. [http://dx.doi.org/10.1016/j.jacc.2005.06.067] [PMID: 16226184]

[117] Tassi EM, Continentino MA, Nascimento EM, Pereira BdeB, Pedrosa RC. Relationship between fibrosis and ventricular arrhythmias in Chagas heart disease without ventricular dysfunction. Arq Bras Cardiol 2014; 102(5): 456-64. [http://dx.doi.org/10.5935/abc.20140052] [PMID: 24918912]

[118] Fabbro DL, Danesi E, Olivera V, *et al.* Trypanocide treatment of women infected with *Trypanosoma cruzi* and its effect on preventing congenital Chagas. PLoS Negl Trop Dis 2014. [http://dx.doi.org/10.1371/journal. pntd.0003312]

[119] Pinazo MJ, Muñoz J, Posada E, *et al.* Tolerance of benznidazole in treatment of Chagas' disease in adults. Antimicrob Agents Chemother 2010; 54(11): 4896-9. [http://dx.doi.org/10.1128/AAC.00537-10] [PMID: 20823286]

[120] Tornheim JA, Lozano Beltran DF, Gilman RH, *et al.* Improved completion rates and characterization of drug reactions with an intensive Chagas disease treatment program in rural Bolivia. PLoS Negl Trop Dis 2013; 7(9)e2407 [http://dx.doi.org/10.1371/journal.pntd.0002407] [PMID: 24069472]

[121] Botoni FA, Poole-Wilson PA, Ribeiro AL, *et al.* A randomized trial of carvedilol after renin-angiotensin system inhibition in chronic Chagas cardiomyopathy. Am Heart J 2007; 153(4): 544.e1-8. [http://dx.doi.org/10.1016/j.ahj.2006.12.017] [PMID: 17383291]

[122] Miranda CH, Figueiredo AB, Maciel BC, Marin-Neto JA, Simões MV. Sustained ventricular tachycardia is associated with regional myocardial sympathetic denervation assessed with 123I-metaiodobenzylguanidine in chronic Chagas cardiomyopathy. J Nucl Med 2011; 52(4): 504-10. [http://dx.doi.org/10.2967/jnumed.110.082032] [PMID: 21441532]

[123] Mello RP, Szarf G, Schvartzman PR, *et al.* Delayed enhancement cardiac magnetic resonance imaging can identify the risk for ventricular tachycardia in chronic Chagas' heart disease. Arq Bras Cardiol 2012; 98(5): 421-30. [http://dx.doi.org/10.1590/S0066-782X2012005000031] [PMID: 22460166]

[124] Ribeiro AL, Rocha MO, Terranova P, Cesarano M, Nunes MD, Lombardi F. T-wave amplitude variability and the risk of death in Chagas disease. J Cardiovasc Electrophysiol 2011; 22(7): 799-805. [http://dx.doi.org/10.1111/j.1540-8167.2010.02000.x] [PMID: 21235679]

[125] Barbosa MPT, da Costa Rocha MO, Neto ES, Brandão FV, Lombardi F, Ribeiro ALP. Usefulness of microvolt T-wave alternans for predicting outcome in patients with Chagas disease with implantable cardioverter defibrillators. Int J Cardiol 2016; 222: 80–85. [http://dx.doi.org/10.1016/j.ijcard. 2016.07.148]

[126] Martinelli M, Rassi A Jr, Marin-Neto JA, *et al.* CHronic use of Amiodarone aGAinSt Implantable cardioverter-defibrillator therapy for primary prevention of death in patients with Chagas cardiomyopathy Study: rationale and design of a randomized clinical trial. Am Heart J 2013; 166(6): 976-982.e4. [http://dx.doi.org/10.1016/j.ahj.2013.08.027] [PMID: 24268211]

[127] Santangeli P, Muser D, Maeda S, *et al.* Comparative effectiveness of antiarrhythmic drugs and catheter ablation for the prevention of recurrent ventricular tachycardia in patients with implantable cardioverter-defibrillators: A systematic review and meta-analysis of randomized controlled trials. Heart Rhythm 2016; 13(7): 1552-9. [http://dx.doi.org/10.1016/j.hrthm.2016.03.004] [PMID: 26961297]

[128] Sapp JL, Wells GA, Parkash R, *et al.* Ventricular tachycardia ablation versus escalation of antiarrhythmic drugs. N Engl J Med 2016; 375(2): 111-21. [http://dx.doi.org/10.1056/NEJMoa1513614] [PMID: 27149033]

[129] Moya P, Basso B, Moretti E. Congenital Chagas disease in Córdoba, Argentina: epidemiological, clinical, diagnostic, and therapeutic aspects. Experience of 30 years of follow up. Rev Soc Bras Med Trop 2005; 38 (Suppl. 2): 33-40. [PMID: 16482811]

[130] Pinazo MJ, Miranda B, Rodríguez-Villar C, *et al.* Recommendations for management of Chagas disease in organ and hematopoietic tissue transplantation programs in nonendemic areas. Transplant Rev (Orlando) 2011; 25(3): 91-101. [http://dx.doi.org/10.1016/j.trre.2010.12.002] [PMID: 21530219]

[131] Chin-Hong PV, Schwartz BS, Bern C, *et al.* Screening and treatment of chagas disease in organ transplant recipients in the United States: recommendations from the chagas in transplant working group. Am J Transplant 2011; 11(4): 672-80. [http://dx.doi.org/10.1111/j.1600-6143.2011.03444.x] [PMID: 21401868]

[132] Diez M, Favaloro L, Bertolotti A, *et al.* Usefulness of PCR strategies for early diagnosis of Chagas' disease reactivation and treatment follow-up in heart transplantation. Am J Transplant 2007; 7(6): 1633-40. [http://dx.doi.org/10.1111/j.1600-6143.2007.01820.x] [PMID: 17511688]

[133] Bestetti RB, Theodoropoulos TA. A systematic review of studies on heart transplantation for patients with end-stage Chagas' heart disease. J Card Fail 2009; 15(3): 249-55. [http://dx.doi.org/10.1016/j.cardfail.2008.10.023] [PMID: 19327627]

[134] Kransdorf EP, Czer LS, Luthringer DJ, *et al.* Heart transplantation for Chagas cardiomyopathy in the United States. Am J Transplant 2013; 13(12): 3262-8. [http://dx.doi.org/10.1111/ajt.12507] [PMID: 24165397]

[135] Fiorelli AI, Santos RH, Oliveira JL Jr, *et al.* Heart transplantation in 107 cases of Chagas' disease. Transplant Proc 2011; 43(1): 220-4. [http://dx.doi.org/10.1016/j.transproceed.2010.12.046] [PMID: 21335192]

[136] Morillo CA, Marin-Neto JA, Avezum A, *et al.* BENEFIT Investigators. BENEFIT Investigators. Randomized trial of benznidazole for chronic Chagas' cardiomyopathy. N Engl J Med 2015; 373(14): 1295-306. [http://dx.doi.org/10.1056/NEJMoa1507574] [PMID: 26323937]

[137] Fabbro DL, Streiger ML, Arias ED, Bizai ML, del Barco M, Amicone NA. Trypanocide treatment among adults with chronic Chagas disease living in Santa Fe city (Argentina), over a mean follow-up of 21 years: parasitological, serological and clinical evolution. Rev Soc Bras Med Trop 2007; 40(1): 1-10.
[http://dx.doi.org/10.1590/S0037-86822007000100001] [PMID: 17486245]

[138] Dumonteil E, Bottazzi ME, Zhan B, *et al.* Accelerating the development of a therapeutic vaccine for human Chagas disease: rationale and prospects. Expert Rev Vaccines 2012; 11(9): 1043-55.
[http://dx.doi.org/10.1586/erv.12.85] [PMID: 23151163]

[139] Gupta S, Garg NJ. TcVac3 induced control of *Trypanosoma cruzi* infection and chronic myocarditis in mice. PLoS One 2013; 8(3)e59434.
[http://dx.doi.org/10.1371/journal.pone.0059434] [PMID: 23555672]

[140] Nakayasu ES, Sobreira TJ, Torres R Jr, *et al.* Improved proteomic approach for the discovery of potential vaccine targets in *Trypanosoma cruzi*. J Proteome Res 2012; 11(1): 237-46.
[http://dx.doi.org/10.1021/pr200806s] [PMID: 22115061]

[141] Quijano-Hernandez I, Dumonteil E. Advances and challenges towards a vaccine against Chagas disease. Hum Vaccin 2011; 7(11): 1184-91.
[http://dx.doi.org/10.4161/hv.7.11.17016] [PMID: 22048121]

[142] Vázquez-Chagoyán JC, Gupta S, Garg NJ. Vaccine development against *Trypanosoma cruzi* and Chagas disease. Adv Parasitol 2011; 75: 121-46.
[http://dx.doi.org/10.1016/B978-0-12-385863-4.00006-X] [PMID: 21820554]

[143] Berneman A, Montout L, Goyard S, *et al.* Combined approaches for drug design points the way to novel proline racemase inhibitor candidates to fight Chagas' disease. PLoS One 2013; 8(4)e60955.
[http://dx.doi.org/10.1371/journal.pone.0060955] [PMID: 23613764]

CHAPTER 9

Non-Compaction Cardiomyopathy from Infancy to Adulthood

Iroegbu Chukwuemeka Daniel[1], Jiang Bo[2], Jindong Liu[3], Zhou Zhongxin[2] and **Jinfu Yang[1,*]**

[1] *Department of Cardiovascular Surgery, The Second Xiangya Hospital, Central South University, Middle Renmin Road 139, 410011 Changsha, China*

[2] *Department of Thoracic and Cardiovascular Surgery, Affiliated Hospital of Xuzhou Medical University, Xuzhou, 99 Huaihai Road West Xuzhou, Jiangsu Province 221000, China*

[3] *Department of Anesthesiology, Affiliated Hospital of Xuzhou Medical University, Xuzhou, 99 Huaihai Road West Xuzhou, Jiangsu Province 221000, China*

Abstract: Accepted as an unclassified cardiomyopathy by the American Heart Association or a genetic cardiomyopathy by the European Society of Cardiology, left ventricular non-compaction is an intriguing, but poorly understood condition characterized by the presence of a non-compacted extensive myocardial layer lining the cavity of the left ventricle which potentially leads to malignant arrhythmias, cardiac failure, and thromboembolism. Whether it is distinct cardiomyopathy or a morphological heterogeneous clinical condition with phenotypic morphologic traits often overlapping other types of cardiomyopathies remains very much debated. Ventricular trabeculation and compaction are two of the many essential steps for generating a functionally competent ventricular wall whereas, hyper trabeculation and the lack of ventricular wall compaction (non-compaction) are also one of the significant cardio-embryogenic defects associated with left ventricular non-compaction. This chapter aims to discuss in detail the current knowledge on embryology, epidemiology, clinical spectrum, genetics as both an isolated trait, and as part of other cardiac diseases or complex syndromes. It also explains the physiology, and the present pathophysiological concepts of non-compaction cardiomyopathy, provide an up-to-date view on imaging and also reevaluate the current diagnostic criteria and its impact on overdiagnosis of left ventricular non-compaction as well as the available data on prognosis, and therapy. The chapter will even go further to describe the challenges, and uncertainties facing the medical community, and the future directions in diagnosing left ventricular non-compaction.

Keywords: Cardiomyopathy, Congenital heart disease, Cardiac magnetic resonance, Cardiac computed tomography, Counseling, Diagnosis, Diagnostic

* **Corresponding author Jinfu Yang:** Department of Cardiovascular Surgery, The Second Xiangya Hospital, Central South University, Middle Renmin Road 139, 410011 Changsha, China; E-mails: yjf19682005@csu.edu.cn, Dr.iroegbu_daniel@yahoo.com and Dr.iroegbu_daniel@csu.edu.cn

Jinfu Yang & Iroegbu Chukwuemeka Daniel (Eds.)

accuracy, Epidemiology, Echocardiography, Genetics, Genetic testing, Heart failure, Heart ventricles, Imaging, Left ventricular non-compaction, Myocardium, Myocardial fibrosis, Mitochondrial myopathies, Non-compaction, Pathology, Pregnancy, Prognosis, Right ventricular non-compaction, Spongy myocardium, Trabeculae.

INTRODUCTION

Non-compaction cardiomyopathy (NCM) is a myocardial disorder with a characteristic distinct ("spongy") morphological appearance of the left ventricle (LV) thought to occur due to compaction failure during embryogenesis [1, 2]. Based on the frequency of occurrence, non-compaction pertains to the LV but may also involve the right ventricle (RV), as either biventricular or an isolated right variant [3, 4]. By definition, the European Society of Cardiology (ESC) classification defines LVNC as a non-classified entity [5], while the American Heart Association (AHA) classification defines LVNC as a genetic cardiomyopathy [1]. The recent MOGE(S) (morpho-functional, organ involvement, genetic or familial inheritance pattern, and etiological annotation of details of the genetic disease or underlining cause) nosology proposes a simple description of the trait in subjects with either normal LV size and wall thickness and preserved systolic/diastolic function, or in combination with dilated cardiomyopathy (DCM), restrictive cardiomyopathy (RCM), hypertrophic cardiomyopathy (HCM), or arrhythmogenic right ventricular cardiomyopathy (ARVC) [6]. The LVNC trait may be non-familial (sporadic) or familial (inherited). Sporadic LVNC can be acquired, as in highly-trained athletes [7], pregnant women [8], and sickle cell anemia patients [9]. Non-familial forms are, however, diagnosed when LVNC is proven absent in relatives [10]. LVNC may be an isolated finding or associated with other congenital heart anomalies, such as complex cyanotic congenital heart diseases.

The terminology of this entity has been variable, being known as 'spongy myocardium' or 'persistent embryonic myocardium,' but more frequently known as 'LV non-compaction'(LVNC) or NCM. An intriguing, new, and a poorly understood condition, NCM is a recently recognized cardiomyopathy with an estimated prevalence of 0.011% to 0.18% [11] characterized by prominent LV trabeculae, deep intertrabecular recesses which communicate with the ventricular cavity but not with the coronary circulation [12, 13], thickened myocardial wall with a thin compacted epicardial layer and a thickened non-compacted endocardial layer. However, there is still ongoing controversy surrounding the differentiation from normal LV trabeculation, and the relationship with other cardiomyopathies, such as HCM and DCM, which may share the same genetic basis and be associated with NCM. The process of the compaction progresses from epicardium to endocardium, and from the base of the heart to the apex. The overlapping features of LVNC with other cardiomyopathies, morphologic variations of the endomyocardial recesses, and the trabecular outpouchings present the medical community with a diagnostic puzzle till date. The clinical features are heterogeneous, and the patient could either be asymptomatic or symptomatic. Symptomatic patients usually present with heart failure resulting from systolic and diastolic dysfunction, primarily of the LV. Systolic dysfunction is as the result of relative ischemia of the myocardium due to the mismatch of myocardial oxygen supply and demand [14]. Mechanisms implicated in the diastolic dysfunction are as a result of the abnormalities phased in both ventricular relaxation and restriction secondary to the prominence of intracavitary trabeculations [14]. Heart failure variability with age exists from infancy to adulthood, due to the degree of myocardial trabeculations and the chronic myocardial ischemic effects. Other manifestations include ventricular and atrial tachyarrhythmias [15], conduction abnormalities (mainly bundle branch block) [16], and thromboembolic events.

This chapter aims to discuss in detail the current knowledge on embryology, epidemiology, clinical spectrum, genetics as both an isolated trait, and as part of other cardiac diseases or complex syndromes. It also, explains the physiology, and the present pathophysiological concepts of LVNC, provide an up-to-date view on imaging and also reevaluate the current diagnostic criteria and its impact on overdiagnosis of LVNC as well as the available data on prognosis, and therapy. The chapter will even go further to describe the challenges, and uncertainties facing the medical community, and the future directions in diagnosing left ventricular non-compaction.

HISTORICAL ASPECT

Grant was the first to describe in his publication in 1926 [17, 18], the sponge-like appearance of the myocardium in a variety of congenital heart defects (CHDs). However, it was Dusek *et al.* [19], who was credited for bringing the term "spongy myocardium" as a disease entity into clinical focus, though, completely and entirely different in representation on how it has been described today. As time went on, Engberding [20] became the first to publish and illustrate the disease as a rare isolated sponge-like myocardium without other structural anomalies. The Zurich group, however, published case reports which confirmed Engberding's clinical findings by describing their reports with anatomical, pathological, echo-graphical, and angiographical findings [21, 22]. Be it as it may, these early reports describing the persistence of embryonic myocardial structures, Chin *et al.* [12], recognized the underlying arrest of the normal compaction process during embryogenesis hence, they introduced the term "isolated non-compaction of the left ventricular myocardium."

TERMINOLOGIES

Since the first description of the disease as persistent trabeculated spongy myocardium, other terms have been used to describe the disease entity, in general, such as non-compaction, hyper trabeculation, and persistent sinusoids, *etc*. The first descriptive term "spongy myocardium" used in the field is described based on the morphological appearance of the affected myocardium which resembled a loosely interwoven mesh of trabeculated muscle fibers seen in both embryo and cold-blooded vertebrates. However, some of these terminologies used to describe the disease are entirely wrong, misleading, and non-descriptive of the underlying disease itself. The term "non-compaction first introduced by Chin *et al.*, was and remained the proper descriptive term of the disease. Apart from its early description (spongy myocardium) by Grant and Dusek *et al.*, which still has the virtue of precedence as their term, however, underscores the hypothesis of an arrest of the normal compaction process of the loosely interwoven mesh of muscle fibers in the embryo. Also, some hearts with a sponge-like myocardium are heavily trabeculated but it does not mean that all hearts with a spongy myocardium have heavy trabeculations in the affected ventricle.

Furthermore, the term "Hypertraberculation" is not correct as it implies an increased number of customarily formed trabeculations, and the term "persistent sinusoids" is not right either as it describes an intertrabecular space connecting the ventricular cavity with the epicardial coronary artery system through the capillary bed or a ventricular-coronary arterial communication. Myocardial failure during embryogenesis and impaired compaction (trabecular remodeling failure) is best descriptive of the disease [2, 12, 18] as both hyper trabeculation, and persistent sinusoids have an entirely different histologic appearance from that of non-compaction, and the disease morphogenesis. Hence, scientific statements using the term "non-compaction" entirely and duly acknowledges its myocardial morphogenesis.

EPIDEMIOLOGY

Once considered a rare form of cardiomyopathy, its true prevalence varies considerably and to an extent unknown, which is largely due to the study design used, different inclusion criteria's, and significant selection bias. Non-compaction of the myocardium occurs in infants (0.81 per 100,000 infants/year), children (0.12 cases per 100,000 children/year) [23], and adults (prevalence 0.014%) [11]. Non-compaction can involve either ventricle, and its prevalence also described based on the anatomic variant of ventricular structure involved [24, 25]. It can also be associated with other cardiomyopathies, such as DCM, RCM, HCM, and ARVC, congenital heart diseases, as an isolated myocardial trait [26], and/or complex syndromes affecting multiple organs and tissues, including mitochondrial diseases caused by mutations in both nuclear [27], and mitochondrial genes [28].

NORMAL CARDIAC STRUCTURE

Cardiac muscle fibers comprise of small units of myocytes connected in series [29]. Each myocyte is surrounded by sarcolemma, and its inferior contains bundles of longitudinally arranged myofibrils. Each myocyte is joined at each other's end adjacent to the intercalated disc. In contrast to skeletal muscle fibers, cardiac fibers are not assembled in parallel arrays but rather bifurcate and recombine to form a complex three-dimensional network. The intercalated discs are gap and mechanical junctions containing connexins, desmocollin, desmoglein, desmoplakin, and desmins. The basic contractile units of cardiac muscle consist of an interdigitating thin (actin) and thick (myosin) filaments (with additional C, H, and X myosin-binding protein) which are formed by repeating sarcomeres giving the cardiac muscle its striated appearance [30, 31]. The thin filaments, however, are composed of cardiac actin, a-tropomyosin (a-TM), and troponins T, I, and C (cTnT, cTnI, cTnC). Also, the myofibrils contain a third filament formed by the giant filamentous titin and protein which extends from the Z disc to the M line and acts as a molecular template for the layout of the sarcomere. The Z disc at the borders of the sarcomere is formed by interdigitating proteins maintaining the core of the structure by cross-linking the antiparallel thin and titin filaments from the adjacent sarcomeres. Other proteins in the Z disc include capZ, telethonin/T-cap, nebulette, Cypher/ZASP, a-actinin, myopalladin, filamin, FATZ, myotilin, and muscle LIM protein (MLP) [30, 31]. The chemical and mechanical transmission of signals within and between the cells is provided with the support of the sarcolemma and the extracellular matrix (ECM) a complex network of proteins in the extrasarcomeric cytoskeleton composed of microfilaments, intermyofibrillar intermediate filaments, and microtubules [32]. The complex networks microfilaments form costameres which are sites of interconnections between various cytoskeletal networks linking sarcomere and sarcolemma serving as anchors for stabilization. The Costameres contain three principal components (dystrophin/dystrophin-associated protein complex, spectrin-based complex, and focal adhesion-type complex) [33]. The C-terminus of dystrophin binds b-dystroglycan which in turn interacts with a-dystroglycan to link to the ECM *via* a-2-laminin while the N-terminus of dystrophin interacts with actin.

ETIOLOGY, PATHOLOGY, AND PATHOPHYSIOLOGY

The embryonic myocardium in humans is composed of a fine loosed meshwork of interwoven fibers separated by deep recesses, which communicates with the LV cavity, giving room for a myocardial surface area increase and an exchange of diffusion in the cavity. From fifth to eight weeks of embryogenesis, the developing coronary vasculature coming from the epicardium coincides with LV trabecular compaction. The entire stage and process coincide with the maturation of the myocardium, which is stimulated by hypoxia in the subepicardial layer of the compacted myocardium [2]. Trabecular compaction, which is the background face of NCM, is hypothesized to occur as a result of the arrest during the phase of embryogenesis. This arrest results in a two-layered myocardium, consisting of an epicardial compacted layer and an extended trabeculated loosed network of interwoven fibers (non-compacted layer), and a deep endomyocardial recess which communicates with the LV cavity but not with the coronary bed. The compaction, however, progresses from the base of the heart to its apex and from the epicardium to the endocardium (Fig. **1 A & B**). Moreover, Ischemia also plays an essential role in the pathology and the pathophysiology of NCM [34] due to the underlying abnormalities found in the capillary bed associated with the increased stress on the compacted thin layer causing perfusion irregularities [13].

A **B**

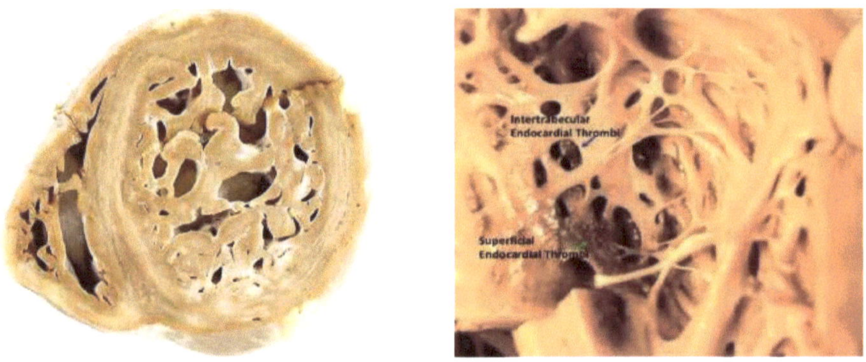

Fig. (1 A & B). [A] Trabeculation and sinusoidal invaginations of The Left Ventricle **[B]** High-Magnification View of Intertrabecular and Endocardial Thrombotic Stratification. Blue arrow (intertrabecular thrombotic stratification). The green arrow (endocardial thrombotic stratification).

RIGHT VENTRICULAR NONCOMPACTION

Quite evidently, right ventricular non-compaction [RVNC] is not frequently diagnosed as that of the LV. However, there has been a handful of reported cases. RVNC has been published in newborns with CHDs, and also in adult patients presenting with neurological symptoms [35]. Isolated RVNC is also an uncommon occurrence in adults, and it usually coexists with LVNC [36]. Although there are still yet no established diagnostic criteria for RVNC, the diagnosis has traditionally been made using 3D echocardiography, which helps to identify the dilated hypokinetic RV and prominent trabeculations [37].

LEFT VENTRICULAR NONCOMPACTION

LVNC can occur as a random genetic mutation, or it can be familiar with an autosomal dominant mode of transmission [18] (discussed in detail further in the chapter). The most common mutations occur in the cardiac sarcomere proteins, such as beta-myosin heavy chain [38]. They possess an extended range of expressivity, and individuals who have these sarcomeric mutations go on to display an early onset of lethal disease to no evidence of cardiomyopathy. This variable expression and the genotype-to-phenotype heterogenicity is the reason why LVNC diagnosis remains elusive and challenging.

DEVELOPMENTAL CONSIDERATIONS

A compound knowledge on the ontogenetic myocardial development is essential to appreciate the morphological appearance of NCM better. Cardiac development follows the same pattern in all vertebrates from fish to humans undergoing complex changes during the evolutionary development;

I. Early heart tube

II. Emergence of trabeculations

III. Trabecular remodeling and

IV. Development of the multilayered spiral system.

Therefore, the emergence of trabeculations and trabecular remodeling is of utmost importance in elucidating the NCM disease (Fig. **2**).

Emergence of Trabeculations

Trabeculations emerge after primitive heart tube looping at the end of the fourth week of gestation in the human embryo [2]. The trabeculation is ventricle specific, profound in the LV, thicker, and the intertrabecular spaces are more substantial at this embryonic stage. Persistence of this myocardial pattern postnatally over time will strongly resemble the spongy myocardium seen in non-mammalian vertebrates like reptiles, and amphibians [18] (Fig. **3**).

Trabecular Remodeling

Remodeling starts at eight weeks of gestation (in humans) after the completion of the ventricular septum. However, endocardial trabeculation rearrangement is specie, and ventricle specific. Luminal trabeculations in the mammalian heart coalesce to form posterior, and anterior papillary muscles of the mitral valve. The apical trabeculations further transform into fine honeycomb-like reliefs in the inner ventricular surface [2] (Fig. **3**).

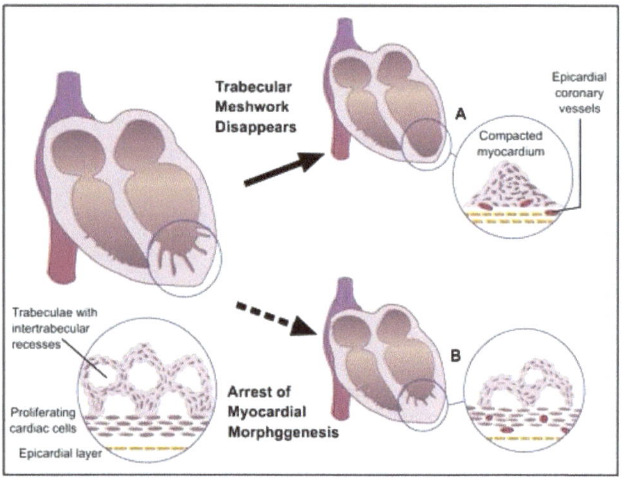

Fig. 2. Embryonic Development of LVNC. The myocardium starts as a meshwork of fibers that regress at weeks 5 to 8 to form compacted outer and inner smooth muscle layers **(A)**. In left ventricular non-compaction (LVNC), there is retarded myocardial morphogenesis and persistence of the trabecular meshwork **(B)**.

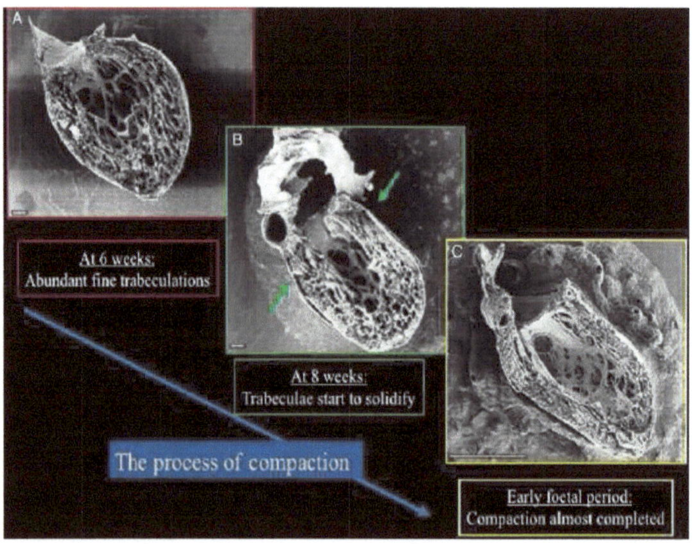

Fig. 3. Parietal view of sagittally dissected human embryonic left ventricles showing the process of normal trabecular compaction. **(A)** Abundant fine trabeculations present at six weeks. **(B)** The trabeculae start to solidify at the base of the heart, contributing to the added thickness of the compacted layer; initiation of this process coincides with the development of the epicardial coronary system. **(C)** The thick layer forms most of the myocardium mass after completion of compaction in the early fetal period.

EMBRYOGENIC AND NON-EMBRYOGENIC HYPOTHESIS

The etiological bases for NCM are multiple as it can occur as an isolated trait or disease; associated with congenital defects and other genetic diseases; transient or permanent [8]; acquired or sporadic in pathologic [9] or physiological conditions [7]. It can, however, also originate during the embryonic development or be acquired later in life.

Embryogenic Hypothesis

The two hypotheses supporting the morpho-embryogenic pathogenesis state that:

I. NCM occurs as a result of the inhibiting embryogenic structures as sponginess would occur due to the loosed cells or cell bundles. The non-compaction produced is as a result of a total mismatch between the compacted myocyte layers and the non-compacted trabeculae [11].

II. Myocardial morphogenesis leading to NCM occurs as a result of an arrest during cardiac development, when myocyte organization fails to evolve from the immature phase (spongiform) to a somewhat mature state (compact one) [3]. Although both ventricles are involved, LV is generally more affected than the right, which is the same for the first hypothesis too.

Data is supporting the embryogenic hypothesis of NCM mainly comes from experimental studies. However, in a recent echocardiographic survey carried out by Arunamata *et al.* [39], and studies done on identical twins [40] helps to elucidate the embryogenic hypothetic mechanism of NCM precisely that of LVNC. Experimental study models suggest that the process of cardiac trabeculation begins after the cardiac looping stage. Cardiac trabeculae formation beings with the emerging myocytes through the delamination from the compacted myocardium [41]. Although, other emerging evidence on ventricular trabeculation suggests that it arises from an entirely different clonal origin in the cardiac wall [41, 42]. The myocytes covered by the endocardial layer radially projects into the ventricular cavity. This radial projection pattern provides adequate perfusion to the myocytes by increasing the surface contact between the myocytes, and the LV cavity, while the coronary bed is yet to develop which is later fully developed as the proliferating myocytes, and the epicardium enters the myocardial wall hence, forming the coronary vasculature [23, 43]. The intertrabecular spaces are, however, been transformed into capillary vessels. It is at this stage where failure leads to the formation of elongated thin trabecular projections which are separated by deep recesses.

Non-Embryogenic Hypothesis

There is an emerging evidence which supports the hypothesis that increased trabeculation or non-compaction may occur later in adulthood, leading to an acquired right or left NCM. In young athletic individuals, an increased LV trabeculation may represent signs of cardiac remodeling as the trabeculations become more prominent over a long period. T-wave inversion and reduced basal systolic indices are shown during electrocardiographic (ECG), and echocardiographic readings in these highly trained athletes are diagnostic of LVNC [7]. Moreover, increased LV trabeculations in sickle cell anemia patients represent a myocardial exaggerated myocardial response to an increased cardiac preload [9], and also increased LV loading conditions or other physiological adaptation mechanisms in pregnant women [8]. These, in general, support the phenotypic characteristics of non-embryonic genesis in NCM as can be seen in pregnant women, athletes, and sick-cell anemic patients.

CLINICAL SPECTRUM AND OUTCOME

The clinical spectrum and outcomes vary and depend on many factors: whether NCM is studied in an adult or pediatric population, diagnosed in an asymptomatic patient during family screening or if isolated or associated with a syndrome, CHDs, or other diseases. Typical triad involves ventricular arrhythmias, heart failure, and systemic embolization, which may all, however, occur at any age. NCM in severe neonatal form presents with the typical triad and inevitably lead to sudden cardiac death [12]. The natural history and outcomes are so far challenging to ascertain as most studies use distinct methods and are retrospective.

NONCOMPACTION CARDIOMYOPATHY CLASSIFICATION AND SUBTYPES

By definition, the European Society of Cardiology (ESC) classification defines LVNC as a non-classified entity [5], while the American Heart Association (AHA) classification defines LVNC as genetic cardiomyopathy [1]. The 1995 World Health Organization (WHO)/International Society and Federation of Cardiology Task Force, however, did not classify NCM but rather grouped it as unclassified cardiomyopathy. Notwithstanding, the appealing initiative and idea to provide a generic classification applicable to all cardiomyopathies with the recently proposed novel classification system (MOGES) by Arbustini *et al.* [44] endorsed by the World Heart Federation, NCM remains a challenge potentially limiting its use. These uncertainties make NCM diagnosis difficult, and the MOGE(S) classification system imperfect. With the increasing number of physicians recognizing the clinical features of NCM, its significantly essential to identify the different phenotypes and the different phenotypic outcomes. The subtypes include the following:

Isolated Form

Here in this subtype, the ventricular thickness and size are reasonable with no evidence of arrhythmias. Clinically, this particular subgroup in childhood is benign and approximately 20-25% in all patient. Medical therapy and activity restrictions are not typical of this subgroup.

Isolated Form with Arrhythmias

This subtype is similar to that of the isolated form with normal function on echocardiography, but an arrhythmia is predominantly expressed in patients typically tachyarrhythmias. Unlike the Isolated subtype, patients in this group require a structured follow-up system and therapeutic interventions (either medications or an implantable defibrillator) as they seem to have an increased risk of unexpected events depending on the specific of arrhythmia and associated symptoms.

Hypertrophic Form

This subtype mimics HCM and has similar outcomes Follow-up in this group is typically identical to patients with pure HCM. Another differentiating clinical feature of this subtype is its undulating phenotypic ability to change its characteristic cardiac appearance to any other cardiomyopathy such as DCM and revert to HCM-like phenotype.

Dilated Form

This subtype mimics DCM and has similar outcomes. Follow-up in this group is typically identical to patients with pure DCM. Another differentiating clinical feature of this subtype is its undulating phenotypic ability to change its characteristic appearance to any other cardiomyopathy such as HCM and revert to DCM-like phenotype.

Restrictive Form

Although a rare form as compared to other subtypes, it's diagnostically challenging as it mimics RCM. Adults and children in this subgroup are typical candidates for a heart transplant after diagnosis is confirmed.

Mixed Form

The mixed form is the worse clinical subtype, which, in many cases, is associated with hypotonia and neuromuscular diseases. Infants and children are most affected, particularly if they have any form of metabolic disorder. An essential differentiating clinical feature of this subtype is its undulating phenotypic ability to change its characteristic appearance to either HCM or DCM and revert to HCM-dilated phenotype. ECGs taken in infants or children show pre-excitation with or without a severe increase in voltage.

Non-Compaction with CHDs

This subtype can occur in conjunction with any form of CHD. The most common form includes septal defects, although, rare associations like heterotaxy syndrome and single ventricle are likely possible.

OVERLAPPING ASSOCIATION WITH NEUROMUSCULAR DISORDERS

The Vienna group [6] over time has thoroughly investigated the association of NCM with neuromuscular diseases such as myotonic dystrophy, Becker's muscular dystrophy, Leber's hereditary optic neuropathy, Duchenne muscular dystrophy, and metabolic myopathy. However, the pathogenic relationship of these neuromuscular associations remains elusive, though, a strong predictor of adverse prognosis.

GENETICS

Non-compaction of the ventricular myocardium is a complex genetical disorder with a familial and sporadic form [11, 12, 15]. The familiar form is transmitted in an autosomal dominant inheritance pattern with incomplete penetrance as an autosomal recessive, and as X-linked traits. Sporadic cases are also common though limited due to its study design. Several disease loci have been identified to date. It can be linked to mutations in sarcomeric proteins, cytoskeletal, Z-line, and mitochondrial [45] (Fig. **4**). The genetic basis of NCM was first recognized in Barth syndrome, characterized by DCM with NCM. It is an X-linked disease with mutations in the G4.5 gene, located at Xq28, which encodes a family of proteins (tafazzins) with acetyltransferase functions in the mitochondria. α-dystrobrevin, a cytoskeletal protein component of dystrophin, another mutation associated with glycogen complex which links the ECM to the muscle fiber of the dystrophin cytoskeleton. Mutations in the Z-line protein Cypher/ ZASP found in the cytoplasm of skeletal and cardiac muscle, which maintains the myocyte architecture is associated with NCM and DCM and their phenotypic severity.

Also, NCM phenotype has been reported with an associated mutation in the Lamin A/C protein, which is further linked with conduction system disease, DCM, and muscular dystrophy.

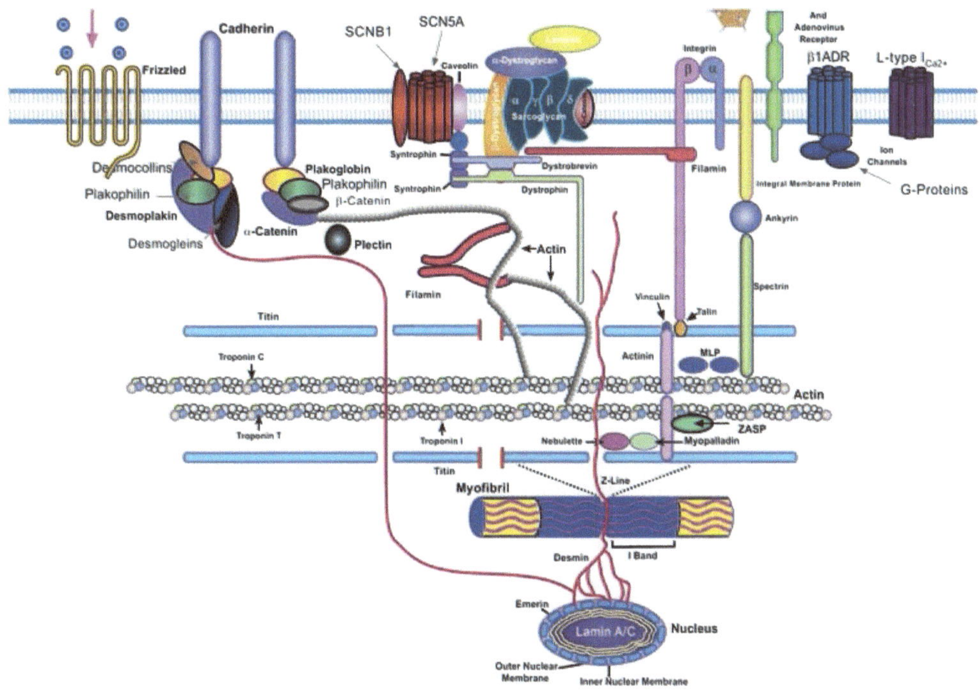

Fig. (4). Variable expressions and common pathways involved.

UNANSWERED QUESTIONS AND LINGERING DOUBTS

Despite significant advances in the genetic background and understanding of the etiology of cardiomyopathies, there is a poor understanding between genotype-phenotype correlation and many unanswered questions yet and lingering doubts (the fear of the known or the unknown) regarding the phenotypic expression of the same gene defect such as (Table **1**):

I. Is non-Compaction distinct cardiomyopathy?

II. LVNC as an isolated and non-isolated trait or disease and

III. Is non-compaction of the myocardium acquired or congenital?

Indeed, the morphological appearance of the myocardium in patients with NCM is characteristic and suggests distinct cardiomyopathy. However, the same mutations can cause different cardiomyopathic phenotypes as NCM can be associated with different CHDs (*e.g.*, ventricular septal defect, aortic stenosis, Ebstein anomaly, and pulmonary atresia) and can also be found with genetic syndromes, and metabolic diseases (*e.g.*, Barth syndrome, and Noonan syndrome). Furthermore, evolutionary changes during morphogenesis strongly suggest that NCM reflects an arrested or impaired compaction in the early developmental stages of the myocardium. However, a series of echocardiographic studies suggest that NCM develops where LVNC was not present at initial diagnosis but became evident on subsequent examinations. Correspondingly, LVNC can also be regarded as a fundamental trait which can contribute to LV dysfunction in coexisting morpho-functional disorders such as CHDs, or as a separate entity found in cardiac and non-cardiac diseases. It can also be used as a marker to suggest a specific diagnosis, such as tafazzin opathies usually seen in males with dilated hypokinetic phenotype [46, 47].

DIAGNOSIS (TABLE 2)

Electrocardiography

ECG readings are typical, particularly in asymptomatic, and young patients. Changes expressed in an ECG reading are usually non-specific but which however include repolarization abnormalities, LV hypertrophy, and left bundle branch block which is although, relatively common in patients with LV dysfunction. The presence of Wolff-Parkinson syndrome in patients also indicates an arrest in the embryogenic process and is more frequent in pediatric cases.

Table 1. Unanswered Questions and Lingering Doubts (The Fear of The Known or The Unknown).

The role of genetics on the non-compaction process: the same mutation associated with cardiomyopathies
Is non-Compaction distinct cardiomyopathy?
Which additional modifier factors may intervene in the embryogenesis arrest process?
Is non-compaction of the myocardium acquired or congenital?
Differentiation of non-compaction patterns from normal left ventricle trabeculations.
The natural history and outcomes of NCM
To identify appropriate therapeutic strategies for early prevention of complications.
Which are the perfect diagnostic imaging method and the most accurate diagnostic criteria?
LVNC as an isolated and non-isolated trait or disease
Does genetics play a role in the clinical picture and prognosis?

Echocardiography

This modality allows the detection, location, and confirmation of the widely used criterion (ratio of non-compacted and compacted myocardium >2.0 in end-systole) (Fig. **5**) [13, 15], showing both broad trabeculae and deep intertrabecular recesses in the LV myocardium (Fig. **6**). This technique is the first line for diagnosing NCM in both index patients and family members, a bedside modality, and readily available. Although, if the image is inadequate, it can, however, be confused for apical cardiomyopathy [48], fibroelastosis, or a thrombus as its inherent limitation in evaluating the LV apex still poses a diagnostic issue in the medical community today. Thus, it is essential that one must keep in mind quite high interobserver and intraobserver variability as a limitation.

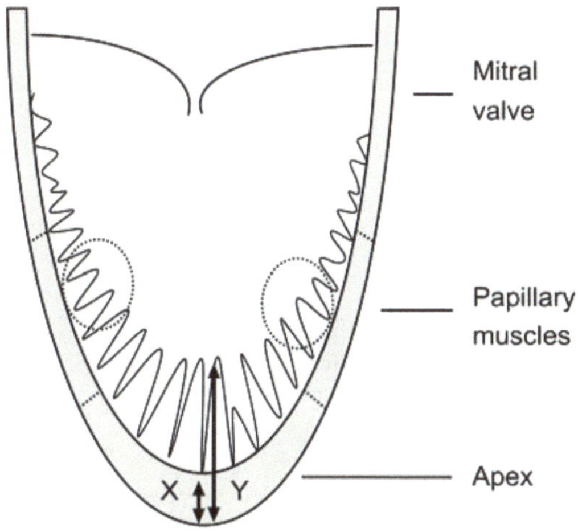

Fig. (5). Method of determining X-to-Y ratio according to Chin *et al.*,12 X represents the distance between the epicardial surface and the trough of the recesses and Y represents the distance between the epicardial surface and the peak of the trabeculations. X-to-Y ratios were measured at the level of the apex, papillary muscles, and mitral valve.

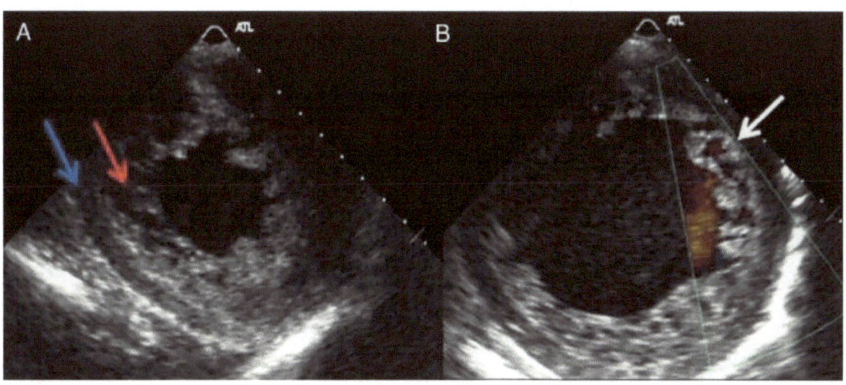

Fig. (6). Echocardiographic short-axis apical views of the left ventricle in a patient with non-compaction cardiomyopathy. (**A**) End-systolic image, showing the compacted layer (red arrow) with 6.3 mm thickness and the non-compacted layer (blue arrow) with 14.4 mm (ratio non-compacted/compacted >2). (**B**) Diastolic image depicting Doppler color flow in the intertrabecular recesses (white arrow).

***Contrast Echocardiography*:** This imaging modality is helpful when conventional echocardiographic images are inadequate or diagnosis uncertain. In patients with lung disease expressing poor acoustic windows, or an obese patient, the use of traditional echocardiography as a diagnostic modality tool will pose a significant amount of limitation as the diagnosis can easily be missed due to poor imaging, especially at the apical region of the heart. But with the use of contrast imaging with various agents would, however, enhance the endocardial border, and avoid a misdiagnosis (Fig. **7 A**, **B**, **C**, **D**).

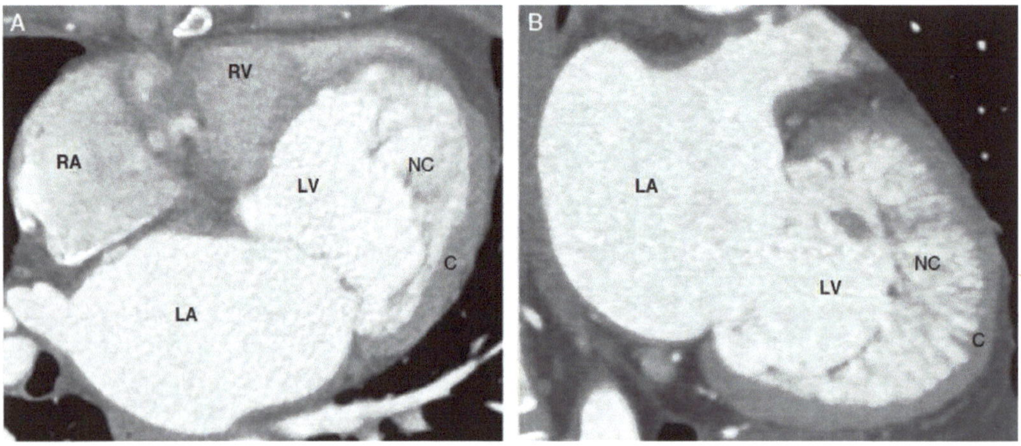

Fig. (7 A). Contrast-enhanced CT. **(A)** 4-chamber view of the heart and **(B)** a long-axis view of the heart. There is a clear distinction between compacted **(C)** and non-compacted myocardium (NC). LA indicates left atrium; RA, right atrium; RV, right ventricle.

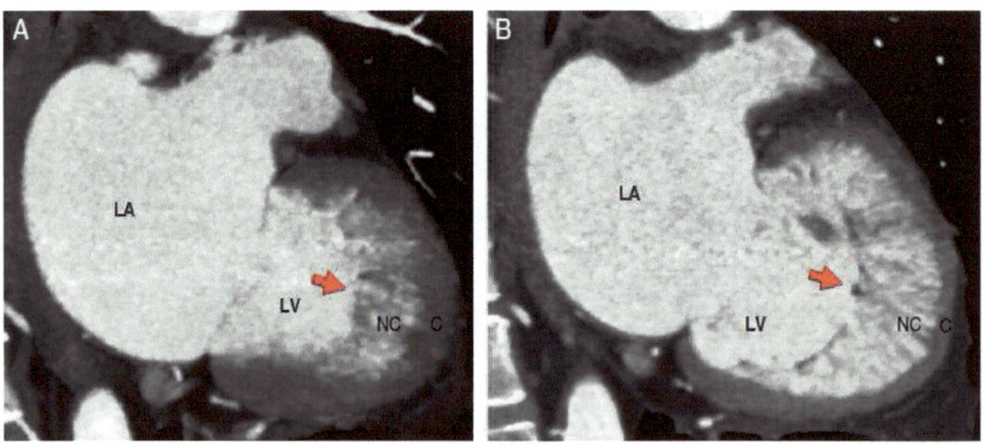

Fig. (7 B). Contrast-enhanced CT scan. **A** Long-axis view of the heart in systole showing two layers of the heart [non-compacted (NC) and compacted (C)] in a patient with LVNC. **B**, long-axis view in end-diastole. Red arrows point toward the non-compacted myocardium. LA indicates a left atrium.

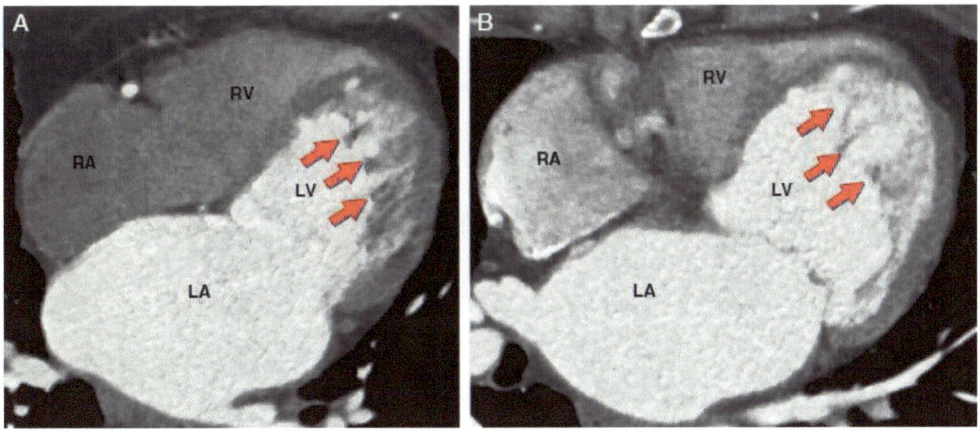

Fig. (7 C). Contrast-enhanced CT scan. Four-chamber view in systole (**A**) and diastole (**B**). Two layers of the heart can be seen in these views. Red arrows point toward the compacted myocardium. LA indicates left atrium; RA, right atrium; RV, right ventricle.

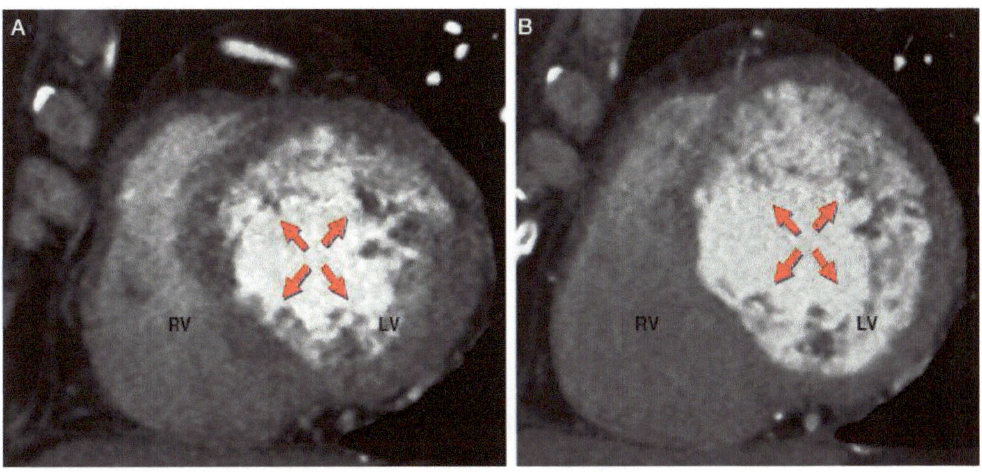

Fig. (7 D). Contrast-enhanced CT scan. Short-axis view showing the right ventricle (RV) and LV in systole (**A**) and diastole (**B**). Red arrows point toward the non-compacted myocardium.

Cardiac Magnetic Resonance Imaging

Cardiac magnetic resonance (CMR) imaging help to accurately describe and diagnose NCM and distinguish true LVNC from the prominent hyper trabeculation that can be seen in healthy hearts and individuals [49] (Fig. **8**). This diagnostic modality helps to confirm the presence of NCM anatomic features, as well as an accurate and reproducible measurement of the compacted and non-compacted myocardial layers. CMR reveals a broader extent of the disease with a high-resolution imaging technique without any form of acoustic limitations at the poorly observed segments, particularly at the LV apex, which is often problematic with echocardiography.

The careful evaluation of LV function is an additional advantage offered by CMR. The use of CMR also helps in diagnosing biventricular NCM as echocardiography presents inherent difficulties in analyzing this chamber.

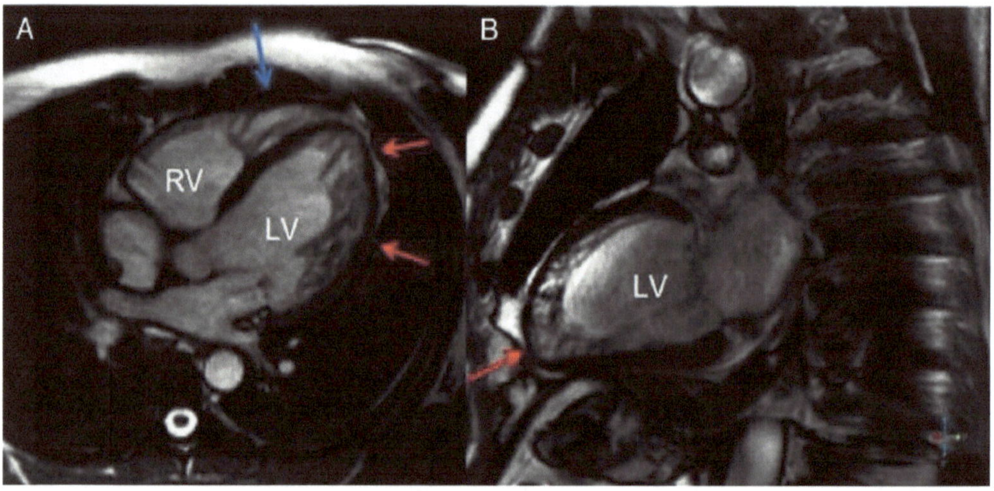

Fig. (8). End-diastolic cardiac magnetic resonance representative images from a patient with familial non-compaction cardiomyopathy. (**A**) Four chamber plane showing the non-compacted left ventricle (LV) myocardium at the apical segment and lateral wall (red arrows) and hyper-trabeculated right ventricle, suggestive of biventricular non-compaction (blue arrow); the maximum ratio non-compacted/ compacted layer is 4.5. (**B**) Two-chamber planes, depicting the non-compacted myocardium at the apical (red arrow) and the mid-anterior and inferior segments. RV, right ventricle.

Genetic Assessment

Following the imaging assessment, genetic assessment is also vital as it helps in the characterization of the myocardial phenotype of genetic mutations and the genotype-phenotype correlation. According to current guidelines following the identification of NCM causative mutation index in an individual, mutation-specific genetic testing is, however, recommended for family members and appropriate relatives (Fig. **9**).

EMERGING ECHOCARDIOGRAPHIC TECHNIQUES

The new echocardiographic techniques provide a quantitative and more objective assessment of NCM. The new methods include; speckle tracking, Doppler imaging, and strain rate imaging [50 - 52] as myocardial strain values are usually abnormal with LVNC patients even in the presence of a normal LV systolic/diastolic function.

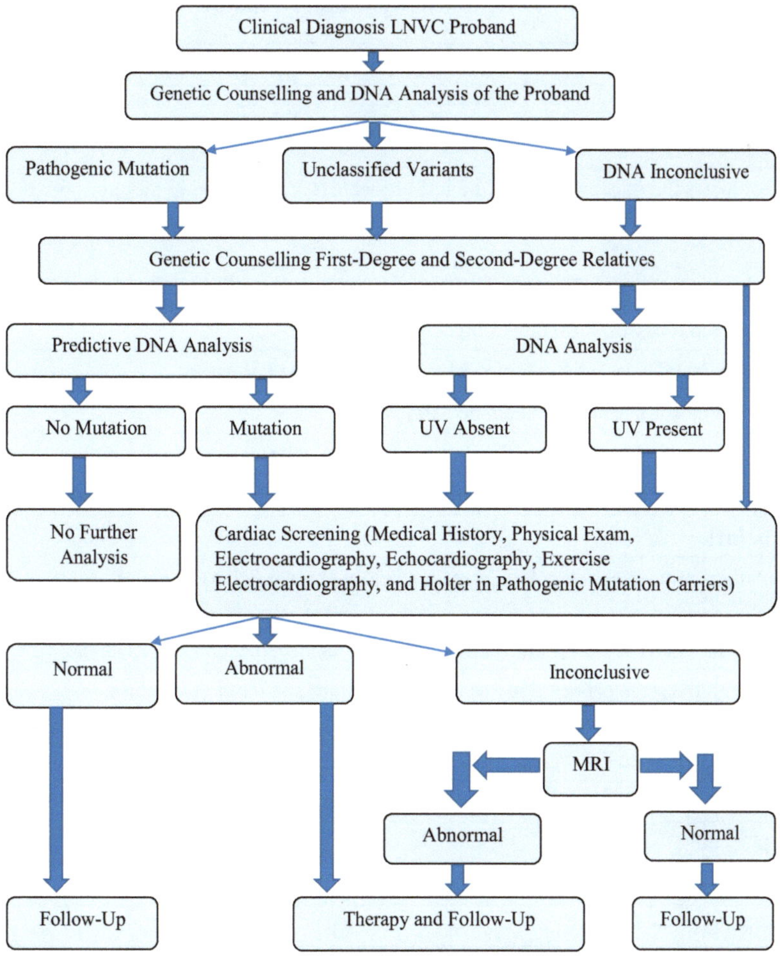

Fig. (9). Left Ventricular Non-Compaction Flow chart for family screening.

DIFFERENTIAL DIAGNOSIS AND DIAGNOSTIC CHALLENGES

The differential diagnosis between DCM and LVNC is quite challenging, especially in dilated ventricles. Other well-known differential diagnosis includes apical thrombus or tumors [53, 54], HCM, DCM, abnormal chords, epicardial fibroelastosis, eosinophilic heart disease, and a combination of both apical cardiomyopathy and LVNC. However, the diagnosis of NCM, especially LVNC, is daunting and imperative given the fact that there is no diagnostic gold standard, and LVNC shares to many features with other cardiomyopathies, such as DCM, and HCM. The distinction of these overlapping cardiomyopathies can be ambiguous, despite the use of all possible diagnostic modalities.

Table 2. Diagnostic Criteria Used in Non-Compaction Cardiomyopathy.

Echocardiographic Criteria
Chin ***et al*** **[12]**
» Ratio of X*/Y† <0.5
» Acquisition: evaluates the trabeculations at the left ventricle (LV) apex, using the short axis and apical views and the free wall, at end-diastole
Jenni ***et al*** **[13]**
» Bilayered LV myocardium, with a thin compacted layer and a thick non-compacted layer, with trabeculations and deep recesses; ratio non-compacted/compacted >2.0
» Evidence of intratrabecular recesses filled by blood flow from the LV cavity
» Absence of coexisting cardiac structural abnormalities
» Predominant localization of non-compaction in the lateral, apical or inferior walls of the LV
» Acquisition: short axis view; end-systolic acquisition
Stöllberger ***et al*** **[61]**
» Three trabeculations protruding from the LV wall, apically to the papillary muscles, visible in one image plane
» Intertrabecular spaces perfused from the ventricular cavity as visualized on color Doppler imaging
» Trabeculations with the same echogenicity as the myocardium and moving synchronously with ventricular contractions
» Acquisition: oblique views to differentiate false chords, aberrant bands and trabeculations
Cardiac Magnetic Resonance Criteria
Petersen ***et al*** **[62]**
» Ratio non-compacted/compacted >2.3
» Acquisition: end-diastolic
Jacquier ***et al*** **[63]**
» Trabecular LV mass >20% of global LV mass
» Acquisition: end-diastolic
*X, the distance between the epicardial surface and trough of a trabecular recess; †Y, the distance between the epicardial surface and peak of the trabeculation

PREGNANCY AND NONCOMPACTION CARDIOMYOPATHY

Pregnancy and childbirth can easily be successfully managed in NCM patients same as in other cardiac conditions if diagnosis, echocardiography, and other appropriate interventions are carried out early as there could be possibilities of giving birth to NCM babies [55].

THERAPEUTIC MANAGEMENT

Till date, there are no specific treatment guidelines for the management of NCM. However, the clinical management of NCM depends on the absence or presence of cardiac arrhythmias or dysfunction. Symptomatic patients with LV hypertrophy or dysfunction should be clinically managed according to phenotype, whereas, patients with normal LV size and function should be clinically monitored. Further echocardiographic screening of family members is mandatory to

better manage treatments effectively and improve prognosis. Be it as it may, we the authors, however, recommend the application of the current guidelines for the management of heart failure to manage NCM patients too rather than managing patients according to phenotypic type which might put patients at significant potential risk of heart failure and/or sudden death (SCD) [56, 57]. Because deep intertrabecular recesses with sluggish blood flow perpetuate thrombus formation, and the prevention of embolic complications is an important therapeutic goal, we recommend anticoagulation (target INR 2.0-3.0) in patients with impaired systolic function (LV ejection fraction, 35%) but should be individual specific after the assessment of the risk and benefits. Correspondingly, we also recommend the use of the current practice guidelines on ICD's and biventricular pacing [58, 59] for the prevention of SCD in NCM patients presenting with severely impaired LV systolic function (LVEF 35%), symptomatic ventricular arrhythmias, or syncope.

CONCLUSION AND FUTURE DIRECTIONS

The knowledge and understanding about the etiology, natural history, embryogenesis of the myocardium, genetic background, diagnosis and outcome still remain unclear, and controversial leading to overdiagnosis, poor prevalence, and weak epidemiological stratification with only limited improvements in the field so far. The current diagnostic criteria using echocardiography and CMR though useful, tend to over-diagnose NCM and also present with limitations of interobserver, and intraobserver variability. Keeping this in mind, physicians, and echocardiographers should remain careful and cautioned not to overdiagnose NCM as there remains a grey zone between a pathological myocardial structure with clinical relevance and a standard variant. Nevertheless, whether Non-compaction in isolation or associated with other pathologies, such as CHDs has a similar or completely different genetic/molecular basis, natural course, pathobiology, and whether different mechanisms, yet unknown modifiers, characteristic morphological appearance, and environmental factors accounting for various entities remain a matter of future research. To minimize issues related to the diagnosis of NCM, we, the authors suggest a comprehensive diagnostic workup which should include a systematic genetic screening of all first-degree relatives by a multidisciplinary team and multimodality imaging to determine whether NCM is a phenotypic variant or just a morphological expression of other cardiomyopathies of a primarily genetic disorder. We suggest and hope that the ESC, AHA, and the WHO form a working group shortly and agree on guidelines to specifically define:

I. The role of NCM as a marker for addressing genetic and clinical diagnostic hypotheses.

II. NCM as primary pathology, which can be associated with another cardiomyopathy (DCM, HCM, RCM) or isolated.

III. The risk of thrombosis in patients, especially when LV size and function are normal and also implore the collection of genetic, and imaging electronic health record data [60] and

IV. Reproducible and unified imaging-based diagnostic criteria for NCM.

Despite the steady improvements made so far in tissue harmonics, and echocardiography, there are still many unanswered questions, discrepancy, and limitations among the available published criteria diagnosis of NCM. Future multicenter collaboration research is required to build up an extensive international registry of patients with NCM to improve the understanding of this complicated cardiomyopathy.

LIST OF ABBREVIATIONS

AHA American Heart Association

ARVC Arrhythmogenic Right Ventricular Cardiomyopathy

CHDs Congenital Heart Defects

CMR Cardiac Magnetic Resonance

ECM Extracellular Matrix

ECG Electrocardiography

ESC European Society of Cardiology

LV Left Ventricle

LVNC Left Ventricular Non-Compaction

NCM Noncompaction Cardiomyopathy

RV Right Ventricle

RVNC Right Ventricular Non-Compaction

SCD Sudden Cardiac Death

WHO World Health Organization

CONSENT FOR PUBLICATION

Not applicable.

CONFLICT OF INTEREST

The authors confirm that this chapter contents have no conflict of interest.

ACKNOWLEDGEMENTS

Declared none.

REFERENCES

[1] Maron BJ, Towbin JA, Thiene G, *et al.* Contemporary definitions and classification of the cardiomyopathies: an American Heart Association Scientific Statement from the Council on Clinical Cardiology, Heart Failure and Transplantation Committee; Quality of Care and Outcomes Research and Functional Genomics and Translational Biology Interdisciplinary Working Groups; and Council on Epidemiology and Prevention. Circulation 2006; 113(14): 1807-16. [http://dx.doi.org/10.1161/CIRCULATIONAHA.106.174287] [PMID: 16567565]

[2] Sedmera D, Pexieder T, Vuillemin M, Thompson RP, Anderson RH. Developmental patterning of the myocardium. Anat Rec 2000; 258(4): 319-37. [http://dx.doi.org/10.1002/(SICI)1097-0185(20000401)258:4<319::AID-AR1>3.0.CO;2-O] [PMID: 10737851]

[3] Ulusoy RE, Kucukarslan N, Kirilmaz A, Demiralp E. Noncompaction of ventricular myocardium involving both ventricles. Eur J Echocardiogr 2006; 7(6): 457-60. [http://dx.doi.org/10.1016/j.euje.2005.07.011] [PMID: 16140587]

[4] Ranganathan A, Ganesan G, Sangareddi V, Pillai AP, Ramasamy A. Isolated noncompaction of right ventricle--a case report. Echocardiography 2012; 29(7): E169-72. [http://dx.doi.org/10.1111/j.1540-8175.2012.01671.x] [PMID: 22404341]

[5] Elliott P, Andersson B, Arbustini E, *et al.* Classification of the cardiomyopathies: a position statement from the european society of cardiology working group on myocardial and pericardial diseases. Eur Heart J 2008; 29(2): 270-6. [http://dx.doi.org/10.1093/eurheartj/ehm342] [PMID: 17916581]

[6] Arbustini E, Narula N, Dec GW, *et al.* The MOGE(S) classification for a phenotype-genotype nomenclature of cardiomyopathy: endorsed by the World Heart Federation. J Am Coll Cardiol 2013; 62(22): 2046-72. [http://dx.doi.org/10.1016/j.jacc.2013.08.1644] [PMID: 24263073]

[7] Gati S, Chandra N, Bennett RL, *et al.* Increased left ventricular trabeculation in highly trained athletes: do we need more stringent criteria for the diagnosis of left ventricular non-compaction in athletes? Heart 2013; 99(6): 401-8. [http://dx.doi.org/10.1136/heartjnl-2012-303418] [PMID: 23393084]

[8] Gati S, Papadakis M, Papamichael ND, *et al.* Reversible de novo left ventricular trabeculations in pregnant women: implications for the diagnosis of left ventricular noncompaction in low-risk populations. Circulation 2014; 130(6): 475-83. [http://dx.doi.org/10.1161/CIRCULATIONAHA.114.008554] [PMID: 25006201]

[9] Gati S, Papadakis M, Van Niekerk N, *et al.* Increased left ventricular trabeculation in individuals with sickle cell anemia: physiology or pathology? Int J Cardiol 2013;168:1658-60.noncompaction in low-risk populations.

[10] Zaragoza MV, Arbustini E, Narula J. Noncompaction of the left ventricle: primary cardiomyopathy with an elusive genetic etiology. Curr Opin Pediatr 2007; 19: 619-27.

[11] Oechslin EN, Attenhofer Jost CH, Rojas JR, Kaufmann PA, Jenni R. Long-term follow-up of 34 adults with isolated left ventricular noncompaction: a distinct cardiomyopathy with poor prognosis. J Am Coll Cardiol 2000; 36(2): 493-500.
[http://dx.doi.org/10.1016/S0735-1097(00)00755-5] [PMID: 10933363]

[12] Chin TK, Perloff JK, Williams RG, Jue K, Mohrmann R. Isolated noncompaction of left ventricular myocardium. A study of eight cases. Circulation 1990; 82(2): 507-13.
[http://dx.doi.org/10.1161/01.CIR.82.2.507] [PMID: 2372897]

[13] Jenni R, Oechslin E, Schneider J, Attenhofer Jost C, Kaufmann PA. Echocardiographic and pathoanatomical characteristics of isolated left ventricular non-compaction: a step towards classification as a distinct cardiomyopathy. Heart 2001; 86(6): 666-71.
[http://dx.doi.org/10.1136/heart.86.6.666] [PMID: 11711464]

[14] Agmon Y, Connolly HM, Olson LJ, Khandheria BK, Seward JB. Noncompaction of the ventricular myocardium. J Am Soc Echocardiogr 1999; 12(10): 859-63.
[http://dx.doi.org/10.1016/S0894-7317(99)70192-6] [PMID: 10511656]

[15] Ritter M, Oechslin E, Sütsch G, Attenhofer C, Schneider J, Jenni R. Isolated noncompaction of the myocardium in adults. Mayo Clin Proc 1997; 72(1): 26-31.
[http://dx.doi.org/10.4065/72.1.26] [PMID: 9005281]

[16] Robida A, Hajar HA. Ventricular conduction defect in isolated noncompaction of the ventricular myocardium. Pediatr Cardiol 1996; 17(3): 189-91.
[http://dx.doi.org/10.1007/BF02505211] [PMID: 8662034]

[17] Grant RT. An unusual anomaly of the coronary vessels in the malformed heart of a child. Heart 1926; 13: 273-83.

[18] Freedom RM, Yoo SJ, Perrin D, Taylor G, Petersen S, Anderson RH. The morphological spectrum of ventricular noncompaction. Cardiol Young 2005; 15(4): 345-64.
[http://dx.doi.org/10.1017/S1047951105000752] [PMID: 16014180]

[19] Dusek J, Ostádal B, Duskova M. Postnatal persistence of spongy myocardium with embryonic blood supply. Arch Pathol 1975; 99(6): 312-7.
[PMID: 1147832]

[20] Engberding R, Bender F. Identification of a rare congenital anomaly of the myocardium by two-dimensional echocardiography: persistence of isolated myocardial sinusoids. Am J Cardiol 1984; 53(11): 1733-4.
[http://dx.doi.org/10.1016/0002-9149(84)90618-0] [PMID: 6731322]

[21] Goebel N, Jenni R, Grüntzig AR. Persistierende myokardiale Sinusoide. RoFo Fortschr Geb Rontgenstr Nuklearmed 1985; 142(6): 692-3.
[http://dx.doi.org/10.1055/s-2008-1052740] [PMID: 2988072]

[22] Jenni R, Goebel N, Tartini R, Schneider J, Arbenz U, Oelz O. Persisting myocardial sinusoids of both ventricles as an isolated anomaly: echocardiographic, angiographic, and pathologic anatomical findings. Cardiovasc Intervent Radiol 1986; 9(3): 127-31.
[http://dx.doi.org/10.1007/BF02577920] [PMID: 3089618]

[23] Risebro CA, Riley PR. Formation of the ventricles. Scientific World Journal 2006; 6: 1862-80.
[http://dx.doi.org/10.1100/tsw.2006.316] [PMID: 17205193]

[24] Kawel N, Nacif M, Arai AE, *et al.* Trabeculated (noncompacted) and compact myocardium in adults: the multi-ethnic study of atherosclerosis. Circ Cardiovasc Imaging 2012; 5(3): 357-66.
[http://dx.doi.org/10.1161/CIRCIMAGING.111.971713] [PMID: 22499849]

[25] Peters F, Dos Santos C, Essop R. Isolated left ventricular non-compaction with normal ejection

fraction. Cardiovasc J Afr 2011; 22(2): 90-3.
[http://dx.doi.org/10.5830/CVJA-2010-035] [PMID: 21556452]

[26] Stähli BE, Gebhard C, Biaggi P, *et al.* Left ventricular non-compaction: prevalence in congenital heart disease. Int J Cardiol 2013; 167(6): 2477-81.
[http://dx.doi.org/10.1016/j.ijcard.2012.05.095] [PMID: 22704867]

[27] Gassmann M, Casagranda F, Orioli D, *et al.* Aberrant neural and cardiac development in mice lacking the ErbB4 neuregulin receptor. Nature 1995; 378(6555): 390-4.
[http://dx.doi.org/10.1038/378390a0] [PMID: 7477376]

[28] Jones FE, Golding JP, Gassmann M. ErbB4 signaling during breast and neural development: novel genetic models reveal unique ErbB4 activities. Cell Cycle 2003; 2(6): 555-9.
[http://dx.doi.org/10.4161/cc.2.6.598] [PMID: 14504474]

[29] Schwartz SM, Duffy JY, Pearl JM, Nelson DP. Cellular and molecular aspects of myocardial dysfunction. Crit Care Med 2001; 29(10) (Suppl.): S214-9.
[http://dx.doi.org/10.1097/00003246-200110001-00003] [PMID: 11593064]

[30] Gregorio CC, Antin PB. To the heart of myofibril assembly. Trends Cell Biol 2000; 10(9): 355-62.
[http://dx.doi.org/10.1016/S0962-8924(00)01793-1] [PMID: 10932092]

[31] Clark KA, McElhinny AS, Beckerle MC, Gregorio CC. Striated muscle cytoarchitecture: an intricate web of form and function. Annu Rev Cell Dev Biol 2002; 18: 637-706.
[http://dx.doi.org/10.1146/annurev.cellbio.18.012502.105840] [PMID: 12142273]

[32] Capetanaki Y. Desmin cytoskeleton: a potential regulator of muscle mitochondrial behavior and function. Trends Cardiovasc Med 2002; 12(8): 339-48.
[http://dx.doi.org/10.1016/S1050-1738(02)00184-6] [PMID: 12536120]

[33] Sharp WW, Simpson DG, Borg TK, Samarel AM, Terracio L. Mechanical forces regulate focal adhesion and costamere assembly in cardiac myocytes. Am J Physiol 1997; 273(2 Pt 2): H546-56.
[PMID: 9277468]

[34] Jenni R, Wyss CA, Oechslin EN, Kaufmann PA. Isolated ventricular noncompaction is associated with coronary microcirculatory dysfunction. J Am Coll Cardiol 2002; 39(3): 450-4.
[http://dx.doi.org/10.1016/S0735-1097(01)01765-X] [PMID: 11823083]

[35] Ying ZQ, Xu G, Chen S, Ma J, You XD. Cerebral infarction in an adult patient with right ventricular hypertrabeculation/noncompaction. Int J Cardiol 2008; 127(3): e150-1.
[http://dx.doi.org/10.1016/j.ijcard.2007.04.148] [PMID: 17706303]

[36] Leung SW, Elayi CS, Charnigo RJ Jr, Syed MA. Clinical significance of right ventricular dysfunction in left ventricular non-compaction cardiomyopathy. Int J Cardiovasc Imaging 2012; 28(5): 1123-31.
[http://dx.doi.org/10.1007/s10554-011-9925-z] [PMID: 21792620]

[37] Song ZZ. A possible diagnosis of isolated right ventricular hypertrabeculation /noncompaction in an elderly man by three-dimensional echocardiography. Int J Cardiol 2011; 147(1): e4-7.
[http://dx.doi.org/10.1016/j.ijcard.2008.12.212] [PMID: 19185368]

[38] Hoedemaekers YM, Caliskan K, Michels M, *et al.* The importance of genetic counseling, DNA diagnostics, and cardiologic family screening in left ventricular noncompaction cardiomyopathy. Circ Cardiovasc Genet 2010; 3(3): 232-9.
[http://dx.doi.org/10.1161/CIRCGENETICS.109.903898] [PMID: 20530761]

[39] Arunamata A, Punn R, Cuneo B, Bharati S, Silverman NH. Echocardiographic diagnosis and prognosis of fetal left ventricular noncompaction. J Am Soc Echocardiogr 2012; 25(1): 112-20.
[http://dx.doi.org/10.1016/j.echo.2011.09.019] [PMID: 22014428]

[40] Vinograd CA, Srivastava S, Panesar LE. Fetal diagnosis of left-ventricular noncompaction cardiomyopathy in identical twins with discordant congenital heart disease. Pediatr Cardiol 2013; 34(6): 1503-7.
[http://dx.doi.org/10.1007/s00246-012-0406-5] [PMID: 22695766]

[41] Liu J, Bressan M, Hassel D, *et al.* A dual role for ErbB2 signaling in cardiac trabeculation. Development 2010; 137(22): 3867-75. [http://dx.doi.org/10.1242/dev.053736] [PMID: 20978078]

[42] Gupta V, Poss KD. Clonally dominant cardiomyocytes direct heart morphogenesis. Nature 2012; 484(7395): 479-84. [http://dx.doi.org/10.1038/nature11045] [PMID: 22538609]

[43] Sedmera D, Thompson RP. Myocyte proliferation in the developing heart. Dev Dyn 2011; 240(6): 1322-34. [http://dx.doi.org/10.1002/dvdy.22650] [PMID: 21538685]

[44] Arbustini E, Narula N, Tavazzi L, *et al.* The MOGE(S) classification of cardiomyopathy for clinicians. J Am Coll Cardiol 2014; 64(3): 304-18. [http://dx.doi.org/10.1016/j.jacc.2014.05.027] [PMID: 25034069]

[45] Sen-Chowdhry S, McKenna WJ. Left ventricular noncompaction and cardiomyopathy: cause, contributor, or epiphenomenon? Curr Opin Cardiol 2008; 23(3): 171-5. [http://dx.doi.org/10.1097/HCO.0b013e3282fdc939] [PMID: 18382203]

[46] Chen R, Tsuji T, Ichida F, *et al.* Noncompaction study collaborators. Mutation analysis of the G4.5 gene in patients with isolated left ventricular noncompaction. Mol Genet Metab 2002; 77(4): 319-25. [http://dx.doi.org/10.1016/S1096-7192(02)00195-6] [PMID: 12468278]

[47] Ferreira C, Thompson R, Vernon H. Barth syndrome.GeneReviews Seattle, WA. Seattle: University of Washington 1993. http://www.ncbi.nlm.nih.gov/books/NBK247162/

[48] Jorge C, Marques JS, Miltenberger-Miltényi G, Pinto FJ. Hypertrophic cardiomyopathy or non-compaction? How the first impression can be wrong. Int J Cardiol 2012; 158(3): e53-4. [http://dx.doi.org/10.1016/j.ijcard.2011.10.110] [PMID: 22078399]

[49] Peritz DC, Vaughn A, Ciocca M, Chung EH. Hypertrabeculation *vs.* left ventricular noncompaction on echocardiogram: a reason to restrict athletic participation? JAMA Intern Med 2014; 174(8): 1379-82. [http://dx.doi.org/10.1001/jamainternmed.2014.1066] [PMID: 24911984]

[50] Bellavia D, Michelena HI, Martinez M, *et al.* Speckle myocardial imaging modalities for early detection of myocardial impairment in isolated left ventricular non-compaction. Heart 2010; 96(6): 440-7. [http://dx.doi.org/10.1136/hrt.2009.182170] [PMID: 19966109]

[51] van Dalen BM, Caliskan K, Soliman OI, *et al.* Left ventricular solid body rotation in non-compaction cardiomyopathy: a potential new objective and quantitative functional diagnostic criterion? Eur J Heart Fail 2008; 10(11): 1088-93. [http://dx.doi.org/10.1016/j.ejheart.2008.08.006] [PMID: 18815069]

[52] van Dalen BM, Caliskan K, Soliman OI, *et al.* Diagnostic value of rigid body rotation in noncompaction cardiomyopathy. J Am Soc Echocardiogr 2011; 24(5): 548-55. [http://dx.doi.org/10.1016/j.echo.2011.01.002] [PMID: 21345651]

[53] Chukwuemeka Daniel. Iroegbu, Zhou, Zhongxin, Hao, Zhang, Liu, Jindong Mitral Valve Insufficiency, a Constituent of Left Atrial Myxoma: Pathobiology, Physiopathology, and Pathophysiology of Left Atrial Myxoma. Are Long-Term Results Still Feasible 2018.

[54] Iroegbu DC, Zhou Z. Huge pedunculated left atrial myxoma with mitral valve replacement due to annular dilatation and concomitant coronary artery disease: A literature review. Ital J Vasc Endovasc Surg 2017; 24: 70-5. [http://dx.doi.org/10.23736/S1824-4777.17.01289-X]

[55] Rehfeldt K, Pulido J, Mauermann W, *et al.* Left ventricular hypertrabeculation/noncompaction in a patient with peripartum cardiomyopathy Int J Cardiol 2008; 2008: 025.

[56] Dickstein K, Cohen-Solal A, Filippatos G, *et al.* ESC Committee for Practice Guidelines (CPG). ESC

Guidelines for the diagnosis and treatment of acute and chronic heart failure 2008: the Task Force for the Diagnosis and Treatment of Acute and Chronic Heart Failure 2008 of the European Society of Cardiology. Developed in collaboration with the Heart Failure Association of the ESC (HFA) and endorsed by the European Society of Intensive Care Medicine (ESICM). Eur Heart J 2008; 29(19): 2388-442.
[http://dx.doi.org/10.1093/eurheartj/ehn309] [PMID: 18799522]

[57] Hunt SA, Abraham WT, Chin MH, *et al.* 2009 Focused update incorporated into the ACC/AHA 2005 Guidelines for the Diagnosis and Management of Heart Failure in Adults A Report of the American College of Cardiology Foundation/American Heart Association Task Force on Practice Guidelines Developed in Collaboration With the International Society for Heart and Lung Transplantation. J Am Coll Cardiol 2009; 53(15): e1-e90.
[http://dx.doi.org/10.1016/j.jacc.2008.11.013] [PMID: 19358937]

[58] Epstein AE, DiMarco JP, Ellenbogen KA, *et al.* ACC/AHA/HRS 2008 Guidelines for Device-Based Therapy of Cardiac Rhythm Abnormalities: a report of the American College of Cardiology/American Heart Association Task Force on Practice Guidelines (Writing Committee to Revise the ACC/AHA/NASPE 2002 Guideline Update for Implantation of Cardiac Pacemakers and Antiarrhythmia Devices) developed in collaboration with the American Association for Thoracic Surgery and Society of Thoracic Surgeons. J Am Coll Cardiol 2008; 51(21): e1-e62.
[http://dx.doi.org/10.1016/j.jacc.2008.02.032] [PMID: 18498951]

[59] Wilkoff BL, Auricchio A, Brugada J, *et al.* HRS/EHRA expert consensus on the monitoring of cardiovascular implantable electronic devices (CIEDs): description of techniques, indications, personnel, frequency and ethical considerations. Heart Rhythm 2008; 5(6): 907-25.
[http://dx.doi.org/10.1016/j.hrthm.2008.04.013] [PMID: 18551743]

[60] Rasmussen LV. The electronic health record for translational research. J Cardiovasc Transl Res 2014; 7(6): 607-14.
[http://dx.doi.org/10.1007/s12265-014-9579-z] [PMID: 25070682]

[61] Stöllberger C, Finsterer J, Blazek G. Left ventricular hypertrabeculation/noncompaction and association with additional cardiac abnormalities and neuromuscular disorders. Am J Cardiol 2002; 90(8): 899-902.
[http://dx.doi.org/10.1016/S0002-9149(02)02723-6] [PMID: 12372586]

[62] Petersen SE, Selvanayagam JB, Wiesmann F, *et al.* Left ventricular non-compaction: insights from cardiovascular magnetic resonance imaging. J Am Coll Cardiol 2005; 46(1): 101-5.
[http://dx.doi.org/10.1016/j.jacc.2005.03.045] [PMID: 15992642]

[63] Jacquier A, Thuny F, Jop B, *et al.* Measurement of trabeculated left ventricular mass using cardiac magnetic resonance imaging in the diagnosis of left ventricular non-compaction. Eur Heart J 2010; 31(9): 1098-104.
[http://dx.doi.org/10.1093/eurheartj/ehp595] [PMID: 20089517]

CHAPTER 10

Takotsubo Cardiomyopathy

Jeremiah Ong'achwa Machuki[1], **Iroegbu Chukwuemeka Daniel**[2,*] and **Jinfu Yang**[2]

[1] *Department of Biochemistry, University of Nairobi, P.O. Box 30197-001000, Nairobi, Kenya*

[2] *Department of Cardiovascular Surgery, The Second Xiangya Hospital, Central South University, Middle Renmin Road 139, 410011 Changsha, China*

Abstract: Takotsubo syndrome is one of the few heart conditions that have witnessed an increasing incidence in modern clinical practice. It is an acute syndrome that presents with various clinical symptoms and etiological factors. Since its first description in the early 1990s, much progress has been made in many aspects of the condition including its treatment approaches, clinical investigations, prognosis, clinical presentation, complications, pathophysiology, epidemiology, triggers, anatomical variants, primary and secondary clinical subtypes, diagnosis, definition, and terminology. In addition to clinical studies, many pre-clinical and basic research platforms and technologies have been developed to help advance our understanding of this syndrome. This chapter presents a comprehensive discussion on what is the current state of knowledge concerning this disease. By so doing, we provide the clinical and non-clinical scientists as well as general readers with new diagnostic approaches, sub-types classification, and management tools for Takotsubo. New algorithms to facilitate decision-making by a cardiologist are provided as well as grey areas for further research.

The sex preference of Takotsubo and the role of estrogen and catecholamines are brought to focus on providing the future research outlook of this condition. The available treatments and proposed mechanisms are also summarized. Although Takotsubo is generally considered to have a good prognosis, some complications of severe nature may occur in a subset of patients, *e.g.*, dangerous ventricular arrhythmias, cardiogenic shock, pulmonary edema, which can cause damage to the myocardium which transcends the recovery phase of the left ventricular ballooning.

Keywords: Acute coronary syndrome, Cardiomyopathies, Catecholamine toxicity, Cardiac remodeling, Drug-induced cardiomyopathy, Heart failure, Heart syndromes, Menopausal diseases, Multi-vessel coronary spasm, Microvascular angina, Pathophysiological mechanisms, Risk stratification, Reversible cardiac

* **Corresponding author Iroegbu Chukwuemeka Daniel:** Department of Cardiovascular Surgery, The Second Xiangya Hospital, Central South University, Middle Renmin Road 139, 410011 Changsha, China;
E-mails: yjf19682005@csu.edu.cn, dr.iroegbu_daniel@yahoo.com, dr.iroegbu_daniel@csu.edu.cn

syndrome, Stress cardiomyopathy, Stress-induced cardiomyopathy, Takotsubo syndrome, Takotsubo cardiomyopathy, Variant Angina.

HISTORY OF TAKOTSUBO AND EPIDEMIOLOGY

The term 'Takotsubo' was first coined by H. Sato in 1990 to refer to the dysfunction of the left ventricle (LV) following a multi-vessel coronary spasm [1]. This name indicates the geometrical features of the heart, resembling a traditional Japanese octopus trap which has a round base and a narrow neck (Fig. **1**). Several other terms referring to this condition were proposed later on, such as apical ballooning syndrome [2] and 'ampulla cardiomyopathy' [3], but this name became mainstream only in the aftermath of the documentation of 5 patients who were suspected for myocardial infarction (MI) in 1991 by K. Dote *et al.* The patients presented with electrocardiographic abnormalities and chest pain resembling the patients with acute MI [4]. Examinations by left ventriculography demonstrated the presence of hyperkinesis in the basal segments, but with akinesis in the diaphragmatic, anterolateral segments and apical parts of the LV. Interestingly, these features disappeared within seven days. Based on the angiographic examination, two patients had diffuse multi-vessel spasms, including two others who received ergonovine. One patient showed decreased R waves while the other 4 had ST elevation, and one patient had Q waves. However, none of the patients had coronary artery stenosis [4]. A significant milestone that followed these findings was the multi-center, retrospective study performed in 2001 by K. Tsuchihashi *et al.* involving 88 patients (76 women and 12 men). This study was critical, as it revealed a high prevalence of Takotsubo in women than in men [2]. A magnetic resonance imaging performed in 239 patients showed four types of 'ampulla cardiomyopathy': basal (1%), midventricular (17%), biventricular (34%), and apical (82%) [5]. Classification by the American Heart Association described Takotsubo syndrome as a category of stress-induced cardiomyopathy in 2006 [6].

EPIDEMIOLOGY

Following its discovery, an explosion of studies has been witnessed beginning the first papers published outside Japan [7, 8] Currently, a search on PubMed database with the search terms 'Takotsubo cardiomyopathy' yields more than 3335 publications between 2008 and 2018 December. It has been reported that about 2% of patients manifesting with acute coronary syndrome are likely to develop Takotsubo [9]. Indeed, there are diagnostic challenges when distinguishing patients with takotsubo from those with the acute coronary syndrome, which is due to the similarity in symptomatology between these two conditions at the initial stage [10]. Initially, patients with the takotsubo present with electrocardiographic changes, wall motion abnormalities, elevated cardiac enzymes and chest pain, all of which are quite similar with patients with acute coronary syndrome. Therefore, there exist challenges on how to apply differential diagnosis to differentiate these conditions, partly due to the lack of reliable and conventional electrocardiographic criteria.

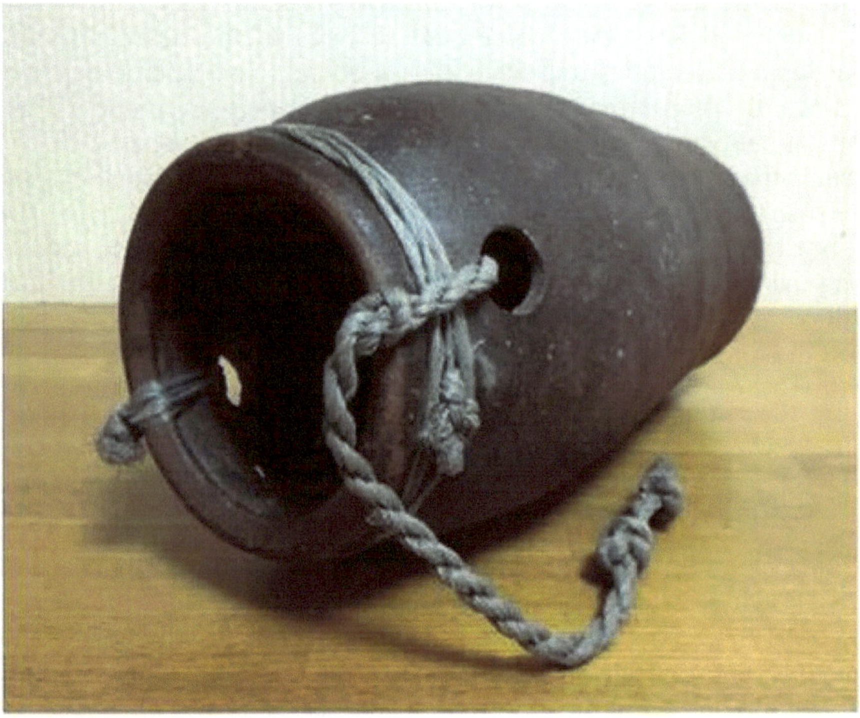

Fig. (1). A traditional Japanese Fishing pot.

In this aspect, diagnosis by ECG is limited because of differences in anatomical presentation of takotsubo, variations in ECG parameters that vary with race and patient features, time from symptoms onset, triggers and wall motion abnormalities [11]. Although it was initially thought to be a benign syndrome, recent statistics indicate that takotsubo may lead to significantly high in-patient morbidity and with cases of deaths [12]. So far, the reported prevalence of takotsubo is about 2% [13]. However, it has been found that it is more prevalent in postmenopausal women averaging approximately 67.7 years old. For instance, it was recognized that among 1750 takotsubo patients, almost 90% were postmenopausal women who are over 67 years [14]. Takotsubo has been diagnosed in patients of all races, although it has been noted that it is rare among African American and Hispanics [15]. The prevalence of this condition is underrepresented due to a significant lack of awareness about this condition. Many cases are now being reported based on the initial diagnosis with coronary angiography, as is evidenced by the rising number of studies on Takotsubo, as shown in Fig. (**2**).

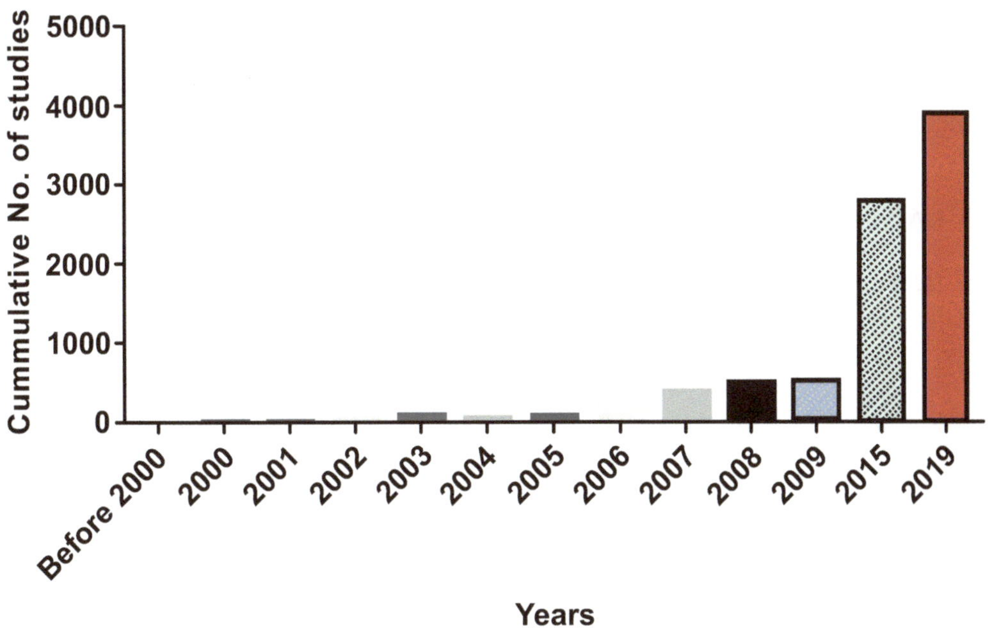

Fig. (2). A publication trend for studies on Takotsubo from discovery.

About 20-fold increase of cases was recorded between 2012 and 2006 [10]. Similarly, between 2007 and 2012, the number of cases reported increased by 3-fold in the USA alone [16] which has been accompanied by high levels of hospitalization and mortality due to takotsubo [17, 18]. Among 24,700, takotsubo patients hospitalized, the mortality rate was 4.2% [19]. Among them, male patients had a higher death rate than females (8.4% *vs.* 3.6%). The recurrence rate for takotsubo was reported to be 1.5% by Singh *et al.* [20]. Most recurrences were found to occur in the first 5 years after the first episode, with a recurrence rate of about 6% [21]. For instance, the recurrence rate in cases where takotsubo is triggered by pheochromocytoma was estimated to be about 18% [22].

IMPACT OF MALIGNANCIES ON TAKOTSUBO

Many studies have investigated the association between neurohormonal activation, inflammation, emotional stress, and cancer [23]. Indeed, reversible cardiac dysfunction precipitated by catecholamine has been reported due to increased catecholamines levels [24]. The findings from a collaborative review comprising 1109 patients with takotsubo found that the rate of fatalities in such patients was between 4-29% [25]. Also, takotsubo patients were more likely to have histories of malignancy in a study that comprised 24,701 [26]. Burgdorf *et al.* also recognized that takotsubo patients are likely to have a previous diagnosis with malignancy relative to acute myocardial infarction [27]. High levels of mortality, CRP, leukocyte, and BNP were found in takotsubo patients with malignancies [28]. It might, however, provide the basis for the link between malignancy and takotsubo. Other studies have shown that there exists a causal relationship between cancer, emotional stress, and takotsubo [29].

SEX LANDSCAPE OF TAKOTSUBO

Statistical data from the international Takotsubo registry shows a higher prevalence of takotsubo in postmenopausal females with a ratio of men-to-women of 1:9. In terms of the clinical manifestations, some differences exist such as; high ventricular arrhythmia, sepsis, use of catecholamines, in-hospital complications in men compared to women takotsubo patients. Also, emotional triggers are more frequent in women, while physical and acute neurological disorders are common in men [30]. Based on the long-term prognosis of takotsubo, men had higher levels of adverse events and mortality rate after 30 days. Similarly, major adverse cardiac events (MACE) are frequently higher in women than in men [31].

GENETIC BASIS OF TAKOTSUBO

Several investigations have been carried out to explore the genetic basis of Takotsubo [32, 33]. Recent findings that indicate the presence of various genetic variants in specific genes involved in heat physiology points to the genetic predisposition in Takotsubo [34, 45]. More evidence for the existence of the genetic basis for takotsubo comes from some studies that identified familial cases of takotsubo [35, 36]. Moreover, up to 10% of takotsubo patients are likely to have a recurrence indicating a genetic susceptibility. Also, not all postmenopausal women who suffer from stress experience takotsubo, suggesting that there are genetic factors regulating predisposition. In this regard, a study by Citro *et al.* demonstrated that some genes such as Bcl2-associated athanogene (BAG3) [36].

The severity of cardiac dysfunction in pheochromocytoma and subarachnoid hemorrhage has been linked to differential adrenergic variant genes [37]. But the results investigating the genetics of adrenergic receptors in Takotsubo have been explicit with some reporting no differences in ADRB1 and ADRB2 polymorphism [38]. And, other studies indicate that GRK5-Gln4Ileu and ADRB1-Gly389Arg are highly expressed in takotsubo patients [39, 40]. Therefore, although the condition is primarily thought to be genetic cardiomyopathy, the current clinical data points to a specific pool of genetic risk factors. But such findings have been based on a small number of subjects. Much more largescale genetic screening might help resolve these inconsistencies.

PATHOPHYSIOLOGY

The development of takotsubo is multifactorial encompassing systemic physiological responses to emotional or physical triggers. Catecholamines are thought to play a crucial role in the initiation and progress of Takotsubo patients often present with symptoms of sympathetic activation following an emotional or physical stress trigger. Some of the key mechanisms prosed include the left ventricular outlet tract obstructions (LVOTO), myocardial ischemia, catecholamine cardiotoxicity, epinephrine triggered β2AR-Gs/Gi signal trafficking and hyperactive sympathetic nervous system. It, therefore, implies that two main pathways account for these pathomechanisms, *i.e.*, the response of cardiovascular elements such as myocardial cells, peripheral vascular tissues and coronary arteries to high blood catecholamines and the brain-hypothalamic-pituitary adrenal (HPA) axis regulation [41]. Fig. (**3**) summarizes the pathomechanisms of Takotsubo.

MULTIVESSEL CORONARY ARTERY VASOSPASMS

Following the discovery of Takotsubo by Sato and Dote [42], it was then considered to be a form of myocardial stunning caused by multivessel coronary vasospasms as examined by the coronary angiography. To date, up to 10% proportion of spontaneous coronary vasospasm has been reported, which suggests that the prevalence of spontaneous vasospasms is very low [43]. Myocardial stunning caused by ischemia as a result of the coronary atherosclerotic condition is thought to exert card protection against further injuries due to recurrent ischemia episodes by suppressing cardiac metabolic and contractile activities [44]. Considering the transient nature of myocardial ischemia arising from coronary artery occlusion and reperfusion, it is primarily observed that coronary perfusion is normal or slightly enhanced in Takotsubo patients [45]. Some studies have demonstrated that regional myocardial metabolism of glucose or fatty acids is impaired during the acute phase of ischemia. In line with this, there is metabolic dysregulation in apical regions of the left ventricle in takotsubo patients, which, however, returns to normal level after recovery [46].

Moreover, the diagnosis of normal perfusion but impaired metabolism in the left ventricle dysfunction in takotsubo supports the involvement of myocardial stunning in this disease [47]. Several factors have been proposed to contribute to myocardial stunning such as coronary bridging, coronary vasospasm, and aborted myocardial infarction [48]. The concept of myocardial stunning may explain the different types of takotsubo patients such as inverted type depending on the vascular territory affected. Based on nine cohort studies, it was reported that stimuli-induced vasospasms were found in 34 of 123 study subjects (27.6%) [49]. It was also recognized that vasospasm triggered by acetylcholine-induced acute apical dysfunction, underscoring the influence of multivessel vasospasm in a subset of takotsubo patients with apical variant [50]. Endothelin is a potent vasoconstrictor and is increased in takotsubo patients [51]. Thus, the high level of Endothelin may precipitate multivessel vasospasm. It is also likely that high circulating catecholamines may induce oxidative stress and further endothelial dysfunction, which may lead to the induction of vasospasm of peripheral and coronary arteries.

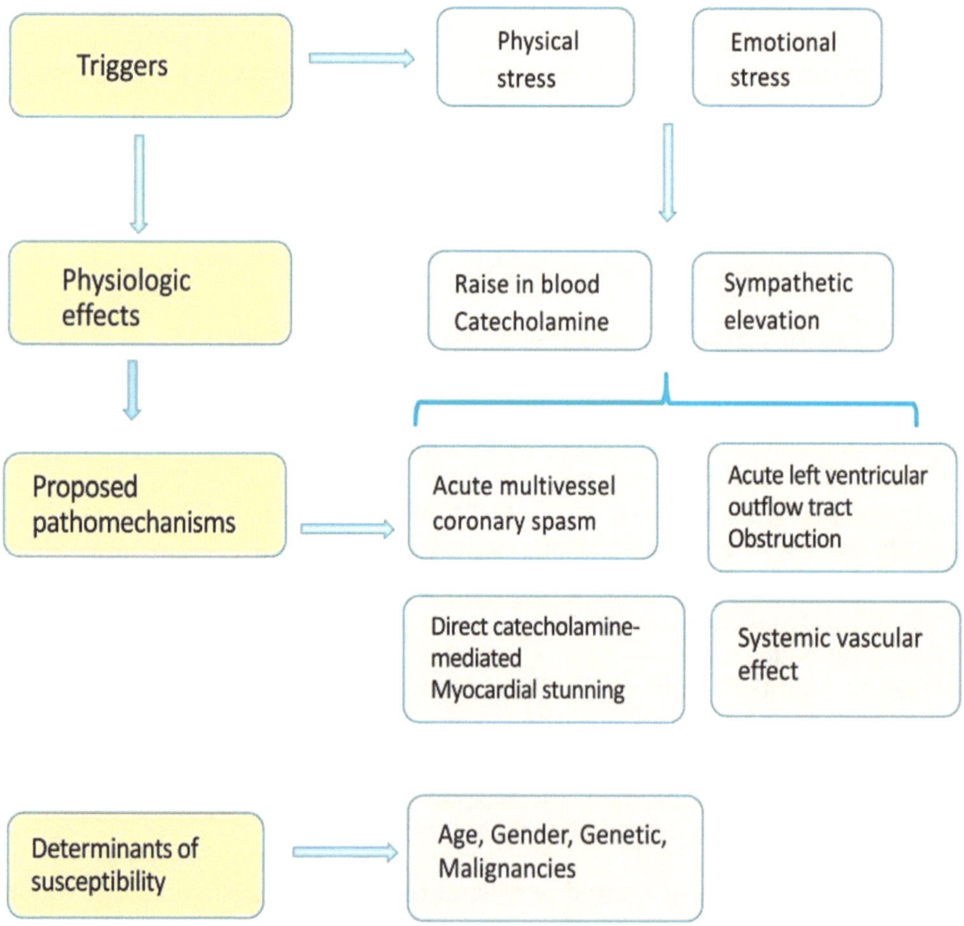

Fig. (3). Summary of pathomechanisms of Takotsubo.

Left Ventricular Outlet Tract Obstruction (LVOTO)

Clinical observations have revealed the existence of LVOTO takotsubo patients. It has, however, been associated with the occurrence of cardiogenic shock and hypotension in takotsubo patients. In a study involving 32 takotsubo patients, it was found that the prevalence of LVOTO was 25% [52]. The authors postulated that patients with the small left ventricle and a localized sigmoid septum are susceptible to severe mid-cavity obstruction when subjected to extreme stimulation of sympathetic nerves. In theory, LVOTO may cause apical subendocardial ischemia and a high-pressure difference between the base and apex of the left ventricle leading to ballooning. It is essential to note that a large proportion of takotsubo patient does not present with LVOTO [52]. LVOTO may not fully account for the basal patterns and apical-sparing of takotsubo, a key feature in many takotsubo patients [53]. It also does not account for the occurrence of right ventricular in about 1/3 of the patients [54]. Therefore, the diagnosis of LVOTO in a subset of takotsubo subjects may imply that LVOTO is a complication and not a cause of the LVWMA.

DIRECT CATECHOLAMINES-TRIGGERED MYOCARDIAL STUNNING

Several studies have proposed that the sudden increase in the blood concentration of catecholamines may directly trigger the apical ballooning pattern observed in the left ventricle. One of the hypotheses proposed earlier [55], is that β2AR signal trafficking from Gαs to Gαi. This proposition is based on the typical findings of apical-basal gradients of βARs and sympathetic nerve endings in the hearts [55]. It has been found that the basal segment of the left ventricle has a higher number of sympathetic nerves relative to the apex segment [56]. Therefore, it implies the cardiac sympathetic innervation patterns cannot explain the decreased contraction observed in the apical portion. Instead, this innervation pattern describes the inverted or basal takotsubo variant.

Interestingly, many animal heart studies show that β2ARs are more in the apical segment of the left ventricle, implying that this renders this segment more responsive to catecholamines [57]. This concept has not been validated in the human heart. The different patterns of βAR gradients and apical-basal sympathetic innervation keeps cardiac responses to catecholamine stimulation in balance in normal level sympathetic activation, *e.g.*, during mild stress or exercise. But, in situations of extreme stress, adrenal glands produce supernormal levels of epinephrine into the blood. Following this phenomenon, the resultant left ventricular response is determined by the βAR receptor gradient.

Although epinephrine triggers positive inotropy, this true at medium or low doses, many investigations have shown that the cardiac contractile response is bell-shaped, in which the contraction decreased at the highest epinephrine concentration mediated by β2AR [58, 59]. A pharmacological phenomenon of β2AR referred to as stimulus trafficking, in which high epinephrine doses triggers a shift from the Gαs stimulatory to the cardioinhibitory Gαi G proteins in cardiac myocytes [55, 59]. This switch is thought to be cardioprotective as β2AR-Gαi signaling is known to activate pathways that prevent apoptosis [60]. Thus β2AR-Gαi suppress the negative consequence of excessive catecholaminergic stimulation, pressure-induced injury, and vasospastic ischemia to the myocardial cells. Nevertheless, the outcomes of the β2AR-Gαi pathway have not been elucidated in the human heart during acute takotsubo syndrome, although they have been shown in chronic heart failure of human hearts. In a rat model of stress-induced cardiomyopathy, Gαi protein inhibitor pertussis toxin was found to prevent catecholamine triggered decrease in left apical ventricle [57]. A similar outcome was obtained in another animal experiment, although treatment with the pertussis toxin resulted in a high number of deaths [61].

CLINICAL SUBTYPES

In the clinical setup, takotsubo patients manifest diverse clinical contexts. Based on characteristics, Takotsubo cases are categorized as being either primary or secondary. The primary takotsubo syndrome refers to cases where the main reason for such patients being referred to specialized care is the presence of acute cardiac symptoms, often indicated by primary care physician, critical cardiac services or from emergency medical services. At the initial encounter with such patients, it is not clear whether they have an emotional trigger. Other underlying diseases may seem to be predisposing risk factors, although they are not the primary triggers of the increase in catecholamine. Such patients are considered to have primary takotsubo, and their treatment is given in consideration to their specific symptoms. In secondary takotsubo, many patients presenting with this type of takotsubo often have other medical conditions such as psychiatric, obstetric, anesthetic, or surgical cases. Some are, therefore, already hospitalized due to such situations. The development of takotsubo in such patients is often a secondary complication trigger by the presence of the underlying condition. The medical conditions trigger the production of catecholamines or hyperactivation of the sympathetic nervous system, which then precipitates takotsubo. Hence, the treatment of secondary takotsubo should address symptoms of Takotsubo but also the underlying primary trigger. Some of the medical contexts that have been found to trigger secondary takotsubo are shown in (Table **1**).

Table 1. Triggers for secondary Takotsubo syndrome [62].

Endocrine, hyperglycemic hyperosmolar state, hyponatremia, severe hypothyroidism, Addison's disease, adrenocorticotropin hormone deficiency, autoimmune polyendocrine syndrome II, autoimmune polyendocrine syndrome II
Neurological and neurosurgical
Acute neurosurgical emergencies (*e.g.*, subarachnoid hemorrhage, severe head injury, severe spinal injury)
Acute neuromuscular crises, especially if involving acute ventilatory failure (*e.g.*, severe myasthenia gravis, acute Guillain–Barré syndrome)
Epileptic seizures, limbic encephalitis, ischemic stroke, posterior reversible encephalopathy syndrome
Respiratory
Acute exacerbation of asthma or COPD (especially with excessive use of inhaled β2-agonists)
Acute pulmonary embolism
Acute pneumothorax
Obstetric, *e.g.* miscarriage, labor, emergency Caesarean section
Psychiatric
Acute anxiety attack/panic disorder
Attempted suicide
Drug-withdrawal syndromes
Electroconvulsive therapy
Gastrointestinal, *e.g.*, acute cholecystitis, biliary colic, acute pancreatitis, severe vomiting, severe diarrhea, pseudomembranous colitis, peritonitis
Infection
Severe sepsis
Babesiosis
Cardiological
Dobutamine stress echocardiography
Radiofrequency arrhythmia ablation
Pacemaker implantation
Electrical DC cardioversion for atrial fibrillation
Post-cardiac arrest including ventricular fibrillation
Hematological
Blood transfusions
Thrombotic thrombocytopenic purpura
Surgical

(Table 1) cont.....

Many cases have been reported during induction of general anesthesia or during non-cardiac surgery or interventional procedures under local or general anesthesia (*e.g.*, cholecystectomy, hysterectomy, rhinoplasty, Caesarean section, radiofrequency liver ablation, radiotherapy, colonoscopy, difficult urinary catheterization, carotid endarterectomy)
Medication and illicit drugs
Epinephrine injection
Nortriptyline overdose, venlafaxine overdose, albuterol, flecainide, metoprolol withdrawal, 5-fluorouracil, duloxetine
Cocaine abuse

RIGHT VENTRICLE INVOLVEMENT

Although Takotsubo primarily affects the left ventricle, it is estimated that about 34% of the patients experience some level of right ventricular involvement, it may, however, not be noticed at clinical presentation [62]. The involvement of the right ventricle can be imaged using MRI and echocardiography. Based on various observational retrospective investigations, the main segments of the right ventricle that are frequently affected include inferior walls, antero-lateral, and apical-lateral [63]. Other studies have shown that RV involvement may correlate with a cardiovascular complication such as in-hospital mortality, cardiogenic shock, and heart failure [63, 64]. Moreover, RV involvement tends to predominantly occur in older patients with a lower baseline left ventricular ejection fraction, an effect that leads to bilateral pleural effusions [63, 64].

Inverted Forms (Basal Pattern)

This pattern of Takotsubo is prevalent in patients of younger age, especially those who have a physical or emotional triggering event relative to those with a typical pattern [65]. Clinical estimates reveal that complication such as mitral regurgitation and heart failure are not highly prevalent in the inverted forms [65]. In contrast, subarachnoid hemorrhage is frequent in inverted forms [66]. Other studies have shown that some atypical forms, such as the reverse patterns, may lead to worse prognosis [62].

CLINICAL FEATURES

Most of the patients diagnosed with primary takotsubo are aged women who often report a stressful event [67]. In some cases, such patients may present symptoms of the panic disorder of anxiety [68, 69]. Based on studies, most patients do not have a prior history of stress-related psychological conditions. According to the most extensive research, up to 35% of cases did not have a stressful trigger, and up to 10% of takotsubo patients were younger women or men [68]. Therefore, it implies that stressful triggers, menopausal status, and sex are not mandatory characteristics and indeed, they are not listed as the criteria for diagnosis in the 2015 Heart Failure Association of the European Society of Cardiology (HFA) Takotsubo Syndrome Diagnostic Criteria. The most common features are acute chest pain of cardiac origin (angina), arrhythmia-triggered palpitations, or breathlessness. Left LVOTO, syncope or pre-syncope caused by ventricular tachyarrhythmias, or cardiogenic shock are diagnosed in severe cases. The occurrence of a pressure wave originating from the chest to the neck and into the head is diagnosed.

It is recommended that a resting 12-lead ECG should be acquired and such patients should be evaluated urgently. In less severe cases, where patients do not have pain, but with apparent takotsubo symptoms based on cardiac imaging, coronary computed tomography angiography may be performed [67]. For severe cases, based on symptoms, a coronary angiography test may be applied in some cases, and acute coronary syndrome management should be initiated using the European Society of Cardiology guidelines [70]. After confirmation of takotsubo using catheterization laboratory, testing for cardiac biomarkers and use of cardiac imaging can be applied to exclude myocardial infarction and to assess the risk. Because of the diverse nature of anatomical and clinical features of takotsubo, some borderline cases exist. In such cases, CMR imaging with late gadolinium enhancement (LGE) may be helpful [71, 72]. To examine the presence of complications and facilitate risk classification, CMR imaging can be applied to complement echocardiography and is highly sensitive for identifying left ventricular apical thrombus.

DIAGNOSIS OF TAKOTSUBO

Cardiac Magnetic Resonance (CMR)

CMR is an effective method of exploring the anatomical patterns, which is a powerful diagnostic tool used even during follow-up [73, 74]. Using CMR, it is proposed that the presence of the following features aid in the diagnosis of takotsubo [2]:

I. Abnormally high uptake of early myocardial gadolinium (reflected by an early EGE ratio ≥4.0 [optimal cutoff values may vary between scanners]);
II. No high-signal regions on LGE images (cutoff value of >5 standard deviations above the mean are defined as significant);
III. Transmural myocardial edema, which is a high signal intensity area on T2-weighted CMR collocated with a regional wall motion abnormality (edema should be verified by a quantitative signal intensity [SI] analysis, and it is best

to calculate the SI ratio between the myocardium and skeletal muscle [T2 SI ratio]; a cutoff value of $\geq$1.9 should be used to define edema); and

IV. Extreme dysfunction of the left ventricle without a non-coronary regional distribution pattern.

Moreover, many of these features may disappear during the chronic phase. The lack of LGE in takotsubo is a useful feature that distinguishes takotsubo from myocardial infarction as well as other myocarditis. But it is in some cases minor LGE may be observed in takotsubo patients [74].

Coronary Computed Tomography and Angiography Coronary Angiography

Based on coronary angiography, takotsubo patients may not present with coronary artery lesions, which may reflect left ventricular wall motion abnormalities and ST-segment elevation. It should be noted that some patients do have coronary artery lesions, which may indicate the coexistence of coronary artery disease and takotsubo [75]. In addition to this, coronary artery stenosis may not necessarily be present in patients with myocardial infarction. Coronary angiography should be urgently performed in cases where the patients manifest with ST-segment elevation and chest pain. With delayed presentation (longer than >48 hours after symptom onset) in a hemodynamically stable patient without chest pain at presentation, coronary computed tomography angiography is useful to differentiate between coronary artery disease and takotsubo [76].

Echocardiography

Another useful diagnostic technique is transthoracic echocardiography. It is a non-invasive imaging tool which enables visualization of cardiac rupture, mitral regurgitation, right ventricular involvement, thrombus formation, LVOTO, and the left ventricular function assessment and morphology when combined with echocardiography with color and tissue Doppler imaging [77]. Although distinguishing takotsubo from AMI is difficult; information derived from echocardiography is essential for achieving differential assessment. Unlike anteroseptal AMI, patients with apical ballooning pattern show symmetrical regional wall motion abnormalities that spread to lateral walls, inferior, and anterior based on transthoracic echocardiography [78]. The information derived from echocardiography also contains some hints that may be used to understand the pathomechanisms of takotsubo. For instance, Leva *et al.* reported a patient who had basal hyperkinesis at the early acute stage, which then transformed into apical ballooning. It, therefore, implies that hypercontraction at left ventricular basal region may increase the intraventricular pressure, triggering apical ballooning [79]. It has been found that severe mitral regurgitation, increased E/e' ratio, and low left ventricular ejection fraction findings from echocardiography are associated with significant adverse outcomes [77, 80].

Biomarkers

Some of the takotsubo patients are misdiagnosed with AMI due to the high levels of cardiac creatinine kinase and troponin found in more than 90% such patients. Moreover, the dynamic changes in troponin levels resemble that of AMI. But unlike AMI, the levels of creatinine kinase and troponin in takotsubo is small, which matches with the widespread wall motion abnormality. In the acute phase of takotsubo, the peak concentration of creatinine kinase is 500 U/La, and troponin is one ng/mL [81 - 83]. Other biomarkers found to be increased in sera of patients with takotsubo include cardiac natriuretic peptide which is known to be increased relative to patients with the acute coronary syndrome who have the same age and sex [84]. Moreover, the elevated concentration of troponin and BNP/NT-proBNP suggests poor prognosis and correlates with the severity of ventricular wall motion abnormalities [82, 83].

Electrocardiography

Up to 95% of takotsubo patients show electrocardiographic abnormalities [85, 86]. Within twelve hours after the appearance of first symptoms, left bundle branch block and ST-segment elevation and depression are diagnosed, this is accompanied with strong QT prolongation, deep and widespread T-wave inversions at 24–48 hours after symptoms onset. Significant QTc prolongation (>500 ms) is present, which leads to ventricular fibrillation and torsade de pointes (TdP) [86]. Since it appears the clinical manifestation of the symptoms changes from the onset, distinguishing this condition from ST-segment-elevation myocardial infarction (STEMI) at the initial stage is challenging. Thus, emergent coronary angiography is recommended to cases where there is ST-segment elevation on ECG. To this end, the ECG method is a basic diagnostic approach that can distinguish takotsubo cases from AMI [87, 88].

It was found that patients with anterior AMI had ST-segment elevation in leads V2–V4, but in those with takotsubo, ST-segment elevation frequently occurred in leads II, III, aVF, aVR, and V5–V6, facing the apical and inferolateral regions as well as the V2–V4 leads. Also, the wall motion abnormalities in takotsubo may also extend to the V1 lead regions. These criteria have a specificity and sensitivity of more than 90% in terms of differentiation takotsubo from anterior AMI based on a previous report [87]. But, whether these criteria are accurate need to be tested through prospective diagnosis.

THERAPEUTICS AND TREATMENT OPTIONS

General Treatment Approach

Since Takotsubo initially presents with symptoms that mimic AMI, the first approach should be geared to treating myocardial ischemia with β-blockers, aspirin, intravenous heparin, and oxygen inhalation. Once the diagnosis of takotsubo is confirmed, and there is no related coronary artery disease, then aspirin can be discontinued. Also, the use of thrombolytic agents may not be required since they may cause bleeding complications, and they offer no benefit to the patients.

Renin-Angiotensin-Aldosterone System Blockers

Majority of the reversible regional wall motion abnormality symptoms (RWMA) resolve spontaneously from few days to 1-2 weeks. Angiotensin-converting enzyme inhibitors or angiotensin II type 1 receptor blockers may be recommended for patients RWMA symptoms.

Beta-Blockers

Until now, the effectiveness of β-blockers for Takotsubo patients has not been clinically proven. In cases where there is no coronary spasm at the initial presentation, it is reasonable to administer β-blockers since high catecholamine levels might be precipitating the disease. If β-blockers are given, care should be taken to address any threating coronary spasm or heart failure that may arise after initiating β-blockers therapy. Indeed, β-blockers can prevent acute complications such as cardiogenic shock caused by ventricular rupture, ventricular arrhythmias, or LVOT obstruction.

Anticoagulation Therapy

Following the diagnosis of takotsubo cardiomyopathy, it is crucial to continue intravenous heparin, if well-tolerated, as a strategy to avoid the occurrence of left ventricular apical thrombosis. Together with warfarin, this therapy should be continued until RWMA resolves in the apical segment. Along with the treatment program, echocardiography should be performed to confirm the resolution of RWMA, after which warfarin can be discontinued.

Prognosis and Course of Takotsubo

Despite the clinical finding that reversible regional wall motion abnormality symptoms often disappear spontaneously within a period of days to a few weeks, it has been recognized that some cases of RWMA may persist even up to 3 months [89]. Similar findings have recently been reported by Lee *et al.* [90] and Shim *et al.* [91] in which some cases of takotsubo cardiomyopathy complicated by apical thrombosis were prolonged beyond the typical few-weeks resolution period. It is, therefore, worth noting that the outcomes of Takotsubo are not identical in patients. Moreover, the exact reasons for this scenario are not well-understood. More clinical studies are required to monitor the progress of the disease to initiate appropriate interventions for patients that do not recover spontaneously. In these cases, long-term management of apical thrombosis or heart failure should be given.

Although Takotsubo was previously thought to have a good prognosis, accumulating evidence shows that the in-hospital death rate ranges from 0% to 8% [92 - 94]. This indicates a favorable prognosis, although, some patients develop life-threatening complications. It has also been stated that ECG or echocardiographic recordings may help in determining short-term prognosis after diagnosis. For instance, Shimizu *et al.* suggested that a J wave, which appears transiently only at a very early stage, may indicate ventricular tachyarrhythmia or cardiac death [95] In their report, Citro et al found that reversible moderate to severe mitral regurgitation, E/e' ratio and left ventricular ejection fraction were independent predictors of major adverse cardiac events [96]. In cases where Takotsubo cardiomyopathy occurs in patients who are critically ill of other medical conditions [92, 97], the clinical outcomes of such patients may be influenced by the underlying disease instead of takotsubo cardiomyopathy itself.

Some Takotsubo patients may experience a recurrence within a few years after symptom remission. The recurrent rates range from 0% to 15% [93, 94, 98]. Four-year recurrence rate and prognosis of the apical ballooning syndrome study reported a recurrence rate of 10% in patients who were followed up to four years. Additionally, the recurrence was highest within the first four years, which decreased after that [98]. It has been shown in many case reports that takotsubo cardiomyopathy may be manifested as typical RWMA in the apical segment at the initial stage and atypical RWMA with apical sparing during a recurrence [99, 100]. Kurisu *et al.* recognized that takotsubo cardiomyopathy might develop even after administration of statins or aspirin, β-blockers, nitrates, or calcium-channel blockers [101]. Other studies found that the recurrence rate was not influenced by whether the patients received aspirin, statins, β-blockers, angiotensin II type 1 receptor blockers, or angiotensin-converting enzyme inhibitors [98]. Currently, there seem to be no conventional treatment or management strategies for long term follow-up. It is largely limited by the fact that the pathophysiology of takotsubo cardiomyopathy is not sufficiently understood [102, 103].

CONCLUSION, EMERGING ISSUES, AND FUTURE OUTLOOKS

Currently, there are no strategies for preventing Takotsubo. Although catecholamines have been implicated in the pathogenesis of Takotsubo, Santoro *et al.* reported that the use of beta-blockers or other drugs did not affect the risk of recurrence [104]. Nonetheless, Lyon *et al.* stated that beta-blockers can still be used for patients presenting with persistent anxiety elevated, ongoing cardiac symptoms, or sympathetic tone [105]. Moreover, one of the potential preventive approaches for stressful triggers is the use of cognitive behavioral therapy or psychological counseling [105]. While the effectiveness of such a strategy in preventing recurrence of Takotsubo has not been determined, it appears reasonable considering the high correlation between this condition and psychiatric disorders [106].

Cardioprotective Effects of Estrogen

Nearly 90% of Takotsubo patients are menopausal women aged above 60 years, which has led to the recognition that sex hormones, especially estrogen, may have a role in modulating susceptibility to stress-induced cardiomyopathy. Indeed, several studies have documented evidence for the regulatory role of estrogen on βeta-adrenergic receptors function during cardiac stress [107]. Some of the cardioprotective effects of estrogen are linked to the prevention of cardiac hypertrophy, reduction of infarct size, prevention of ischemia-reperfusion injury, promotion of blood vessels relaxation, vascular endothelial cell proliferation and migration, reduction of migration and proliferation of vascular smooth muscle cells, reduction of myocardial cholesterol levels and low-density lipoprotein (LDL), and prevention of insulin resistance [107]. Estrogen receptors are widely distributed in many cells of the cardiovascular system and the nervous system. It is therefore expected that future studies are likely to reveal the mechanistic pathways that like estrogen to Takotsubo.

Long-Term Etiology and Link to Heart Failure Hypothesis

Heart failure (HF) is the leading cause of mortality worldwide [108]. Several heart diseases and conditions such as Takotsubo cardiomyopathy, myocardial infarction, hypertrophic cardiomyopathy, and coronary artery disease affect the heart's function leading to HF. On this basis, HF can be thought of as an outcome in the wake of structural or functional cardiac changes associated with the above diseases. Although Takotsubo patients recover entirely within a few weeks [109], some group of Takotsubo patients, fatal complications arise that results in heart failure. Such complications include congestive heart failure and lethal arrhythmias [109]. As mentioned previously, 90% of Takotsubo patients are postmenopausal, while men account for less than 10% [4]. Moreover, the overall incidence of HF is slightly lower in women compared to men, while the prevalence of HF is similar between aged men and women. In this regard, it is conceivable to interpret Takotsubo as an intermediate cardioprotective strategy against progression into HF in women (Fig. **4**).

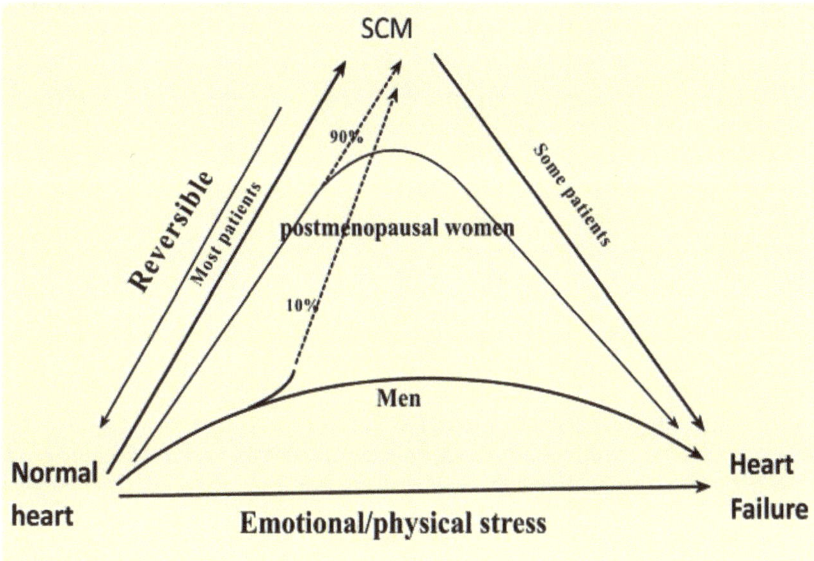

Fig. (4). Possible correlation between Takotsubo and Heart Failure.

It is possible that Takotsubo activates pathways that are intended to preserve the heart function in response to stress. These pathways may include molecular elements such as the emerging role of Non-coding miRNA in Takotsubo. Among the biomarkers of Takotsubo detected by Jaguszewski *et al.* included abnormally high levels of miR-26a and miR-16 relative to STEMI and healthy groups [110]. These findings indicate that there is a wide range of factors that regulate the pathogenesis of this condition.

CONSENT FOR PUBLICATION

Not applicable.

CONFLICT OF INTEREST

The authors confirm that this chapter contents have no conflict of interest.

ACKNOWLEDGEMENTS

Declared none.

REFERENCE

[1] Sato H, Tateishi H, Dote K, Uchida T, Ishihara M. Tako-tsubo-like left ventricular dysfunction due to multivessel coronary spasm.Clinical aspect of myocardial injury: from ischemia to heart failure. Tokyo: Kagakuhyoronsha Publishing Co. 1990; pp. 56-64.

[2] Tsuchihashi K, Ueshima K, Uchida T, *et al.* Transient left ventricular apical ballooning without coronary artery stenosis: a novel heart syndrome mimicking acute myocardial infarction. Angina Pectoris-Myocardial Infarction Investigations in Japan. J Am Coll Cardiol 2001; 38(1): 11-8. [http://dx.doi.org/10.1016/S0735-1097(01)01316-X] [PMID: 11451258]

[3] Kawai S, Suzuki H, Yamaguchi H, *et al.* Ampulla cardiomyopathy ('Takotusbo' cardiomyopathy)--reversible left ventricular dysfunction: with ST segment elevation. Jpn Circ J 2000; 64(2): 156-9. [http://dx.doi.org/10.1253/jcj.64.156] [PMID: 10716533]

[4] Dote K, Sato H, Tateishi H, Uchida T, Ishihara M. [Myocardial stunning due to simultaneous multivessel coronary spasms: a review of 5 cases]. J Cardiol 1991; 21(2): 203-14. [Myocardial stunning due to simultaneous multivessel coronary spasms: a review of 5 cases]. [PMID: 1841907]

[5] Eitel I, von Knobelsdorff-Brenkenhoff F, Bernhardt P, *et al.* Clinical characteristics and cardiovascular magnetic resonance findings in stress (takotsubo) cardiomyopathy. JAMA 2011; 306(3): 277-86. [http://dx.doi.org/10.1001/jama.2011.992] [PMID: 21771988]

[6] Maron BJ, Towbin JA, Thiene G, *et al.* Contemporary definitions and classification of the cardiomyopathies an American heart association scientific statement from the council on clinical cardiology, heart failure and transplantation committee; quality of care and outcomes research and functional genomics and translational biology interdisciplinary working groups; and council on epidemiology and prevention. Circulation 2006; 113(14): 1807-16. [http://dx.doi.org/10.1161/CIRCULATIONAHA.106.174287] [PMID: 16567565]

[7] Sharkey SW, Lesser JR, Zenovich AG, *et al.* Acute and reversible cardiomyopathy provoked by stress in women from the United States. Circulation 2005; 111(4): 472-9. [http://dx.doi.org/10.1161/01.CIR.0000153801.51470.EB] [PMID: 15687136]

[8] Ito K, Sugihara H, Kawasaki T, *et al.* Assessment of ampulla (Takotsubo) cardiomyopathy with coronary angiography, two-dimensional echocardiography and 99mTc-tetrofosmin myocardial single photon emission computed tomography. Ann Nucl Med 2001; 15(4): 351-5. [http://dx.doi.org/10.1007/BF02988242] [PMID: 11577760]

[9] Goh AC, Wong S, Zaroff JG, Shafaee N, Lundstrom RJ. Comparing Anxiety and Depression in Patients With Takotsubo Stress Cardiomyopathy to Those With Acute Coronary Syndrome. J Cardiopulm Rehabil Prev 2016; 32(2): 106-1. [http://dx.doi.org/10.1097/HCR.0000000000000152] [PMID: 26468629]

[10] Zorzi A, Baritussio A, ElMaghawry M, *et al.* Differential diagnosis at admission between Takotsubo cardiomyopathy and acute apical-anterior myocardial infarction in postmenopausal women. Eur Heart J Acute Cardiovasc Care 2016; 5(4): 298-307. [http://dx.doi.org/10.1177/2048872615585515] [PMID: 25964511]

[11] Guerra F, Giannini I, Capucci A. The ECG in the differential diagnosis between takotsubo cardiomyopathy and acute coronary syndrome. Expert Rev Cardiovasc Ther 2017; 15(2): 137-44. [http://dx.doi.org/10.1080/14779072.2017.1276441] [PMID: 28005450]

[12] Isogai T, Matsui H, Tanaka H, Fushimi K, Yasunaga H. Early β-blocker use and in-hospital mortality in patients with Takotsubo cardiomyopathy. Heart 2016; 102(13): 1029-35. [http://dx.doi.org/10.1136/heartjnl-2015-308712] [PMID: 26879240]

[13] Khalid N, Iqbal I, Coram R, Raza T, Fahsah I, Ikram S. Thrombolysis In Myocardial Infarction Frame Count in Takotsubo Cardiomyopathy. Int J Cardiol 2015; 191: 107-8. [http://dx.doi.org/10.1016/j.ijcard.2015.04.192] [PMID: 25965614]

[14] Templin C, Ghadri JR, Diekmann J, *et al.* Clinical features and outcomes of takotsubo (stress) cardiomyopathy. N Engl J Med 2015; 373(10): 929-38.
[http://dx.doi.org/10.1056/NEJMoa1406761] [PMID: 26332547]

[15] Nascimento FO, Larrauri-Reyes MC, Santana O, Pérez-Caminero M, Lamas GA. Comparison of stress cardiomyopathy in Hispanic and non-Hispanic patients. Rev Esp Cardiol (Engl Ed) 2013; 66(1): 67-8.
[http://dx.doi.org/10.1016/j.rec.2012.05.006] [PMID: 22921457]

[16] Minhas AS, Hughey AB, Kolias TJ. Nationwide trends in reported incidence of takotsubo cardiomyopathy from 2006 to 2012. Am J Cardiol 2015; 116(7): 1128-31.
[http://dx.doi.org/10.1016/j.amjcard.2015.06.042] [PMID: 26279109]

[17] Khera R, Light-McGroary K, Zahr F, Horwitz PA, Girotra S. Trends in hospitalization for takotsubo cardiomyopathy in the United States. Am Heart J 2016; 172: 53-63.
[http://dx.doi.org/10.1016/j.ahj.2015.10.022] [PMID: 26856216]

[18] Isogai T, Matsui H, Tanaka H, Fushimi K, Yasunaga H. Early β-blocker use and in-hospital mortality in patients with Takotsubo cardiomyopathy. Heart 2016; 102(13): 1029-35.
[http://dx.doi.org/10.1136/heartjnl-2015-308712] [PMID: 26879240]

[19] Brinjikji W, El-Sayed AM, Salka S. In-hospital mortality among patients with takotsubo cardiomyopathy: a study of the National Inpatient Sample 2008 to 2009. Am Heart J 2012; 164(2): 215-21.
[http://dx.doi.org/10.1016/j.ahj.2012.04.010] [PMID: 22877807]

[20] Singh K, Carson K, Usmani Z, Sawhney G, Shah R, Horowitz J. Systematic review and meta-analysis of incidence and correlates of recurrence of takotsubo cardiomyopathy. Int J Cardiol 2014; 174(3): 696-701.
[http://dx.doi.org/10.1016/j.ijcard.2014.04.221] [PMID: 24809923]

[21] El-Battrawy I, Santoro F, Stiermaier T, *et al.* Incidence and Clinical Impact of Recurrent Takotsubo Syndrome: Results From the GEIST Registry. J Am Heart Assoc 2019; 8(9)e010753
[http://dx.doi.org/10.1161/JAHA.118.010753] [PMID: 31046506]

[22] Agrawal S, Shirani J, Garg L, *et al.* Pheochromocytoma and stress cardiomyopathy: Insight into pathogenesis. World J Cardiol 2017; 9(3): 255-60.
[http://dx.doi.org/10.4330/wjc.v9.i3.255] [PMID: 28400922]

[23] Burgdorf C, Kurowski V, Radke PW. Long-term prognosis of transient left ventricular ballooning syndrome and cancer. Heart Lung 2011; 40(5): 472.
[http://dx.doi.org/10.1016/j.hrtlng.2010.06.005] [PMID: 20723983]

[24] Tara C. Gangadhar, Elisabeth Von der Lohe, Stephen G Sawada, Paul R Helft. Takotsubo cardiomyopathy in a patient with esophageal cancer: A case report J Med Case Reports 2008; 2: 379.
[http://dx.doi.org/10.1186/1752-1947-2-379]

[25] Pelliccia F, Parodi G, Greco C, *et al.* Comorbidities frequency in Takotsubo syndrome: an international collaborative systematic review including 1109 patients. Am J Med 2015; 128(6): 654.e11-9.
[http://dx.doi.org/10.1016/j.amjmed.2015.01.016] [PMID: 25660245]

[26] El-Sayed AM, Brinjikji W, Salka S. Demographic and co-morbid predictors of stress (takotsubo) cardiomyopathy. Am J Cardiol 2012; 110(9): 1368-72.
[http://dx.doi.org/10.1016/j.amjcard.2012.06.041] [PMID: 22819424]

[27] Burgdorf C, von Hof K, Schunkert H, Kurowski V. Regional alterations in myocardial sympathetic innervation in patients with transient left-ventricular apical ballooning (Tako-Tsubo cardiomyopathy). J Nucl Cardiol 2008; 15(1): 65-72.
[http://dx.doi.org/10.1016/j.nuclcard.2007.08.005] [PMID: 18242481]

[28] Sattler K, El-Battrawy I, Lang S, *et al.* Prevalence of cancer in Takotsubo cardiomyopathy: Short and long-term outcome. Int J Cardiol 2017; 238: 159-65.

[http://dx.doi.org/10.1016/j.ijcard.2017.02.093] [PMID: 28318661]

[29] Burgdorf C, Nef HM, Haghi D, Kurowski V, Radke PW. Tako-tsubo (stress-induced) cardiomyopathy and cancer. Ann Intern Med 2010; 152(12): 830-1. [http://dx.doi.org/10.7326/0003-4819-152-12-201006150-00026] [PMID: 20547921]

[30] Dias A, Franco E, Figueredo VM, Hebert K, Quevedo HC. Occurrence of Takotsubo cardiomyopathy and use of antidepressants. Int J Cardiol 2014; 174(2): 433-6. [http://dx.doi.org/10.1016/j.ijcard.2014.04.028] [PMID: 24768456]

[31] Bank IEM, de Hoog VC, de Kleijn DPV, *et al.* Sex-based differences in the performance of the heart score in patients presenting to the emergency department with acute chest pain. J Am Heart Assoc 2017; 6(6)e005373 [http://dx.doi.org/10.1161/JAHA.116.005373] [PMID: 28637780]

[32] Goodloe AH, Evans JM, Middha S, Prasad A, Olson TM. Characterizing genetic variation of adrenergic signalling pathways in Takotsubo (stress) cardiomyopathy exomes. Eur J Heart Fail 2014; 16(9): 942-9. [http://dx.doi.org/10.1002/ejhf.145] [PMID: 25132214]

[33] Adele HG, Jared ME, Middha S, Prasad A, Olson TM. Characterizing genetic variation of adrenergic signaling pathways in Takotsubo (stress) cardiomyopathy exome. Eur J Heart Fail 2014; 16: 942-9. [http://dx.doi.org/10.1002/ejhf.145]

[34] Dorn GW II. Adrenergic signaling polymorphisms and their impact on cardiovascular disease. Physiol Rev 2010; 90(3): 1013-62. [http://dx.doi.org/10.1152/physrev.00001.2010] [PMID: 20664078]

[35] Citro R, d'Avenia M, De Marco M, *et al.* Polymorphisms of the antiapoptotic protein bag3 may play a role in the pathogenesis of tako-tsubo cardiomyopathy. Int J Cardiol 2013; 168(2): 1663-5. [http://dx.doi.org/10.1016/j.ijcard.2013.03.050] [PMID: 23582692]

[36] d'Avenia M, Citro R, De Marco M, *et al.* A novel miR-371a-5p-mediated pathway, leading to BAG3 upregulation in cardiomyocytes in response to epinephrine, is lost in Takotsubo cardiomyopathy. Cell Death Dis 2015; 6(10)e1948. [http://dx.doi.org/10.1038/cddis.2015.280] [PMID: 26512958]

[37] Zaroff JG, Pawlikowska L, Miss JC, *et al.* Adrenoceptor polymorphisms and the risk of cardiac injury and dysfunction after subarachnoid hemorrhage. Stroke 2006; 37(7): 1680-5. [http://dx.doi.org/10.1161/01.STR.0000226461.52423.dd] [PMID: 16728691]

[38] Sharkey SW, Maron BJ, Nelson P, Parpart M, Maron MS, Bristow MR. Adrenergic receptor polymorphisms in patients with stress (tako-tsubo) cardiomyopathy. J Cardiol 2009; 53(1): 53-7. [http://dx.doi.org/10.1016/j.jjcc.2008.08.006] [PMID: 19167638]

[39] Spinelli L, Trimarco V, Di Marino S, Marino M, Iaccarino G, Trimarco B. L41Q polymorphism of the G protein coupled receptor kinase 5 is associated with left ventricular apical ballooning syndrome. Eur J Heart Fail 2010; 12(1): 13-6. [http://dx.doi.org/10.1093/eurjhf/hfp173] [PMID: 20023040]

[40] Handy AD, Prasad A, Olson TM. Investigating genetic variation of adrenergic receptors in familial stress cardiomyopathy (apical ballooning syndrome). J Cardiol 2009; 54(3): 516-7. [http://dx.doi.org/10.1016/j.jjcc.2009.08.008] [PMID: 19944334]

[41] Nef HM, Möllmann H, Akashi YJ, Hamm CW. Mechanisms of stress (Takotsubo) cardiomyopathy. Nat Rev Cardiol 2010; 7(4): 187-93. [http://dx.doi.org/10.1038/nrcardio.2010.16] [PMID: 20195267]

[42] Y-Hassan S, Yamasaki K. History of takotsubo syndrome: is the syndrome really described as a disease entity first in 1990? Some inaccuracies. Int J Cardiol 2013; 166(3): 736-7. [http://dx.doi.org/10.1016/j.ijcard.2012.09.183] [PMID: 23073280]

[43] Akashi YJ, Nef HM, Lyon AR. Epidemiology and pathophysiology of Takotsubo syndrome. Nat Rev

Cardiol 2015; 12(7): 387-97.
[http://dx.doi.org/10.1038/nrcardio.2015.39] [PMID: 25855605]

[44] Dilsizian V, Taillefer R. Journey in evolution of nuclear cardiology: will there be another quantum leap with the F-18-labeled myocardial perfusion tracers? JACC Cardiovasc Imaging 2012; 5(12): 1269-84.
[http://dx.doi.org/10.1016/j.jcmg.2012.10.006] [PMID: 23236979]

[45] Ghadri JR, Wittstein IS, Prasad A, *et al.* International Expert Consensus Document on Takotsubo Syndrome (Part I): Clinical Characteristics, Diagnostic Criteria, and Pathophysiology. Eur Heart J 2018; 39(22): 2032-46.
[http://dx.doi.org/10.1093/eurheartj/ehy076] [PMID: 29850871]

[46] Matsuo S, Nakajima K, Kinuya S, Yamagishi M. Diagnostic utility of 123I-BMIPP imaging in patients with Takotsubo cardiomyopathy. J Cardiol 2014; 64(1): 49-56.
[http://dx.doi.org/10.1016/j.jjcc.2013.10.019] [PMID: 24331764]

[47] Dilsizian V. 18F-FDG uptake as a surrogate marker for antecedent ischemia. J Nucl Med 2008; 49(12): 1909-11.
[http://dx.doi.org/10.2967/jnumed.108.053892] [PMID: 18997055]

[48] Taegtmeyer H, Dilsizian V. Imaging cardiac metabolism.Atlas of nuclear Cardiology. 4th ed. New York: Springer 2013; pp. 289-321.
[http://dx.doi.org/10.1007/978-1-4614-5551-6_8]

[49] Pilgrim TM, Wyss TR. Takotsubo cardiomyopathy or transient left ventricular apical ballooning syndrome: A systematic review. Int J Cardiol 2008; 124(3): 283-92.
[http://dx.doi.org/10.1016/j.ijcard.2007.07.002] [PMID: 17651841]

[50] Angelini P. Transient left ventricular apical ballooning: A unifying pathophysiologic theory at the edge of Prinzmetal angina. Catheter Cardiovasc Interv 2008; 71(3): 342-52.
[http://dx.doi.org/10.1002/ccd.21338] [PMID: 18288755]

[51] Cowburn PJ, Cleland JG, McArthur JD, *et al.* Endothelin-1 has haemodynamic effects at pathophysiological concentrations in patients with left ventricular dysfunction. Cardiovasc Res 1998; 39(3): 563-70.
[http://dx.doi.org/10.1016/S0008-6363(98)00084-4] [PMID: 9861298]

[52] El Mahmoud R, Mansencal N, Pilliére R, *et al.* Prevalence and characteristics of left ventricular outflow tract obstruction in Tako-Tsubo syndrome. Am Heart J 2008; 156(3): 543-8.
[http://dx.doi.org/10.1016/j.ahj.2008.05.002] [PMID: 18760139]

[53] Y-Hassan S. YH S. Clinical features and outcome of pheochromocytoma- induced takotsubo syndrome: analysis of 80 published cases. Am J Cardiol 2016; 117(11): 1836-44.
[http://dx.doi.org/10.1016/j.amjcard.2016.03.019] [PMID: 27103159]

[54] Y-Hassan S, Tornvall P. Epidemiology, pathogenesis, and management of takotsubo syndrome. Clin Auton Res 2018; 28(1): 53-65.
[http://dx.doi.org/10.1007/s10286-017-0465-z] [PMID: 28917022]

[55] Lyon AR, Rees PS, Prasad S, Poole-Wilson PA, Harding SE. Stress (Takotsubo) cardiomyopathy - A novel pathophysiological hypothesis to explain catecholamine-induced acute myocardial stunning. Nat Clin Pract Cardiovasc Med 2008; 5(1): 22-9.
[http://dx.doi.org/10.1038/ncpcardio1066] [PMID: 18094670]

[56] Kawano H, Okada R, Yano K. Histological study on the distribution of autonomic nerves in the human heart. Heart Vessels 2003; 18(1): 32-9.
[http://dx.doi.org/10.1007/s003800300005] [PMID: 12644879]

[57] Paur H, Wright PT, Sikkel MB, *et al.* High levels of circulating epinephrine trigger apical cardiodepression in a β2-adrenergic receptor/Gi-dependent manner: a new model of Takotsubo cardiomyopathy. Circulation 2012; 126(6): 697-706.

[http://dx.doi.org/10.1161/CIRCULATIONAHA.112.111591] [PMID: 22732314]

[58] Heubach JF, Blaschke M, Harding SE, Ravens U, Kaumann AJ. Cardiostimulant and cardiodepressant effects through overexpressed human beta2-adrenoceptors in murine heart: regional differences and functional role of beta1-adrenoceptors. Naunyn Schmiedebergs Arch Pharmacol 2003; 367(4): 380-90. [http://dx.doi.org/10.1007/s00210-002-0681-4] [PMID: 12690430]

[59] Heubach JF, Ravens U, Kaumann AJ. Epinephrine activates both Gs and Gi pathways, but norepinephrine activates only the Gs pathway through human beta2-adrenoceptors overexpressed in mouse heart. Mol Pharmacol 2004; 65(5): 1313-22. [http://dx.doi.org/10.1124/mol.65.5.1313] [PMID: 15102960]

[60] Chesley A, Lundberg MS, Asai T, *et al.* The beta(2)-adrenergic receptor delivers an antiapoptotic signal to cardiac myocytes through G(i)-dependent coupling to phosphatidylinositol 3′-kinase. Circ Res 2000; 87(12): 1172-9. [http://dx.doi.org/10.1161/01.RES.87.12.1172] [PMID: 11110775]

[61] Shao Y, Redfors B, Scharin Täng M, *et al.* Novel rat model reveals important roles of β-adrenoreceptors in stress-induced cardiomyopathy. Int J Cardiol 2013; 168(3): 1943-50. [http://dx.doi.org/10.1016/j.ijcard.2012.12.092] [PMID: 23357048]

[62] Lyon AR, Bossone E, Schneider B, *et al.* Current state of knowledge on Takotsubo syndrome: a Position Statement from the Taskforce on Takotsubo Syndrome of the Heart Failure Association of the European Society of Cardiology. Eur J Heart Fail 2016; 18(1): 8-27. [http://dx.doi.org/10.1002/ejhf.424] [PMID: 26548803]

[63] Templin C, Ghadri JR, Diekmann J, *et al.* Clinical Features and Outcomes of Takotsubo (Stress) Cardiomyopathy. N Engl J Med 2015; 373(10): 929-38. [http://dx.doi.org/10.1056/NEJMoa1406761] [PMID: 26332547]

[64] Ghadri JR, Cammann VL, Napp LC, *et al.* Differences in the clinical profile and outcomes of typical and atypical takotsubo syndrome: data from the international takotsubo registry. JAMA Cardiol 2016; 1(3): 335-40. [http://dx.doi.org/10.1001/jamacardio.2016.0225] [PMID: 27438117]

[65] Angelini P. Reverse, or inverted, transient Takotsubo cardiomyopathy: terms and status of an open discussion. Tex Heart Inst J 2013; 40(1): 60-3. [PMID: 23468584]

[66] Elgendy AY, Elgendy IY, Mansoor H, Mahmoud AN. Clinical presentations and outcomes of Takotsubo syndrome in the setting of subarachnoid hemorrhage: A systematic review and meta-analysis. Eur Heart J Acute Cardiovasc Care 2018; 7(3): 236-45. [http://dx.doi.org/10.1177/2048872616679792] [PMID: 27852798]

[67] Otalvaro L, Zambrano JP, Fishman JE. Takotsubo cardiomyopathy: utility of cardiac computed tomography angiography for acute diagnosis. J Thorac Imaging 2011; 26(3): W83-5. [http://dx.doi.org/10.1097/RTI.0b013e3181eebc2d] [PMID: 20921912]

[68] Deshmukh A, Kumar G, Pant S, Rihal C, Murugiah K, Mehta JL. Prevalence of Takotsubo cardiomyopathy in the United States. Am Heart J 2012; 164(1): 66-71.e1. [http://dx.doi.org/10.1016/j.ahj.2012.03.020] [PMID: 22795284]

[69] Summers MR, Prasad A. Takotsubo cardiomyopathy: definition and clinical profile. Heart Fail Clin 2013; 9(2): 111-122, vii. [vii.]. [http://dx.doi.org/10.1016/j.hfc.2012.12.007] [PMID: 23562112]

[70] Steg PG, James SK, Atar D, *et al.* ESC Guidelines for the management of acute myocardial infarction in patients presenting with ST-segment elevation. Eur Heart J 2012; 33(20): 2569-619. [http://dx.doi.org/10.1093/eurheartj/ehs215] [PMID: 22922416]

[71] Haghi D, Athanasiadis A, Papavassiliu T, *et al.* Right ventricular involvement in Takotsubo cardiomyopathy. Eur Heart J 2006; 27(20): 2433-9.

[http://dx.doi.org/10.1093/eurheartj/ehl274] [PMID: 17000628]

[72] Bratis K. Cardiac Magnetic Resonance in Takotsubo Syndrome. Eur Cardiol 2017; 12(1): 58-62. [http://dx.doi.org/10.15420/ecr.2017:7:2] [PMID: 30416553]

[73] Iacucci I, Carbone I, Cannavale G, *et al.* Myocardial oedema as the sole marker of acute injury in Takotsubo cardiomyopathy: a cardiovascular magnetic resonance (CMR) study. Radiol Med (Torino) 2013; 118(8): 1309-23. [http://dx.doi.org/10.1007/s11547-013-0931-1] [PMID: 23716287]

[74] Gaikwad N, Butler T, Maxwell R, *et al.* Late gadolinium enhancement does occur in Tako-tsubo cardiomyopathy - A quantitative cardiac magnetic resonance and speckle tracking strain study. Int J Cardiol Heart Vasc 2016; 12: 68-74. [http://dx.doi.org/10.1016/j.ijcha.2016.07.009] [PMID: 28616546]

[75] Gaibazzi N, Ugo F, Vignali L, Zoni A, Reverberi C, Gherli T. Tako-Tsubo cardiomyopathy with coronary artery stenosis: a case-series challenging the original definition. Int J Cardiol 2009; 133(2): 205-12. [http://dx.doi.org/10.1016/j.ijcard.2007.12.037] [PMID: 18313156]

[76] Bossone E, Lyon A, Citro R, *et al.* Takotsubo cardiomyopathy: an integrated multi-imaging approach. Eur Heart J Cardiovasc Imaging 2014; 15(4): 366-77. [http://dx.doi.org/10.1093/ehjci/jet167] [PMID: 24128655]

[77] Citro R, Lyon AR, Meimoun P, *et al.* Standard and advanced echocardiography in takotsubo (stress) cardiomyopathy: clinical and prognostic implications. J Am Soc Echocardiogr 2015; 28(1): 57-74. [http://dx.doi.org/10.1016/j.echo.2014.08.020] [PMID: 25282664]

[78] Citro R, Rigo F, Ciampi Q, *et al.* Echocardiographic assessment of regional left ventricular wall motion abnormalities in patients with tako-tsubo cardiomyopathy: comparison with anterior myocardial infarction. Eur J Echocardiogr 2011; 12(7): 542-9. [http://dx.doi.org/10.1093/ejechocard/jer059] [PMID: 21606046]

[79] Ieva R, Santoro F, Ferraretti A, *et al.* Hyper-acute precipitating mechanism of Tako-Tsubo cardiomyopathy: in the beginning was basal hyperkinesis? Int J Cardiol 2013; 167(3): e55-7. [http://dx.doi.org/10.1016/j.ijcard.2013.03.138] [PMID: 23628296]

[80] Citro R, Rigo F, D'Andrea A, *et al.* Echocardiographic correlates of acute heart failure, cardiogenic shock, and in-hospital mortality in tako-tsubo cardiomyopathy. JACC Cardiovasc Imaging 2014; 7(2): 119-29. [http://dx.doi.org/10.1016/j.jcmg.2013.09.020] [PMID: 24412188]

[81] Akashi YJ, Goldstein DS, Barbaro G, Ueyama T. Takotsubo cardiomyopathy: a new form of acute, reversible heart failure. Circulation 2008; 118(25): 2754-62. [http://dx.doi.org/10.1161/CIRCULATIONAHA.108.767012] [PMID: 19106400]

[82] Madhavan M, Borlaug BA, Lerman A, Rihal CS, Prasad A. Stress hormone and circulating biomarker profile of apical ballooning syndrome (Takotsubo cardiomyopathy): insights into the clinical significance of B-type natriuretic peptide and troponin levels. Heart 2009; 95(17): 1436-41. [http://dx.doi.org/10.1136/hrt.2009.170399] [PMID: 19468013]

[83] Fröhlich GM, Schoch B, Schmid F, *et al.* Takotsubo cardiomyopathy has a unique cardiac biomarker profile: NT-proBNP/myoglobin and NT-proBNP/troponin T ratios for the differential diagnosis of acute coronary syndromes and stress induced cardiomyopathy. Int J Cardiol 2012; 154(3): 328-32. [http://dx.doi.org/10.1016/j.ijcard.2011.09.077] [PMID: 22044675]

[84] Gopalakrishnan P, Zaidi R, Sardar MR. Takotsubo cardiomyopathy: Pathophysiology and role of cardiac biomarkers in differential diagnosis. World J Cardiol 2017; 9(9): 723-30. [http://dx.doi.org/10.4330/wjc.v9.i9.723] [PMID: 29081904]

[85] Ogura R, Hiasa Y, Takahashi T, *et al.* Specific findings of the standard 12-lead ECG in patients with 'Takotsubo' cardiomyopathy: comparison with the findings of acute anterior myocardial infarction.

Circ J 2003; 67(8): 687-90.
[http://dx.doi.org/10.1253/circj.67.687] [PMID: 12890911]

[86] Kurisu S, Inoue I, Kawagoe T, *et al.* Time course of electrocardiographic changes in patients with tako-tsubo syndrome: comparison with acute myocardial infarction with minimal enzymatic release. Circ J 2004; 68(1): 77-81.
[http://dx.doi.org/10.1253/circj.68.77] [PMID: 14695470]

[87] Kosuge M, Ebina T, Hibi K, *et al.* Simple and accurate electrocardiographic criteria to differentiate takotsubo cardiomyopathy from anterior acute myocardial infarction. J Am Coll Cardiol 2010; 55(22): 2514-6.
[http://dx.doi.org/10.1016/j.jacc.2009.12.059] [PMID: 20510222]

[88] Kosuge M, Kimura K. Electrocardiographic findings of takotsubo cardiomyopathy as compared with those of anterior acute myocardial infarction. J Electrocardiol 2014; 47(5): 684-9.
[http://dx.doi.org/10.1016/j.jelectrocard.2014.03.004] [PMID: 24735641]

[89] Kurisu S, Inoue I, Kawagoe T, *et al.* Persistent left ventricular dysfunction in takotsubo cardiomyopathy after pacemaker implantation. Circ J 2006; 70(5): 641-4.
[http://dx.doi.org/10.1253/circj.70.641] [PMID: 16636505]

[90] Lee PH, Song JK, Park IK, *et al.* Takotsubo cardiomyopathy: a case of persistent apical ballooning complicated by an apical mural thrombus. Korean J Intern Med (Korean Assoc Intern Med) 2011; 26(4): 455-9.
[http://dx.doi.org/10.3904/kjim.2011.26.4.455] [PMID: 22205847]

[91] Shim IK, Kim BJ, Kim H, Lee JW, Cha TJ, Heo JH. A case of persistent apical ballooning complicated by apical thrombus in takotsubo cardiomyopathy of systemic lupus erythematosus patient. J Cardiovasc Ultrasound 2013; 21(3): 137-9.
[http://dx.doi.org/10.4250/jcu.2013.21.3.137] [PMID: 24198920]

[92] Redfors B, Vedad R, Angerås O, *et al.* Mortality in takotsubo syndrome is similar to mortality in myocardial infarction - A report from the SWEDEHEART registry. Int J Cardiol 2015; 185: 282-9.
[http://dx.doi.org/10.1016/j.ijcard.2015.03.162] [PMID: 25818540]

[93] Sharkey SW, Windenburg DC, Lesser JR, *et al.* Natural history and expansive clinical profile of stress (tako-tsubo) cardiomyopathy. J Am Coll Cardiol 2010; 55(4): 333-41.
[http://dx.doi.org/10.1016/j.jacc.2009.08.057] [PMID: 20117439]

[94] Desmet WJ, Adriaenssens BF, Dens JA. Apical ballooning of the left ventricle: first series in white patients. Heart 2003; 89(9): 1027-31.
[http://dx.doi.org/10.1136/heart.89.9.1027] [PMID: 12923018]

[95] Shimizu M, Nishizaki M, Yamawake N, *et al.* J wave and fragmented QRS formation during the hyperacute phase in Takotsubo cardiomyopathy. Circ J 2014; 78(4): 943-9.
[http://dx.doi.org/10.1253/circj.CJ-13-1296] [PMID: 24500071]

[96] Citro R, Rigo F, D'Andrea A, *et al.* Echocardiographic correlates of acute heart failure, cardiogenic shock, and in-hospital mortality in tako-tsubo cardiomyopathy. JACC Cardiovasc Imaging 2014; 7(2): 119-29.
[http://dx.doi.org/10.1016/j.jcmg.2013.09.020] [PMID: 24412188]

[97] Park JH, Kang SJ, Song JK, *et al.* Left ventricular apical ballooning due to severe physical stress in patients admitted to the medical ICU. Chest 2005; 128(1): 296-302.
[http://dx.doi.org/10.1378/chest.128.1.296] [PMID: 16002949]

[98] Elesber AA, Prasad A, Lennon RJ, Wright RS, Lerman A, Rihal CS. Four-year recurrence rate and prognosis of the apical ballooning syndrome. J Am Coll Cardiol 2007; 50(5): 448-52.
[http://dx.doi.org/10.1016/j.jacc.2007.03.050] [PMID: 17662398]

[99] Migliore F, Zorzi A, Perazzolo Marra M, *et al.* Typical and atypical Takotsubo syndrome in the same patient. Int J Cardiol 2013; 162: e28-e30.

[http://dx.doi.org/10.1016/j.ijcard.2012.05.032]

[100] Xu B, Williams PD, Brown M, Macisaac A. Takotsubo cardiomyopathy: does recurrence tend to occur in a previously unaffected ventricular wall region? Circulation 2014; 129(7): e339-40. [http://dx.doi.org/10.1161/CIRCULATIONAHA.113.007015] [PMID: 24550555]

[101] Kurisu S, Inoue I, Kawagoe T, *et al.* Assessment of medications in patients with tako-tsubo cardiomyopathy. Int J Cardiol 2009; 134: e120-e123. [http://dx.doi.org/10.1016/j.ijcard.2008.01.026]

[102] Suzuki H, Matsumoto Y, Kaneta T, *et al.* Evidence for brain activation in patients with takotsubo cardiomyopathy. Circ J 2014; 78(1): 256-8. [http://dx.doi.org/10.1253/circj.CJ-13-1276] [PMID: 24284957]

[103] Delmas C, Lairez O, Mulin E, *et al.* Anxiodepressive disorders and chronic psychological stress are associated with Tako-Tsubo cardiomyopathy- New Physiopathological Hypothesis. Circ J 2013; 77(1): 175-80. [http://dx.doi.org/10.1253/circj.CJ-12-0759] [PMID: 22987076]

[104] Santoro F, Ieva R, Musaico F, *et al.* Lack of efficacy of drug therapy in preventing takotsubo cardiomyopathy recurrence: a meta-analysis. Clin Cardiol 2014; 37(7): 434-9. [http://dx.doi.org/10.1002/clc.22280] [PMID: 24700369]

[105] Lyon AR, Bossone E, Schneider B, *et al.* Current state of knowledge on takotsubo syndrome: A position statement from the taskforce on takotsubo syndrome of the heart failure association of the european society of cardiology. Eur J Heart Fail 2016; 18(1): 8-27. [http://dx.doi.org/10.1002/ejhf.424] [PMID: 26548803]

[106] Corrigan FE III, Kimmel MC, Jayaram G. Four cases of takotsubo cardiomyopathy linked with exacerbations of psychiatric illness. Innov Clin Neurosci 2011; 8(7): 50-3. [PMID: 21860845]

[107] Machuki JO, Zhang HY, Harding SE, Sun H. Molecular pathways of oestrogen receptors and β-adrenergic receptors in cardiac cells: Recognition of their similarities, interactions and therapeutic value. Acta Physiol (Oxf) 2018; 222(2): e12978. [http://dx.doi.org/10.1111/apha.12978] [PMID: 28994249]

[108] McMurray JJ, Adamopoulos S, Anker SD, *et al.* ESC Guidelines for the diagnosis and treatment of acute and chronic heart failure 2012: The Task Force for the Diagnosis and Treatment of Acute and Chronic Heart Failure 2012 of the European Society of Cardiology. Developed in collaboration with the Heart Failure Association (HFA) of the ESC. Eur Heart J 2012; 33(14): 1787-847. [http://dx.doi.org/10.1093/eurheartj/ehs104] [PMID: 22611136]

[109] Stiermaier T, Moeller C, Oehler K, *et al.* Long-term excess mortality in takotsubo cardiomyopathy: predictors, causes and clinical consequences. Eur J Heart Fail 2016; 18(6): 650-6. [http://dx.doi.org/10.1002/ejhf.494] [PMID: 26990821]

[110] Jaguszewski M, Osipova J, Ghadri JR, *et al.* A signature of circulating microRNAs differentiates takotsubo cardiomyopathy from acute myocardial infarction. Eur Heart J 2014; 35(15): 999-1006. [http://dx.doi.org/10.1093/eurheartj/eht392] [PMID: 24046434]

CHAPTER 11

Endemic Agrestic Cardiomyopathy: Where Negligence leads to Heart Failure, While Pain and Sudden Death Become the New Normal

Iroegbu Chukwuemeka Daniel* and **Jinfu Yang**

Department of Cardiovascular Surgery, The Second Xiangya Hospital, Central South University, Middle Renmin Road 139, 410011 Changsha, China

Abstract: Endomyocardial fibrosis is a neglected tropical heart disease of poverty which carries a poor prognosis with no specific treatment, and the most common restrictive cardiomyopathy worldwide, affecting mainly children and young adults. Since the first description(s) in Uganda in 1948, high-frequency areas for EMF have included Africa, Asia, and South America and more recently, developed eastern European countries. Although, its etiology, pathogenesis and natural history remain unclear, its natural history includes both an active and chronic phase with recurrent flare-ups of inflammation characterized by an impaired diastolic filling of either one or both ventricles as a result of the fibrous tissue deposition on the endocardial surface, variable degree of systolic dysfunction, atrioventricular valve dysfunction, and associated intra-cavitary thrombi. This chapter aims to discuss the current knowledge so far in clinical practice about the etiology, mechanism(s) and natural history of the disease which would improve public awareness in rural endemic areas, leading to early detection and diagnosis of the disease, enhancing therapeutic strategies/treatment, biomolecular and other innovative technologies. The chapter would further go on to explore and highlight critical potential gray areas for future translational research which would enable both basic and clinical researchers, physicians and surgeons recognize and address the many gaps, inconsistencies, flaws, and setbacks encountered with this neglected cardiovascular disease.

Keywords: Africa, Asia, Adolescents, Alcohol, Cardiomyopathy, Causes, Children, Death, Epidemiology, Endomyocardial fibrosis, Echocardiography, Endemic disease, Health Services accountability, Heart failure, Latin America, Mortality, Outcomes, Pathology, Physiology, Prognosis, Restrictive cardiomyopathy, Sudden death, Surgical findings.

* **Corresponding author Iroegbu Chukwuemeka Daniel:** Department of Cardiovascular Surgery, The Second Xiangya Hospital, Central South University, Middle Renmin Road 139, 410011 Changsha, China; E-mails: yjf19682005@csu.edu.cn, Dr,iroegbu_daniel@yahoo.com, Dr.iroegbu_daniel@csu.edu.cn

Jinfu Yang & Iroegbu Chukwuemeka Daniel (Eds.)

INTRODUCTION

Endomyocardial Fibrosis (EMF) initially described during episodes of rapidly progressive heart failure (HF) usually associated with atrioventricular-valve regurgitation or from autopsies of patients who died from an advanced disease [1 - 3], is cardiomyopathy that predominantly affects children and young adults. It is one of the most neglected tropical diseases affecting an estimated ten million people worldwide [4] with a high prevalence rate in Africa [5]. Although its etiology, pathogenesis, and natural history remain unclear, the disease is the most common cause of restrictive cardiomyopathy (RCM), characterized by an impaired diastolic filling of either one or both ventricles as a result of the fibrous tissue deposition on the endocardial surface, variable degree of systolic dysfunction, atrioventricular valve dysfunction, and associated intra-cavitary thrombi. Its physiology leads to the right and left HF, or even both carrying a significantly poor prognosis, with an estimated survival of two years after diagnosis. With no currently specific drug therapy, surgery (valvular repair/replacement) though technically challenging and not available in most endemic areas corrects hemodynamic abnormalities thereby, improving quality of life [6, 7] for all patients in New York Heart Association (NYHA) III or IV and the resection of the thickened endocardium.

The use of Magnetic Resonance Imaging (MRI) helps provide information such as; presence or the absence of thrombi's, and the degree of myocardial involvement given a chance for non-invasive monitoring of the disease's progression and prognostication [8]. However, its availability in endemic areas is meager, where the diagnosis is based on echocardiography. Though endemic and rural, with considerable reports from highly-populated regions of sub-Saharan Africa (Uganda [1], Nigeria [9], and Ivory Coast [10]), Latin America [11], Central South Asia [12, 13], and other regions situated within 15 degrees of the equator, or in general low-income communities, significant cases have been reported in countries outside the tropics, including industrialized nations [14 - 21]. Therefore, irrespective of the part of the world one lives in, EMF remains a challenging and mysterious cardiovascular disease poorly understood since its first description in 1948 with variable phenotypic expression (depending stage at which it is diagnosed) leading to HF and sudden death in children and adolescents [22]. Hence, it is paramount that both time and resources be invested in the research given that, EMF, a current burden for both primary and clinical physicians less often appears on public health agendas of countries where it is endemic nor among scientists from developed countries [23].

This chapter aims to discuss the current knowledge so far in clinical practice about the etiology, mechanism(s) and natural history of the disease which would improve public awareness in rural endemic areas, leading to early detection and diagnosis of the disease, enhancing therapeutic strategies/treatment, biomolecular and other innovative technologies. The chapter would further go on to explore and highlight critical potential gray areas for future translational research which would enable both basic and clinical researchers, physicians and surgeons recognize and address the many gaps, inconsistencies, flaws, and setbacks encountered with this neglected tropical cardiovascular disease.

EPIDEMIOLOGY

A cardiovascular disease mostly affecting children and adolescents with regional variation in incidence [24 - 26] where more than half are diagnosed during the first decade of life [5, 27], its second peak is rather often diagnosed in women of childbearing age [28]. Although, adult preponderance has also been found in young women from Mozambique, and in Uganda, males were more commonly affected while in other studies, both sexes were equally affected [1, 5, 25, 29]. A known rural cardiovascular disease affecting mainly poor people living in resource-deprived areas, EMF is sporadically reported in people from high socio-economic levels after short visits to endemic areas (Fig. **1**) [30, 31].

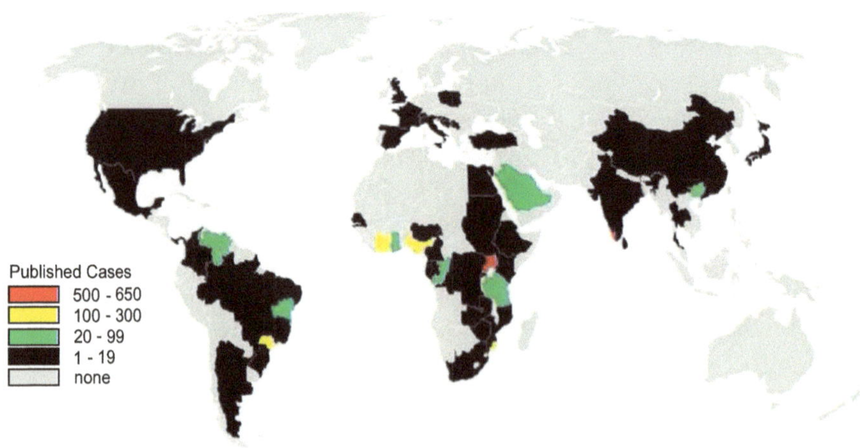

Fig. (1). Distribution by country of published cases of endomyocardial fibrosis between 1950 and 2010. It includes only cases diagnosed at autopsy or confirmed by surgery or cardiac imaging.

NATURAL HISTORY AND PRESENTATION

The natural history of EMF includes an active phase with intermittent flare-ups of inflammation and a transient progressive form leading towards the chronic phase.

Active Phase (Inflammation)

EMF though not completely understood as patients usually present late to medical attention, it often appears to start as a febrile illness that is associated with dyspnea, facial swelling, body itching, periorbital swelling, pancarditis, hypereosinophilia, and thromboembolism [9, 32]. Specific biological marker for EMF does not exist, with eosinophilia varying widely at diagnosis in the range of 0 - 70% [33]. Although higher rates are reported in the early stages with often abnormal morphological eosinophils [33], the resultant acute inflammation of the heart results in myocardial edema, eosinophilic infiltration, subendocardial myofiber necrosis, and vasculitis. As the inflammatory process further declines, eosinophils become undetectable [6, 34] but hypertrophic myocyte and interstitial fibrosis develop leading to myocardial ischemia [35] and cicatricial fibrosis which are mostly observed in chronic phase. Electrocardiographic [ECG] readings are usually nonspecific but may show conduction disturbances, and atrial or ventricular arrhythmias [36]. Echocardiography shows homogeneous infiltrates filling layers of the cardiac walls with pericardial effusion. Mural thrombi frequently occur at this stage along with the endocardial surfaces of the apical and valvular pockets, reducing ventricular cavity size, impeding adequate filling hence, producing its restrictive physiology. Moreover, at this phase, severe atrioventricular regurgitation can be seen due to the moderate-severe large organization of thrombi around the valvular apparatus, causing distortion. A neglected tropical cardiovascular disease and its active phase are quite challenging too due to the difficulties faced in clinically distinguishing its active phase from rheumatic fever especially in rural endemic areas [37] as some cases rapidly evolve to HF and sudden death, whereas others pass through a subacute phase without sequelae [32].

Progressive Transient Phase

Radiological signs and characteristic features in this phase are usually mild, exceptionally revealing the typical linear calcific endocardial lesions, and nonspecific varying degrees of cardiomegaly [5]. As seen echocardiographically at this phase, as the myocardium returns to normal thickness, the affected areas unevenly evolve into endocardial scars. Typically, the fibrotic process stops abruptly just before the ventricular outflow tract, and unlike the interstitial fibrosis seen in the active phase, the progressive restrictive syndrome occurs as a result of dilated atria and chamber distortion with evidence of endomyocardial calcification spots indicating subacute phase sometimes seen in patients in the acute phase of the disease [38]. However, factors responsible for the basis for slow-progression versus fast-progression phenotype, and the entire evolution of the disease remains unclear.

Chronic Phase

The most common presentation observed in the chronic phase includes; jugular venous distension, facial edema and exophthalmos, abdominal swelling, congestive splenomegaly, and gross hepatomegaly all due to long-standing systemic venous hypertension (right ventricular restriction) (Fig. **2**) [23]. Biventricular involvement predominates the chronic phase [5], followed by isolated right or left-sided heart diseases. Atrial fibrillation (AF) [39], and conduction abnormalities such as first-degree atrioventricular block or right bundle-branch block (RBBB) are common characteristics of this phase [40]. Marked ascites out of proportion to peripheral edema is an essential typical feature in chronic phase for both right- and left-sided heart EMF [41]. In some highly severe cases, decreased protein reabsorption, and liver disease with exudative enteropathy can occur [42]. Other keys and non-specific characteristic features seen in this phase include; testicular atrophy, growth retardation, periorbital edema, digital clubbing, hypertrophied parotid gland, cachexia, and proptosis.

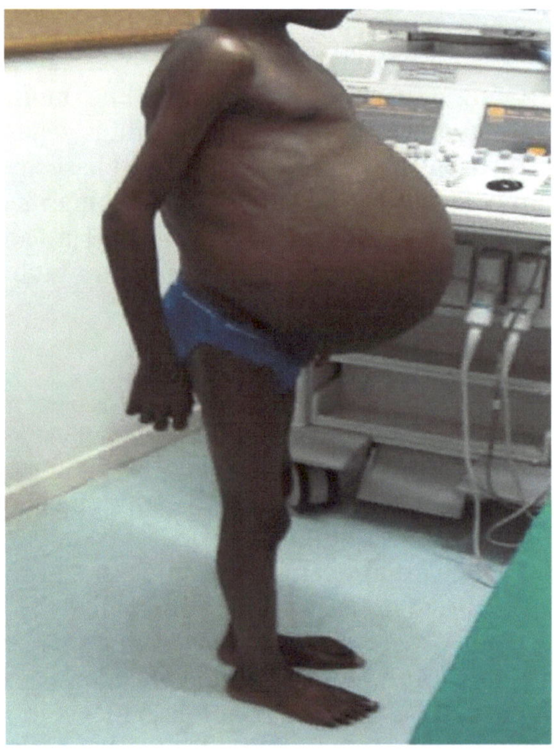

Fig. (2). Typical appearance and clinical profile of the disease (fibrosis tropical endomyocardial) showing striking ascites, regardless of which ventricle is involved, contrasting with little or no peripheral edema.

POSSIBLE ETIOLOGICAL/ETIOPATHOGENIC FACTORS

Though no single proposed factor is yet to explain the occurrence of EMF worldwide, the proposed possible factors frequently implicated in its etiopathogenesis include: (i) ethnicity [24], (ii) toxic agents (plant toxins) and heredity [25], (iii) poverty [28], (iv) malnutrition [43], (v) cerium and vitamin D, infections (viral and parasitic), autoimmunity, eosinophilia [44], (vi) serotonin [45], and (vii) cassava [46] (Fig. **3**). The role of infectious agents has come into the light and seems plausible due to sporadic case reports involving foreigners from temperate areas after short stays in endemic regions [30, 31].

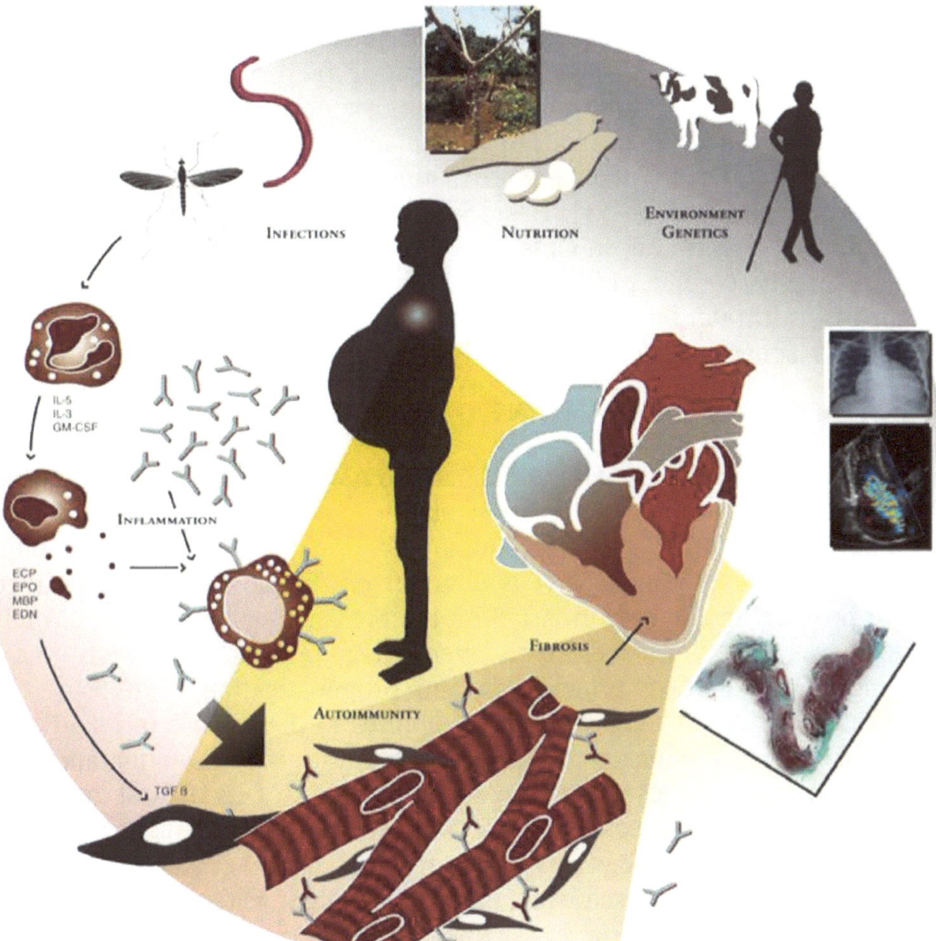

Fig. (3). Potential multifactorial pathogenesis of endomyocardial fibrosis.

Other considered possible causes or triggers for disease include: (i) Helminths [9], (ii) Microfilaria [9], (iii) Schistosoma [47], (iv) Coxsackie B virus, Arboviruses and Toxoplasma Gondi [48], and (v) Plasmodium species [49]. Although still less studied, the demonstration of familial clustering in community-based study cases in Mozambique [5] and the findings of familial cases of EMF in clinical series [44] suggest EMFs genetic predisposition.

PATHOLOGY

The pathological hallmark of an established EMF is diffused or focal endocardial thickening, which is a feature of advanced disease [35]. The endocardial thickening corresponds microscopically to an abnormal stimulation and an increased number of subendocardial cardiac fibroblasts, leading to enhanced collagen synthesis [51, 52]. There is deposition of microscopically dense fibrous tissue in the subendocardial lining with superimposed thrombosis and calcification in advanced stages [6, 50] while macroscopically, its appearance and the ventricular site(s) of involvement are distinctive with no primary involvement of extra-cardiac organs [53, 54]. Basic knowledge about the disease is mostly based on autopsies done on patients [1, 2] in endemic areas due to the lack of open-heart surgery, cardiac catheterization, echocardiography, and MRI [55] with inflammatory infiltrate, interstitial fibrosis, and scars all suggesting the possible likelihood of response to ischemic injury.

MORPHOLOGICAL ASSESSMENT/DIAGNOSIS

The use of chest X-ray (Fig. **4**) and echocardiography helps in the diagnosis of EMF as it gives an optimal delineation of EMF morphology and noninvasive hemodynamics [5, 50]. It is also, comparably available and affordable as compared to MRI. Although, MRI is a preferred diagnostic option as it goes further to provide detailed information on the presence or absence of thrombi's and the degree of myocardial involvement given a chance for non-invasive monitoring of the disease progression and prognostication (Fig. **5**) [8, 56]. Primary criteria used for diagnosing EMF applies to the disease in its advanced stages [57]. However, since then, severity scoring systems, major and minor measures have been suggested to curb several aspects of its natural history and phenotype(s) [5] of the disease as some characteristic clinical features seem to occur before severe chamber/valve distortion (Table **1**). According to this classification, EMF is diagnosed when there is one major criterion with two minor criteria or two major criteria [5]. Other diagnostic modalities include: (i) computed tomography scans (identify endocardial calcifications or intracavitary thrombi's) though more readily available but rarely used, (ii) late-gadolinium-enhancement images which correlate and also, identify fibrosis, (iii) perfusion studies accurately mapping out the hypo-perfused myocardial areas, and (iv) F-18 fluorodeoxyglucose positron emission tomography scan to eliminate sarcoidosis as a differential diagnosis.

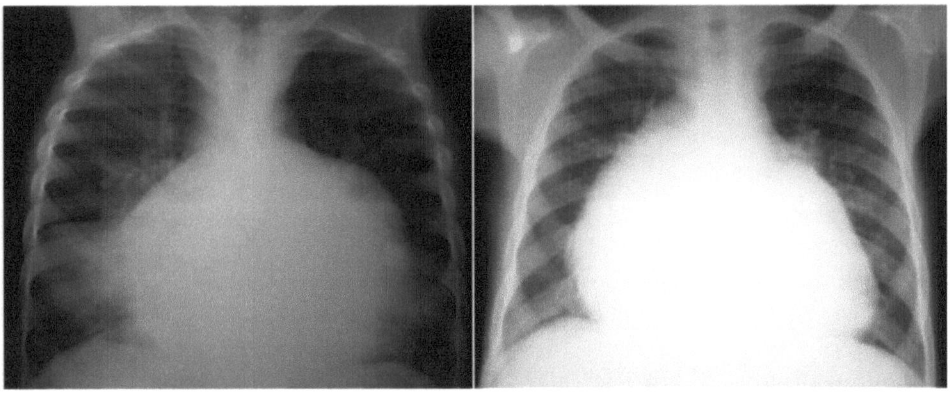

Fig. (4). Chest x-ray features of advanced endomyocardial fibrosis (EMF). Right, cardiomegaly caused by an aneurysmal right atrium in right EMF. Left, severe cardiomegaly secondary to a giant left atrium and massive mitral insufficiency.

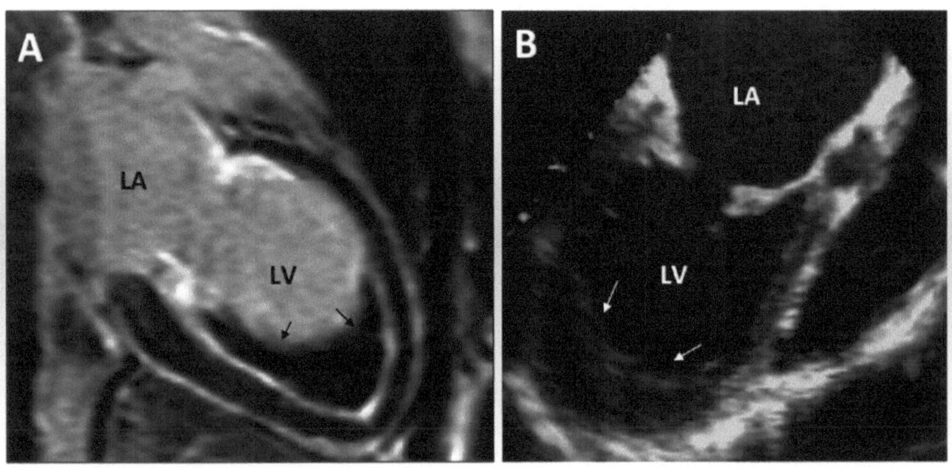

Fig. (5). Cardiac magnetic resonance image (MRI) of endomyocardial fibrosis. Cine cardiac MRI images (A) and transesophageal echocardiography (B) showing a sizeable apical thrombus adhering to the fibrotic endocardium reducing the size of the left ventricular cavity.

DIFFERENTIAL DIAGNOSIS

Evidence of mitral stenosis, aortic valve involvement, and history of rheumatic fever all favor rheumatic heart disease (RHD). Right EMF may mimic Ebstein malformation [58] while dilated cardiomyopathy (DCM) without an underlying known genetic genome or probable cause of HF is a key to exclusion [59]. However, pure mitral insufficiency can be particularly challenging to differentiate from left EMF when endocardial thickening and fibrosis affects valve tissues [3, 60] predominantly. Hence, in endemic areas, a clear distinction should be made from constrictive pericarditis, DCM, RHD, and tuberculous pericarditis.

CURRENT THERAPEUTIC MANAGEMENT STRATEGIES

Medical management consists of ameliorating acute disease, as well as preventing and treating arrhythmias, HF, and thromboembolism. All such medications used in the treatment of the disease (*e.g.*, digitalis, angiotensin-converting enzyme inhibitors, beta-blockers, and diuretics) are offered in combination with anticoagulants given the potential for intracardiac thrombi. In the advanced stage of the disease, large doses of drugs, and frequent admissions to a hospital (either out or inpatient wards) for invasive procedures are required to control arrhythmias and alleviate effusions. However, it is essential to note that, paracentesis either pericardial-pleural windows or pericardial-peritoneal shunts offers short-term relief only, as ascites often rapidly re-accumulates [5]. During the evacuation, an intravenous replacement of albumin at the time of the procedure should be done to compensate for protein loss [27].

SURGICAL MANAGEMENT

Open heart surgery (OHS) increases survival compared to medical treatment/therapy but must be performed before irreversible cardiac and hepatic damage occurs (Fig. **6A**, **6B** & **6C**) [61, 62]. However, asses to an OHS is severely limited in many endemic areas. Low rates of recurrence after OHS have been reported [63] although the real numbers remain uncertain [64] and early postoperative mortality can be high. Surgery consists of mitral valve replacement or repair and conservative endocardectomy [65]. Surgical treatment of EMF should be based on:

I. Feasibility of OHS and endocardectomy
II. The severe hemodynamic derangement caused by atrioventricular regurgitation and restrictive diastolic filling can be corrected
III. The disease is fatal if untreated, and
IV. If decortication (through a relatively well-preserved cleavage plan) can remove fibrotic myocardial tissues and reveal a healthy myocardium.

Table 1. Criteria for Diagnosis and Assessment of the Severity of Endomyocardial Fibrosis (EMF)*.

Criterion	Score
Major Criteria	
Endomyocardial plaques >2 mm in thickness	2
Thin (≤1 mm) endomyocardial patches affecting more than one ventricular wall	3
Obliteration of the RV or LV apex	4
Spontaneous contrast without severe ventricular dysfunction or Thrombi	4
Retraction of the RV apex (RV apical notch)	4
Atrioventricular-valve dysfunction due to adhesion of the valvular apparatus to the ventricular wall	1–4†
Minor Criteria	
Thin endomyocardial patches localized to one ventricular wall	1
Restrictive flow pattern across tricuspid or mitral valves	2
Pulmonary-valve diastolic opening	2
Diffuse thickening of the anterior mitral leaflet	1
Enlarged atrium with normal-size ventricle	2
M-movement of the interventricular septum and flat posterior wall‡	1
The enhanced density of the moderator or other intraventricular bands	1

*A definite diagnosis of EMF was made in the presence of two major criteria or one major criterion associated with two minor criteria. < 8 indicates- mild EMF, 8 to 15- moderate, and >15 severe diseases.
† The assigned score according to the atrioventricular regurgitation severity.
‡ Pattern of movement observed on echocardiography (M-mode) that is thought to be due to obliteration or restriction of the LV apex combined with mitral regurgitation. RV-right ventricular, LV-left ventricular

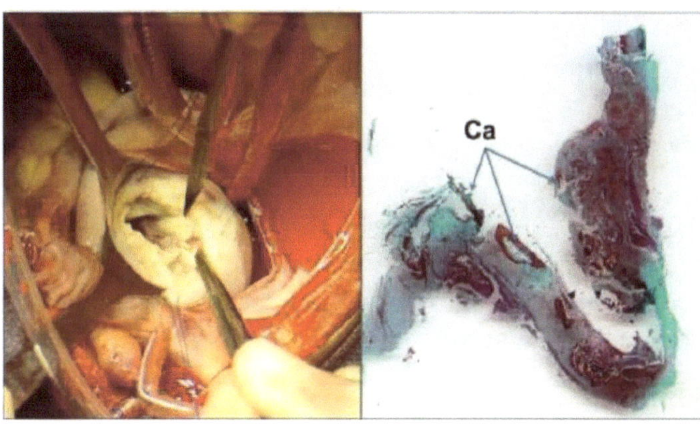

Fig. (6A). Surgical view of ventricular cavity endocardial resection of tropical EMF (left) and a histopathological section showing a thick fibrous shell removed surgically by endocardectomy (Masson trichrome stain) (right).

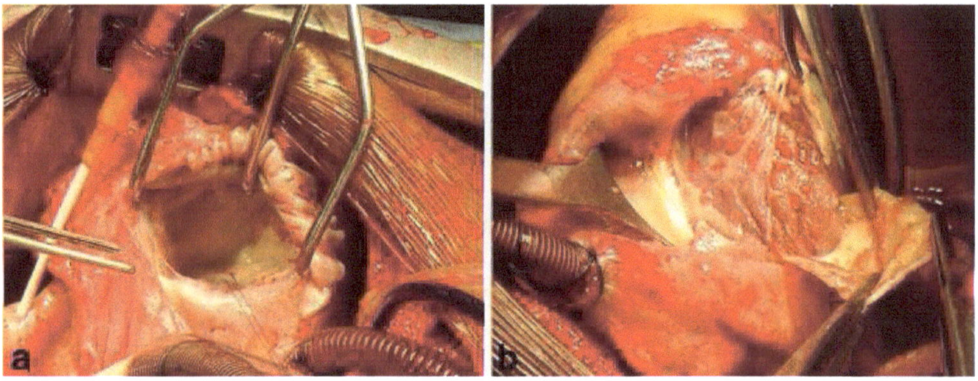

Fig. (6B). Intra-operative findings: A Severe right endomyocardial fibrosis with extensive.

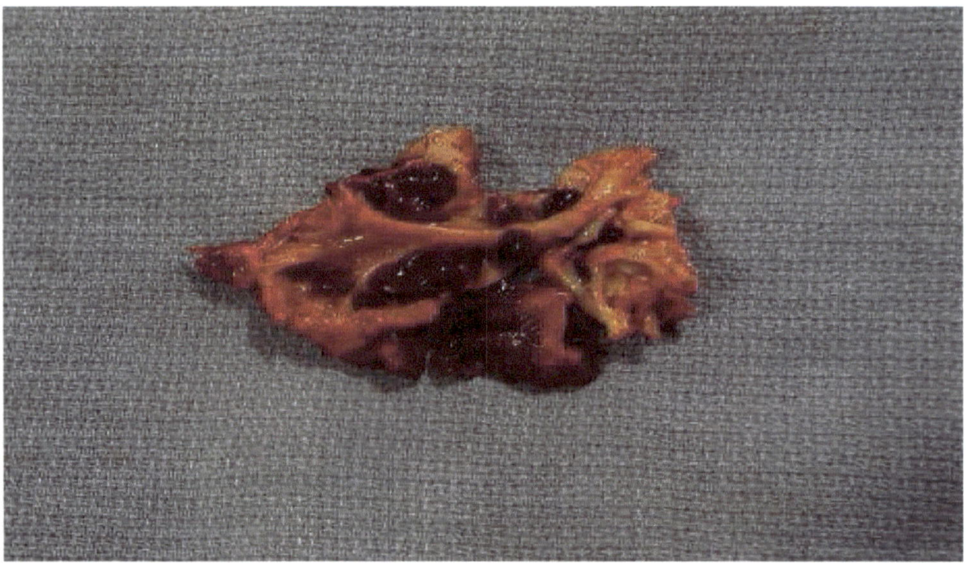

Fig. (6C). Excised right atrial appendage EMF, aneurysmal right atrium and thrombi attached to its wall.

endocardial whitening and thickening seen through the dilated tricuspid annulus. The right ventricular endocardium is shiny and smooth with loss of the trabecular pattern. B Resection of the thickened endocardium reveals healthy-looking myocardium underneath the fibrous tissue

Relative-contraindications for Surgery

I. Inadequate surgical know-how and inappropriate and poor surgical settings for OHS
II. Extreme cachexia

III. Large, long-standing ascites
IV. Right ventricular hypoplasia
V. Extensive endocardial fibrosis or calcification
VI. Chronic pulmonary thromboembolism and
VII. Severe shortening of leaflets and impaired myocardial function with valve replacement being anticipated.

Surgical Approach for Both Right and Left Endomyocardial Fibrosis

- Right EMF should be approached through right atriotomy which would provide conducive access to the RV cavity through a usually marked dilated tricuspid annulus. A combination of both blunt and sharp dissections through a cleavage plan should be applied to excise the thick fibrous endocardial lining hence, separating it from the myocardium at the same time, avoiding the conduction tissues while making sure the tricuspid valve apparatus is conserved [61]. Although tricuspid valve repair is always needed and right atrial reduction and thrombectomy can be performed after that, it is important to note that significant hemodynamic and clinical improvement can be achieved from cavopulmonary anastomosis in patients with right EMF for a planned future OHS endocardectomy months later.
- Left EMF, mitral annulus and the inflow part of the left ventricle can be better exposed through a left atriotomy which would provide a conducive surgical space to access the extent of valve lesions, and the fibrotic distribution. However, ventriculotomy is a better option to evaluate apical lesions and the area of myocardial fibrotic scarring.

Possible Post-Operative Complications

I. Pericardial tamponade
II. Low cardiac output and
III. Complete atrioventricular block

PROGNOSIS

EMF do carry very high morbidity and mortality rate with a mean survival rate of approximately two years [27] even after surgical procedures, which are only correct to some extent, some functional and structural abnormalities. Most deaths associated with EMF are due to arrhythmia, chronic HF, and thromboembolism and the recurrences of EMF lesions on the contralateral ventricle after surgery are high though in variable proportions. In most cases, patients with right-sided EMFs are exercise tolerant and may remain relatively asymptomatic for several years despite associated pericardial effusions and cardiomegaly [66].

SUMMARY AND RESEARCH CHALLENGES

EMF, a neglected cardiovascular disease in tropical regions differs significantly across certain groups and regions especially in some specific geographical pockets of Africa which are due to variations in exposure to known risk factors such as limited access to healthcare, environmental conditions, unhealthy lifestyles, and genetic factors among others. Specific data on the burden of EMF are scant, despite EMF afflicting hundreds of thousands of people in sub-Saharan rural Africa. The dominant factors limiting research in EMF endemic areas are; absence of proper infrastructure, financial constraints, and lack of trained personnel(s). Nevertheless, robust epidemiological population-based studies are urgently needed. It is noteworthy to understand that the Sub-Saharan African Survey (THESUS-HF) [67] study from nine African countries and other similar studies commenting on the prevalence of EMF in sub-Saharan African countries focused on overt HF and carried out in hospital settings or urban areas. Hence, as a disease is often related/attributed to the poor economic standard of living mostly in remote rural areas, its prevalence cannot be adequately ascertained by the aforementioned clinical studies. Therefore, to honestly and effectively access the disease prevalence, prevent, and improve management strategies for EMF, it is strategically important to account for subclinical diseases.

CONCLUSION AND FUTURE DIRECTIONS

An endemic neglected tropical disease of poverty, EMF still remains one of the most poorly understood and mysterious cardiovascular disorders in the field today as there is an urgent need to increase the medical awareness among health workers, policymakers and also, improve both pathogenic and pathophysiologic understanding of the disease, treatment and management strategies which would enhance prognostic features. Structural abnormalities of EMF can accurately be diagnosed by echocardiography, which would lead to early diagnosis and help strengthen epidemiological surveillance, clarify the prognosis and either support or refute the need for systematic screening. Important additional information and knowledge from clinicians and epidemiologists in combination with that from geneticists (if EMF is an acquired condition) and basic science researchers will help direct studies, and address issues of genetic susceptibility [68]. Multicenter investigations into nutritional and environmental factors would help identify common backgrounds across different high-prevalence endemic areas. Moreover, problems of bias and inaccuracies can be overcome with a robust international collaboration from both endemic and non-endemic regions, to third world countries and highly industrialized nations. Furthermore, autoimmunity and potential molecular mimicry pathways and mechanisms involved need to be addressed.

Finally, the role surgery plays in improving the knowledge and understanding of the disease must not and should not be overlooked, despite reduced long-term probabilities and outcomes not until specific environmental factor triggering the pathogenesis and specific treatment/therapies to halt the fibrotic process(s) are identified. Government, insurance agencies and other health care parastatals should aim to provide patients access to surgical treatment especially those in endemic rural areas in order to prevent sudden death, and HF where patients are accustomed to "pain" either from the loss of a loved one or the symptom and burden of the disease itself on them.

LIST OF ABBREVIATIONS

AF Atrial fibrillation

DCM Dilated cardiomyopathy

EMF Endomyocardial fibrosis

ECG Electrocardiography

HF Heart failure

MRI Myocardial resonance imaging

NYHA New York Heart Association

OHS Open heart surgery

RCM Restrictive cardiomyopathy

RHD Rheumatic heart disease

RBBB Right bundle branch block

CONSENT FOR PUBLICATION

Not applicable.

CONFLICT OF INTEREST

The authors confirm that this chapter contents have no conflict of interest.

ACKNOWLEDGEMENTS

Declared none.

REFERENCE

[1] Connor DH, Somers K, Hutt NSR, Manion WC, D'Arbela PGD. Endomyocardial fibrosis in Uganda (Davies' disease) Part I. Am Heart J 1967; 74(5): 687-709. [http://dx.doi.org/10.1016/0002-8703(67)90509-1] [PMID: 4861733]

[2] Connor DH, Somers K, Hutt NSR, Manion WC, D'Arbela P. Endomyocardial fibrosis in Uganda (Davies' disease) Part II. Am Heart J 1968; 74(5): 107-24. [http://dx.doi.org/10.1016/0002-8703(68)90122-1] [PMID: 4229457]

[3] Shaper AG, Hutt MSR, Coles RM. Necropsy study of endomyocardial fibrosis and rheumatic heart disease in Uganda 1950-1965. Br Heart J 1968; 30(3): 391-401.
[http://dx.doi.org/10.1136/hrt.30.3.391] [PMID: 5651254]

[4] Yacoub S, Kotit S, Mocumbi AO, Yacoub MH. Neglected diseases in cardiology: a call for urgent action. Nat Clin Pract Cardiovasc Med 2008; 5(4): 176-7.
[http://dx.doi.org/10.1038/ncpcardio1129] [PMID: 18317476]

[5] Mocumbi AO, Ferreira MB, Sidi D, Yacoub MH. A population study of endomyocardial fibrosis in a rural area of Mozambique. N Engl J Med 2008; 359(1): 43-9.
[http://dx.doi.org/10.1056/NEJMoa0708629] [PMID: 18596273]

[6] Iglezias SD, Benvenuti LA, Calabrese F, *et al.* Endomyocardial fibrosis: pathological and molecular findings of surgically resected ventricular endomyocardium. Virchows Arch 2008; 453(3): 233-41.
[http://dx.doi.org/10.1007/s00428-008-0652-3] [PMID: 18762973]

[7] de Oliveira SA, Pereira Barreto AC, Mady C, *et al.* Surgical treatment of endomyocardial fibrosis: a new approach. J Am Coll Cardiol 1990; 16(5): 1246-51.
[http://dx.doi.org/10.1016/0735-1097(90)90561-3] [PMID: 2229774]

[8] Cheung SC, Chan CWS. Insights of prognostication of Davies disease: What could we learn from serial magnetic resonance imaging studies? Int J Cardiol 2008.
[PMID: 19144428]

[9] Andy JJ, Ogunowo PO, Akpan NA, Odigwe CO, Ekanem IA, Esin RA. Helminth associated hypereosinophilia and tropical endomyocardial fibrosis (EMF) in Nigeria. Acta Trop 1998; 69(2): 127-40.
[http://dx.doi.org/10.1016/S0001-706X(97)00125-3] [PMID: 9588233]

[10] Metras D, Coulibaly AO, Ouattara K. fibrosis: results in 55 patients. Circulation 1985;72: II-274–I--279. Valiathan MS, 7. Balakrishnan KG, Sankarkumar R, Kartha CC. Surgical treatment of endomyocardial fibrosis. Ann Thorac Surg 1987; 43: 68-73.

[11] Moraes F, Lapa C, Hazin S, Tenorio E, Gomes C, Moraes CR. Surgery for endomyocardial fibrosis revisited. Eur J Cardiothorac Surg 1999; 15(3): 309-12.
[http://dx.doi.org/10.1016/S1010-7940(99)00027-5] [PMID: 10333028]

[12] Cherian G, Vijayaraghavan G, Krishnaswami S, *et al.* Endomyocardial fibrosis: report on the hemodynamic data in 29 patients and review of the results of surgery. Am Heart J 1983; 105(4): 659-66.
[http://dx.doi.org/10.1016/0002-8703(83)90491-X] [PMID: 6340450]

[13] Kartha CC. Endomyocardial fibrosis, a case for the tropical doctor. Cardiovasc Res 1995; 30(5): 636-43.
[http://dx.doi.org/10.1016/S0008-6363(96)88509-9] [PMID: 8595606]

[14] Lowenthal MN. Endomyocardial fibrosis: familial and other cases from northern Zambia. Med J Zambia 1978; 12(1): 2-7.
[PMID: 757895]

[15] Gonzalez-Lavin L, Friedman JP, Hecker SP, McFadden PM. Endomyocardial fibrosis: diagnosis and treatment. Am Heart J 1983; 105(4): 699-705.
[http://dx.doi.org/10.1016/0002-8703(83)90508-2] [PMID: 6837430]

[16] Schneider U, Jenni R, Turina J, Turina M, Hess OM. Long-term follow up of patients with endomyocardial fibrosis: effects of surgery. Heart 1998; 79(4): 362-7.
[http://dx.doi.org/10.1136/hrt.79.4.362] [PMID: 9616343]

[17] Hakim JG, Matenga JA, Ternouth I. Endomyocardial fibrosis in Zimbabwe--how rare is it? A report of two cases. Cent Afr J Med 1996; 42(9): 262-5.
[PMID: 8997819]

[18] Yin R. Endomyocardial fibrosis in China. Chin Med Sci J 2000; 15(1): 55-60. [PMID: 12899403]

[19] Niino T, Shiono M, Yamamoto T, *et al.* A case of left ventricular endomyocardial fibrosis. Ann Thorac Cardiovasc Surg 2002; 8(3): 173-6. [PMID: 12479177]

[20] Yie K, Sung S, Kim D, Woo J. Bidirectional cavopulmonary shunt as a rescue procedure for right ventricular endomyocardial fibrosis. Interact Cardiovasc Thorac Surg 2004; 3(1): 86-8. [http://dx.doi.org/10.1016/S1569-9293(03)00189-0] [PMID: 17670184]

[21] Hassan WM, Fawzy ME, Al Helaly S, Hegazy H, Malik S. Pitfalls in diagnosis and clinical, echocardiographic, and hemodynamic findings in endomyocardial fibrosis: a 25-year experience. Chest 2005; 128(6): 3985-92. [http://dx.doi.org/10.1378/chest.128.6.3985] [PMID: 16354870]

[22] Celermajer DS, Chow CK, Marijon E, Anstey NM, Woo KS. Cardiovascular disease in the developing world: prevalences, patterns, and the potential of early disease detection. J Am Coll Cardiol 2012; 60(14): 1207-16. [http://dx.doi.org/10.1016/j.jacc.2012.03.074] [PMID: 22858388]

[23] Mocumbi AO, Ferreira MB. Neglected cardiovascular diseases in Africa: challenges and opportunities. J Am Coll Cardiol 2010; 55(7): 680-7. [http://dx.doi.org/10.1016/j.jacc.2009.09.041] [PMID: 20170795]

[24] Mayanga-Kizza H, Gerwing E, Rutakingirwa M, Mugerwa R, Freers J. Tropical endomyocardial fibrosis in Uganda: the tribal and geographic distribution, and the association with eosinophiliaTropical Cardiology 2000. 26:103, 4548

[25] Bukhman G, Ziegler J, Parry E. Endomyocardial Fibrosis: Still a Mystery after 60 Years. PLoS Negl Trop Dis 2008; 2(2): e97. [http://dx.doi.org/10.1371/journal.pntd.0000097]

[26] Ferreira B, Matsika-Claquin MD, Hausse-Mocumbi AO, Sidi D, Paquet C. [Geographic origin of endomyocardial fibrosis treated at the central hospital of Maputo (Mozambique) between 1987 and 1999]. Bull Soc Pathol Exot 2002; 95(4): 276-9. [PMID: 12596378]

[27] Somers K. Restrictive Cardiomyopathies. In: Pongpanich B, Sueblinvong V, Vongprateep C, Eds. Pediatric Cardiology International Congress Series 906. Amsterdam: Excerpta Medica 1990.

[28] Rutakingirwa M, Ziegler JL, Newton R, Freers J. Poverty and eosinophilia are risk factors endomyocardial fibrosis (EMF) in Uganda. Trop Med Inter Health 1999; 4:3: 229235.

[29] Falase AO. Endomyocardial fibrosis in Africa. Postgrad Med J 1983; 59(689): 170-8. [http://dx.doi.org/10.1136/pgmj.59.689.170] [PMID: 6844202]

[30] Beck W, Schrire V. Endomyocardial fibrosis in Caucasians previously resident in tropical Africa. Br Heart J 1972; 34(9): 915-8. [http://dx.doi.org/10.1136/hrt.34.9.915] [PMID: 5075309]

[31] Brockington IF, Olsen EGJ, Goodwin JF. Endomyocardial Fibrosis in Europeans resident in Africa. Lancet 1967. 289:7490, 583588. [http://dx.doi.org/10.1016/S0140-6736(67)90440-0]

[32] Parry EH, Abrahams DG. The natural history of endomyocardial fibrosis. Q J Med 1965; 34(136): 383-408. [PMID: 5862743]

[33] Vijayaraghavan G, Sadanandan S. Immunological phenomena in tropical endomyocardial fibrosisIndian Heart Journal 1984. 36:2, 8788.

[34] Sasano H, Virmani R, Patterson RH, Robinowitz M, Guccion JG. Eosinophilic products lead to

myocardial damage. Hum Pathol 1989; 20(9): 850-7.
[http://dx.doi.org/10.1016/0046-8177(89)90096-8] [PMID: 2777241]

[35] Mocumbi AO, Falase AO. Recent advances in the epidemiology, diagnosis and treatment of endomyocardial fibrosis in Africa. Heart 2013; 99(20): 1481-7.
[http://dx.doi.org/10.1136/heartjnl-2012-303193] [PMID: 23680893]

[36] Davies J, Spry CJ, Vijayaraghavan G, De Souza JA. A comparison of the clinical and cardiological features of endomyocardial disease in temperate and tropical regions. Postgrad Med J 1983; 59(689): 179-85.
[http://dx.doi.org/10.1136/pgmj.59.689.179] [PMID: 6844203]

[37] Kennedy N, Miller P, Adamczick C, Molyneux E. Endomyocardial fibrosis: the first report from Malawi. Paediatr Int Child Health 2012; 32(2): 86-8.
[http://dx.doi.org/10.1179/1465328111Y.0000000036] [PMID: 22595215]

[38] Vijayaraghavan G, Sivasankaran S. Tropical endomyocardial fibrosis in India: a vanishing disease! Indian J Med Res 2012; 136(5): 729-38.
[PMID: 23287119]

[39] Tharakan JA. Electrocardiogram in endomyocardial fibrosis. Indian Pacing Electrophysiol J 2011; 11(5): 129-33.
[PMID: 21994470]

[40] Zabsonre P, Renambot J, Adoh-Adoh M, N'Dori R, Coulibaly AO, Bertrand E. [Conduction disorders in chronic parietal endocarditis or endomyocardial fibrosis. 170 cases at the Cardiology Institute of Abidjan]. Dakar Méd 2000; 45(1): 15-9. [in French].
[PMID: 14666783]

[41] Freers J, Masembe V, Schmauz R, Mayanja-Kizza H. Endomyocardial fibrosis syndrome in Uganda. Lancet 2000; 355(9219): 1994-5.
[http://dx.doi.org/10.1016/S0140-6736(05)72932-9] [PMID: 10859061]

[42] Grimaldi A, Vermi AC, Alfieri O, *et al.* Calcified left ventricular endomyocardial fibrosis. J Heart Valve Dis 2012; 21(3): 384-6.
[PMID: 22808844]

[43] Mckinney B. Studies on the experimental production of endomyocardial fibrosis and cardiomegaly of unknown origin by dietary meansAm Heart J 1975. 90:2, 206214.
[http://dx.doi.org/10.1016/0002-8703(75)90121-0]

[44] Patel AK, D'Arbela PG, Somers K. Endomyocardial fibrosis and eosinophilia. Br Heart J 1977; 39(3): 238-41.
[http://dx.doi.org/10.1136/hrt.39.3.238] [PMID: 849383]

[45] Ojo GO. The pathogenesis of endomyocardial fibrosis: the question of 5-hydroxytryptamine. Br Heart J 1970; 32(5): 671-4.
[http://dx.doi.org/10.1136/hrt.32.5.671] [PMID: 5470049]

[46] Sezi CL. Effect of protein deficient cassava diet on Cercopithecus aethiops hearts and its possible role in the aetiology and pathogenesis of endomyocardial fibrosis in man. East Afr Med J 1996; 73(5) (Suppl.): S11-6.
[PMID: 8756020]

[47] Victor EG, Lira V, Arruda A, Monteiro I, Lima R. Granulomas cardiacos a ovos de schistosoma e fibrose endomiocardica. Arq Bras Cardiol 1996; 67(4): 259-61.

[48] Ijaola O, Falase AO. Distribution of antibodies against Coxsackie B viruses, arboviruses and Toxoplasma gondii among patients with endomyocardial fibrosis (EMF) compared with normal subjects from EMF endemic and non-endemic zones of Nigeria. Afr J Med Med Sci 1990; 19(2): 93-103.
[PMID: 2165348]

[49] Eling WMC, Jerusalem CR, Heinen-Borries UJ, Hermsen CC, van Run-van Breda JJ. Is malaria involved in the pathogenesis of tropical endomyocardial fibrosis? Acta Leiden 1988; 57(1): 47-52. [PMID: 3072819]

[50] Mocumbi AO, Carrilho C, Sarathchandra P, Ferreira MB, Yacoub M, Burke M. Echocardiography accurately assesses the pathological abnormalities of chronic endomyocardial fibrosis. Int J Cardiovasc Imaging. 2011 Oct;27:7, 955964 [http://dx.doi.org/10.1007/s10554-010-9753-6]

[51] Chopra P, Narula J, Talwar KK, Kumar V, Bhatia ML. Histomorphologic characteristics of endomyocardial fibrosis: an endomyocardial biopsy study. Hum Pathol 1990; 21(6): 613-6. [http://dx.doi.org/10.1016/S0046-8177(96)90007-6] [PMID: 2351390]

[52] Somers K, Hutt MSR, Patel AK, D'Arbela PG. Endomyocardial biopsy in diagnosis of cardiomyopathies. Br Heart J 1971; 33(6): 822-32. [http://dx.doi.org/10.1136/hrt.33.6.822] [PMID: 4107637]

[53] Bijlsma F. Endomyocardial fibrosis and rheumatic heart disease in Mozambique. Trans R Soc Trop Med Hyg 1979; 73(6): 661-2. [http://dx.doi.org/10.1016/0035-9203(79)90015-4] [PMID: 538807]

[54] Ferreira MB, Teixeira R, Damasceno A. Two cases of endomyocardial fibrosis in Mozambique. Rev Port Cardiol 1992; 11(10): 841-5. [In Portuguese.]. [PMID: 1285962]

[55] Santos CL, Moraes CR, Santos FL, Moraes F, Brindeiro Filho D. Endomyocardial fibrosis in childrenCardiol Young 2001. 11:2, 205209. [http://dx.doi.org/10.1017/S1047951101000129]

[56] León D, Martín M, Corros C, Santamarta E, Costilla S, Lambert JL. Usefulness of cardiac MRI in the early diagnosis of endomyocardial fibrosis. Rev Port Cardiol 2012; 31(5): 401-2. [http://dx.doi.org/10.1016/j.repc.2011.12.016] [PMID: 22503434]

[57] Berensztein CS, Piñeiro D, Marcotegui M, Brunoldi R, Blanco MV, Lerman J. Usefulness of echocardiography and doppler echocardiography in endomyocardial fibrosis. J Am Soc Echocardiogr 2000; 13(5): 385-92. [http://dx.doi.org/10.1016/S0894-7317(00)70008-3] [PMID: 10804436]

[58] Vaidyanathan K, Agarwal R, Sahayaraj A, Sankar M, Cherian KM. Endomyocardial fibrosis mimicking Ebstein's anomaly: a diagnostic challenge. Tex Heart Inst J 2009; 36(3): 250-1.

[59] Chimenti C, Pieroni M, Frustaci A. Endomyocardial fibrosis mimicking a dilated cardiomyopathy in a childHeart 2001. 86:1, 73. [http://dx.doi.org/10.1136/heart.86.1.73]

[60] Saraiva LR, Carneiro RW, Arruda MB, Brindeiro D, Lira V. Mitral valve disease with rheumatic appearance in the presence of left ventricular endomyocardial fibrosis. Arq Bras Cardiol 1999; 72(3): 330-2. [http://dx.doi.org/10.1590/S0066-782X1999000300006]

[61] Mocumbi AO, Sidi D, Vouhe P, Yacoub M. An innovative technique for the relief of right ventricular trabecular cavity obliteration in endomyocardial fibrosis. J Thorac Cardiovasc Surg. 2007;134:1070–1072.

[62] Cherian SM, Jagannath BR, Nayar S, Cherian KM. Successful reoperation after 17 years in a case of endomyocardial fibrosis. Ann Thorac Surg 2006; 82(3): 1115-7. [http://dx.doi.org/10.1016/j.athoracsur.2005.12.041] [PMID: 16928558]

[63] Dubost C, Chapelon C, Deloche A, *et al.* Chirurgie des fibroses endomyocardiques: a propos de 32 cas. Arch mal Coeur 1990; 83: 481-6.

[64] Tang A, Karski J, Butany J, David T. Severe mitral regurgitation in acute eosinophilic

endomyocarditis: repair or replacement? Interact Cardiovasc Thorac Surg 2004; 3(2): 406-8. [http://dx.doi.org/10.1016/j.icvts.2004.02.018] [PMID: 17670274]

[65] Uva MS, Jebara VA, Acar C, *et al.* Mitral valve repair in patients with endomyocardial fibrosis. Ann Thorac Surg 1992; 54(1): 89-92. [http://dx.doi.org/10.1016/0003-4975(92)91146-Z] [PMID: 1610260]

[66] Salemi VMC, Rochitte CE, Barbosa MM, Mady C. Clinical and echocardiographic dissociation in a patient with right ventricular endomyocardial fibrosisHeart 2005. 91:11, 1399. [http://dx.doi.org/10.1136/hrt.2005.063610]

[67] Damasceno A, Mayosi BM, Sani M, *et al.* The causes, treatment, and outcome of acute heart failure in 1006 Africans from 9 countries. Arch Intern Med 2012; 172(18): 1386-94. [http://dx.doi.org/10.1001/archinternmed.2012.3310] [PMID: 22945249]

[68] Beaton A, Sable C, Brown J, *et al.* Genetic susceptibility to endomyocardial fibrosis. Glob Cardiol Sci Pract 2014; 2014(4): 473-81. [http://dx.doi.org/10.5339/gcsp.2014.60] [PMID: 25780800]

SUBJECT INDEX

A

Jinfu Yang & Iroegbu Chukwuemeka Daniel (Eds.)

B

D

E

F

G

H

I

J

K

L

M

T

U

V

W

X

www.ingramcontent.com/pod-product-compliance
Lightning Source LLC
LaVergne TN
LVHW070945210926
848482LV00002B/102
* 9 7 8 9 8 1 1 4 3 2 3 3 0 *